Handbook of Antibiotic Resistant Bacteria

Handbook of Antibiotic Resistant Bacteria

Edited by **Sebastian Driussi**

hayle
medical

New York

Published by Hayle Medical,
30 West, 37th Street, Suite 612,
New York, NY 10018, USA
www.haylemedical.com

Handbook of Antibiotic Resistant Bacteria
Edited by Sebastian Driussi

International Standard Book Number: 978-1-63241-236-2 (Hardback)

Printed in the United States of America.

Contents

Preface

Antibiotic Resistant Bacteria are bacteria that cannot be killed or controlled by antibiotics. Most of the infecting bacteria can become resistant to at least one or two antibiotics. Antibiotic resistance can be a serious disease and is currently, a major medical issue faced by scientists all over the world even though preventive, diagnostic and antibiotherapy techniques have improved significantly. In this book, scientists have presented observations from years of research, to provide an updated account on new strategies and methodologies from interventions against antibiotic resistant bacteria. This book deals with all the novel aspects of anti-biotic resistant organisms, providing insight into all recently developed techniques which is a valuable contribution to the progress of medical research such as mechanisms of antibiotic resistance in corynebacterium spp. causing infections in people, AR bacteria in food, assessment of antibiotic resistance in probiotic lactobacilli and susceptibility of probiotic bacteria.

Various studies have approached the subject by analyzing it with a single perspective, but the present book provides diverse methodologies and techniques to address this field. This book contains theories and applications needed for understanding the subject from different perspectives. The aim is to keep the readers informed about the progresses in the field; therefore, the contributions were carefully examined to compile novel researches by specialists from across the globe.

Indeed, the job of the editor is the most crucial and challenging in compiling all chapters into a single book. In the end, I would extend my sincere thanks to the chapter authors for their profound work. I am also thankful for the support provided by my family and colleagues during the compilation of this book.

Editor

Assessment of Antibiotic Resistance in Clinical Relevant Bacteria

.

Antibiotic Resistance: An Emerging Global Headache

Maimoona Ahmed
King Abdul Aziz University Hospital, Jeddah,
Saudi Arabia

1. Introduction

The discovery of antibiotics was one of the greatest achievements of the twentieth century. The subsequent introduction of sulphonamides, penicillin and streptomycin, broad spectrum bacteriostatic antibiotics, bactericidal antibiotics, synthetic chemicals and highly specific narrow spectrum antibiotics to clinical medicine transformed the treatment of bacterial diseases (Baldry, 1976). However, due to the excessive and inappropriate use of antibiotics there has been a gradual emergence of populations of antibiotic –resistant bacteria, which pose a global public health problem (Komolafe, 2003).

According to the WHO, a resistant microbe is one which is not killed by an antimicrobial agent after a standard course of treatment (WHO, 1998). Antibiotic resistance is acquired by a natural selection process. Antibiotic use to combat infection, forces bacteria to either adapt or die irrespective of the dosage or time span. The surviving bacteria carry the drug resistance gene, which can then be transferred either within the species/genus or to other unrelated species (Wise, 1998). Clinical resistance is a complex phenomenon and its manifestation is dependent on the type of bacterium, the site of infection, distribution of antibiotic in the body, concentration of the antibiotic at the site of infection and the immune status of the patient (Hawkey, 1998).

Antibiotic resistance is a global problem. While several pathogenic bacteria are resistant to first line broad spectrum antibiotics, new resistant strains have resulted from the introduction of new drugs (Kunin, 1993, Sack *et al*, 1997, Rahal *et* al, 1997, Hoge, 1998). Penicillin resistant pneumococci initially isolated in Australia and Papua New Guinea is now distributed worldwide (Hansman *et al*, 1974, Hart and Kariuki, 1998). Similarly, multi-drug resistant *Salmonella typhi* was first reported in 1987 and has now been isolated throughout the Indian sub-continent, south-east Asia and sub-Saharan Africa. (Mirza *et al*, 1996) Komolafe *et al* (2003) demonstrated a general broad-spectrum resistance to panels of antibiotics in 20% of the bacterial isolates of burns patients. Multi –drug resistant tuberculosis poses the greatest threat to public health in the new millennium (Kraig, 1998).

2. Molecular epidemiology of resistance genes

Antibiotic resistance in bacteria may be intrinsic or acquired. Intrinsic resistance mechanisms are naturally occurring traits due to the genetic constitution of the organism.

These inherited properties of a particular species are due to lack of either the antimicrobial target site or accessibility to the target site (Schwarz *et al*, 1995). For example, obligate anaerobes are resistant to aminoglycosides as they lack the electron transport system essential for their uptake (Rasmussen, 1997). Gram –negative organisms are resistant to macrolides and certain ß-lactam antibiotics as the drugs are too hydrophobic to traverse the outer bacterial membrane (Nikaido, 1989). Acquired resistance is a trait that is observed when a bacterium previously sensitive to an antibiotic, displays resistance either by mutation or acquisition of DNA or a combination of the two (Tomasz and Munaz, 1995). The methods of acquiring antibiotic resistance are as follows:

- **Spontaneous mutations** – Spontaneous mutations or growth dependent mutations, that occur due to replication errors or incorrect repair of damaged DNA in actively dividing cells may be responsible for generating antibiotic resistance (Krasovec and Jerman, 2003). Point mutations that not only produce antibiotic resistance, but also permit growth are attributed to antibiotic resistance (Woodford and Ellington, 2007). For example, the quinolone resistance phenotype in *Escherichia coli* is due to mutations in seven positions in the *gyrA* gene and three positions in the *parC* gene (Hooper, 1999). As a bacterial cell has several targets, access and protection pathways for antibiotics, mutations in a variety of genes can result in antibiotic resistance. Studies showed that mutations in the genes encoding the targets of rifamicins and fluoroquinolones, i.e. RpoB and DNA-topoisomerases respectively, results in resistance to the compounds (Martinez and Baquero, 2000; Ruiz, 2003). Adewoye *et al* (2002) reported that mutation in *mexR*, in *P. aeruginosa* resulted in upregulation of the *mexA-mexB-oprM* operon, which was associated with resistance to ß-lactams, fluoroquinolones, tetracyclines, chloramphenicol and macrolides. Expression of antibiotic uptake and efflux systems may be modified by mutations in the regulatory gene sequence or their promoter region (Depardieu *et al.*, 2007; Piddock, 2006). Mutations in the *E. coli* mar gene results in up regulation of AcrAB, involved in the efflux of ß-lactams, fluoroquinolones, tetracyclines, chloramphenicol from the cell (Barbosa and Levy, 2000).
- **Hypermutation** – In the last few years, studies have focussed on the association between hypermutation and antibiotic resistance. In the presence of prolonged, non-lethal antibiotic selective pressure, a small population of bacteria enters a brief state of high mutation rate. When a cell in this 'hyper mutable' state acquires a mutation that relieves the selective pressure, it grows, reproduces and exits the state of high mutation rate. While the trigger to enter the hyper mutable state is unclear, it ahs been suggested that it is dependent on a special SOS –inducible mutator DNA polymerase (pol) IV (Krosovec and Jerman, 2003). Hypermutators have been found in populations of *E. coli, Salmonella enterica, Neisseria meningitidis, Haemophilus influenzae, Staphylococcus aureus, Helicobacter pylori, Streptococcus pneumoniae, P. aeruginosa* with frequencies ranging from 0.1 to above 60% (Denamur *et al.*, 2002; LeClerc *et al.*, 1996). It has been observed that the hypermutators isolated from the laboratory as well as from nature have a defective mismatch repair system (MMR) due to inactivation of the *mutS* or *mutL* genes (Oliver *et al*, 2002). The MMR system eliminates biosynthetic errors in DNA replication, maintains structural integrity of the chromosome and prevents recombination between non-identical DNA sequences (Rayssiguier *et al.*, 1989) Studies have shown that the hypermutators play a significant role in the evolution of antibiotic resistance and may also be responsible for the multiresistant phenotype (Martinez and Baquero, 2000; Giraud *et al.*, 2002; Chopra *et al.*, 2003; Blazquez, 2003, Macia *et al.*, 2005).

- **Adaptive mutagenesis** – Recent studies have demonstrated that in addition to spontaneous mutations, mutations occur in non-dividing or slowly dividing cells in the presence of non-lethal selective pressure. These mutations, known as adaptive mutations, have been associated with the evolution of antibiotic resistant mutants under natural conditions (Krasovec and Jerman, 2003; Taddei *et al.*, 1997; Bjedov *et al.*, 2003). Adaptive mutagenesis is regulated by the stress responsive error prone DNA polymerases V (*umuCD*) and IV (*dinB*) (Rosche and Foster, 2000; Sutton *et al.*, 2000). Piddock and Wise (1997) demonstrated that some antibiotics like quinolones induce a SOS mutagenic response and increase the rate of emergence of resistance in *E.coli*.
- **Horizontal gene transfer** – Transfer of genetic material between bacteria, known as horizontal gene transfer is responsible fro the spread of antibiotic resistance. Resistance genes, consisting of a single or multiple mutations, may be transferred between bacteria by conjugation, transformation or transduction, and are incorporated into the recipient chromosome by recombination. These genes may also be associated with plasmids and/or transposons. Simjee and Gill (1997) demonstrated high level resistance to gentamycin and other aminoglycosides (except streptomycin) in enteroccoci. The resistance gene was found to be associated with narrow and broad host range plasmids. Due to the conjugative nature of the plasmids, spread of the resistance gene to other pathogenic bacteria is likely.
- Horizontal transfer of resistance genes is responsible for the dissemination of multiple drug resistance. Gene cassettes are the smallest mobile genetic entities that carry distinct resistance determinants for various classes of antibiotics. Integrons are DNA elements, located on the bacterial chromosome or on broad host range plasmids, with the ability to capture one or more gene cassettes within the same attachment site. Movement of the integron facilitates transfer of the cassette-associated resistance genes from one DNA replicon to another. When an integron is incorporated into a broad host range plasmid, horizontal transfer of the resistance gene may take place. A plasmid with a pre-existing resistance gene cassette can acquire additional resistance gene cassettes from donor plasmids, thereby resulting in multiresistance integrons (Rowe-Magnus and Mazel, 1999; Ploy *et al.*, 2000). Over 40 gene cassettes and three distinct classes of integrons have been identified (Boucher *et al.*, 2007). Dzidic and Bedekovic (2003) investigated the role of horizontal gene transfer in the emergence of multidrug resistance in hospital bacteria and demonstrated the transfer of antibiotic resistance genes between Gram-positive and Gram negative bacilli from the intestine. The fact that bacteria that have been separately evolving for upto 150 million years can exchange DNA, has strong implications with regard to the evolution of antibiotic resistance in bacterial pathogens (Dzidic *et al.*, 2003; Vulic *et al.*, 1997; Normark and Normark, 2002).

3. Mechanisms of resistance

The mechanisms that bacteria exhibit to protect themselves form antibiotic action can be classified into the following types. Table 1 gives an overview of representative antibiotics and their mechanisms of resistance.

- **Antibiotic inactivation** - Inactivation of antibiotic could be a result of either inhibition of activation *in vivo* or due to modification of the parent antibiotic compound, resulting in loss of activity. Loss of enzymes involved in drug activation is a relatively new mechanism of drug resistance. Studies have demonstrated that mutations in the *nfsA* and *nfsB* genes, which encode cellular reductases that reduce members of the nitrofuran family (nitrofurantion, nitrofurazone, nitrofurazolidone, etc.), are associated with nitrofuran resistance (Kumar and Jayaraman, 1991; Zenno *et al.*, 1996; Whiteway *et al.*, 1998).

β-lactamase enzymes cleave the four membered β-lactam ring of antibiotic like penicillin and cephalosporin, thereby rendering the antibiotic inactive. The large number of β-lactamases identified have been classified based on their structure and function. (Bush *et al.*, 1995). The enzymes discovered early (the TEM-1, TEM-2 and SHV-1 β-lactamases) were capable of inactivating penicillin but not cephalosporin. However, subsequent variants with a variety of amino acid substitutions in and around their active sites were identified in many resistant organisms. These have been collectively called 'extended spectrum β-lactamases (ESBLs)' and act on later generation β-lactam antibiotics (Bradford, 2001).

While most of the ESBLs are derivatives of the early enzymes, newer families of ESBLs, like cefotaximases (CTM-X enzymes) and carbapenemases have been discovered recently (Bonnet, 2004; Walther-Ramussen, 2004; Canton and Coque, 2006, Livermore and Woodford, 2000; Nordman and Poirel, 2002; Queenan and Bush, 2007). The CTM-X genes are believed to have descended from progenitor genes present in *Klyuvera* spp. (Decousser *et al.*, 2001; Poirel *et al.*, 2002; Humeniuk *et al.*, 2002). These ESBLs pose a significant threat as they provide resistance against a broad antibacterial spectrum (Bradford, 2001).

Enzymatic acetylation of chloramphenicol is the most common mechanism by which pathogens acquire resistance to the antibiotic (Schwarz *et al.*, 2004). Mosher *et al.* (1995) established that O-phosphorylation of chloramphenicol affords resistance in *Streptomyces venezuelae* ISP 5230.

While the resistance to aminoglycosides due to inhibition of drug uptake in Gram negative organisms is well documented, aminoglycoside inactivating enzymes have been detected in many bacteria and plasmids. The presence of multiple NH_2 and OH groups enables inactivation of aminglycosides. Inactivation occurs through acylation of NH_2 groups and either phosphorylation or adenylation of the OH groups. (Azucena and Mobashery, 2001) Doi and Arakawa (2007) reported a plasmid-mediated mechanism of aminoglycoside resistance involving methylation of 16S ribosomal RNA.

Fluroquinolones (ciprofloxacin, norfloxacin, ofloxacin) inhibit DNA replication by targeting the enzymes, DNA gyrase and topoisomerase IV. Fluoroquinolone resistance occurs either through mutations in the genes coding for the subunits of DNA gyrase (*gyrA* and *gyrB*) and topoisomeraseIV (*parC* and *parE*), drug efflux, or a combination of both mechanisms. (Levy, 1992; Nikaido, 1996; Li and Nikaido, 2004; Ruiz, 2003; Oyamada *et al.*, 2006). However, Robiscek *et al* (2006) and Park *et al* (2006) demonstrated that a gene encoding an aminoglycoside-specific acetylase could mutate further to give an enzyme which could inactivate fluoroquinolones. This is an example to show that genes encoding minor and perhaps unrecognized activities, besides the major activity, could mutate further to gain extended activity and could be selected by appropriate selection pressures.

Type A and type B streptogramins bind to the 50S ribosomal subunit and inhibit translation (Wright, 2007). Resistance to type A streptogramin has been found to be mediated by an enzyme called VatD (virginiamycin acetyl transferase) acetylates the antibiotic (Seoane and Garcia-Lobo, 2000; Suganito and Roderick, 2002). Resistance to type B streptogramin is brought about by the product of the *vgb* gene, a C–O lyase (Mukhtar *et al.*, 2001). Homologues and orthologues of the genes encoding both the enzymes have been detected in a variety of nonpathogenic bacteria, environmental bacteria and plasmids (Wright, 2007).

- **Exclusion from the internal environment** - Alterations in permeability of the outer membrane of bacteria confers antibiotic resistance. This is commonly observed in Gram negative bacteria, such as *Pseudomonas aeruginosa* and *Bacteroides fragilis*. Reports have suggested that the loss or modification of, which are non-specific protein channels spanning the outer membrane, have resulted in antibiotic resistance. (Nikaido, 1989)

Activation of efflux pump, which pump out the antibiotics that enter the cells thereby preventing intracellular accumulation, is also responsible for antibiotic resistance. (Nikaido, 1996; Li and Nikaido, 2004). The AcrAB/TolC system in *E. coli* is the best studied efflux system. The inner membrane protein, Acr B, and outer membrane protein, Tol C are linked by the periplasmic protein, Acr A. When activated, the linker protein is folds upon itself thereby, bringing the Acr B and Tol C proteins in close contact. This results in a channel from inside to the outside of the cell, through which antibiotics are pumped out. In antibiotic-sensitive cells, by the product of *acrR* gene, represses the AcrAB/TolC system. A mutation in *acrR*, causing an arg45cys change, activates expression of the system and consequent drug efflux. (Webber *et al*, 2005). Figure 1 shows the AcrAB/TolC efflux system in *E.coli*.

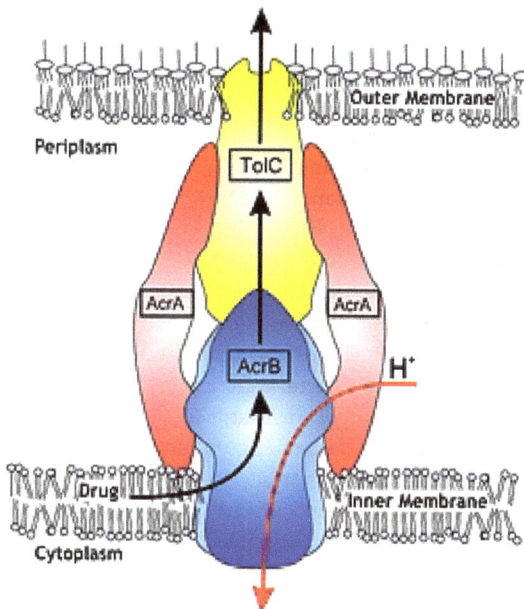

Fig. 1. Efflux system in E. coli (AcrAB/TolC) system (Pos, 2009)

Nine proton-dependent efflux pumps have been identified in *E. coli* so far. These cause the efflux of multiple antibiotics leading to multidrug resistance (Viveiros *et al.*, 2007). Ruiz (2003) demonstrated that although fluoroquinolone resistance occurred commonly due to target mutations, efflux mechanisms were also responsible for the phenomenon.

- **Target alteration** – Structural changes in the target site of the antibiotic prevent interaction of the antibiotic and its target, thus inhibiting the biological activity of the antibiotic. This is exemplified by penicillin resistance due to penicillin binding proteins (PBPs). PBPs are trans-peptidases which catalyse the crosslinking reaction between two peptides each linked to *N*-acetyl-muramic acid residues of the peptidoglycan backbone of the cell wall. Penicillin and other antibiotics which are structurally similar to the cross-linked dipeptide forma stable covalent complex with PBPs, inhibit the crosslinking reaction, resulting in weakening and lysis of the cell. Mutational changes in PBPs, which result in reduction in the affinity of PBPs to penicillin, over expression of endogenous, low-affinity PBPs encoding genes result in penicillin resistance (Zapun *et al.*, 2008).

Vancomycin binds non-covalently to the cell-wall precursors of Gram-positive bacteria. The binding, which occurs through a set of five hydrogen bonds between the antibiotic and the *N*-acyl-D-ala–D-ala dipeptide portion of the stem pentapeptides linked to the *N*-acetyl muramic acid backbone, blocks the crosslinking transpeptidase reaction catalysed by the PBPs. As a result the cell walls are less rigid and more susceptible to lysis. In vancomycin-resistant organisms, the stem peptides terminate in D-lactate as against D-alanine in the sensitive strains. This eliminates the formation of the crucial hydrogen bond and results in a 1000-fold decrease in the affinity for vancomycin and consequent resistance to the same. This process is regulated by a two-component regulatory system involving a set of five genes (*vanR*, *vanS*, *vanH*, *vanA* and *vanX*). *Enterococci* as well as *Staphylococcus aureus* have been shown to acquire resistance to vancomycin by this mechanism, known as vancomycin evasion. (Walsh *et al.*, 1996; Arthur *et al.*, 1996; Courvalin, 2006)

Ruiz (2003) reported that the eight amino acid substitutions in *gyrA* , which have been attributed to fluroquinolone resistance, are predominantly located in the quinolone resistance determining region (QRDR). Rifampicin resistance due to mutation in *rpoB*, the gene encoding the (R)-subunit of RNA polymerase has been observed in rifampicin resistant strains of Mycobacterium *tuberculosis*, laboratory strains of *E. coli*, other pathogens and non pathogens (Jin and Gross, 1988; Anbry-Damon *et al.*, 1998; Padayachee and Klugman, 1999; Somoskovi *et al.*, 2001).

- **Production of alternative target** – Bacteria may protect themselves from antibiotics, by production of an alternative target resistant to inhibition along with the original sensitive target. The alternative target circumvents the effect of the antibiotic and enables survival of the bacteria. In methicillin resistant *Staphylococcus aureus* (MRSA) alternative penicillin binding protein (PBP2a) is produced in addition to penicillin binding protein (PBP). As PBP2a is not inhibited by antibiotics the cell continues to synthesise peptidoglycan and has a structurally sound cell wall. It has been suggested that the evolution of vancomycin resistant enterococci may lead to transfer of genes to *S. aureus* resulting in vancomycin resistant MRSA (Michel and Gutmann, 1997).

Antibiotic Category	Examples	Mode of action	Major mechanisms of resistance
ß-lactams	Penicillin, Cephalosporin, Cetoximes, Carbapenems	Inhibition of cell wall synthesis	Cleavage by ß-lactamases, ESBLs, CTX-mases, Carbapenemases, altered PBPs
Aminoglycosides	Streptomycin, Gentamycin, Tobramycin, Amikacin	Inhibition of protein synthesis	Enzymatic modification, efflux, ribosomal mutations, 16S rRNA methylation
Quinolones	Ciprofloxacin, Ofloxacin, Norfloxacin	Inhibition of DNA	Efflux, modification, target mutations
Glycopeptides	Vancomycin	Inhibition of cell wall synthesis	Altered cell walls, efflux
Tetracyclines	Tetracycline	Inhibition of translation	Efflux
Rifamycins	Rifampicin	Inhibition of transcription	Altered ß-subunit of RNA polymerase
Streptogramins	Virginamycins, Quinupristin, Dalfoprisitin	Inhibition of cell wall synthesis	Enzymatic cleavage, modification, efflux
Oxazolidinones	Linezolid	Inhibition of formation of 70S ribosomal complex	Mutations in 23 S rRNA genes follwed by gene conversion.

Table 1. Representative antibiotics and their mechanisms of resistance. Adapted from Jayaraman, 2009

4. Conclusion

Emergence of antibiotic resistance is driven by repeated exposure of bacteria to antibiotics and access of bacteria to a large antimicrobial resistance pool. Pathogenic and non-pathogenic bacteria are becoming increasingly resistant to conventional antibiotics. While initial studies on antibiotic resistance investigated methicillin resistant *Staphylococcus aureus* and vancomycin resistant *Enterococcus spp.*, the focus has now shifted to multi drug resistant Gram –negative bacteria. The emergence of Gram negative *Enterobacteriaceae* resistant to carbapenem due to New Delhi metallo – ß –lactamase 1 (NDM-1) has been identified as a major global health problem. (Kumarasamy *et al*, 2010). However, it must be noted that resistance selected in non pathogenic or commensal bacteria could act as a reservoir of resistance genes, resulting in emergence of resistance in pathogens. There is a need to review the use and check the misuse of antibiotics and to adopt good infection control practices in order to control antibacterial resistance, since increasing antibiotic resistance has the potential to transport clinical medicine to the pre-antibiotic era.

5. References

Adewoye L, Sutherland A, Srikumar R and Poole K (2002). The *mexR* repressor of the mexAB-oprM multidrug efflux operon in *Pseudomonas aeruginosa*: Characterization of mutations compromising activity. *J. Bacteriol*. 184, 4308–4312.

Anbry-Damon H, Housy CJ and Courvalin P (1998) Characterisation of mutations in *rpo* B that confer rifampicin resistance in *Staphylococcus aureus*. *Antimicrob. Agents Chemother*. 42, 2590–2594

Arthur M, Reynolds PE, Depardieu F, Evers S, Dutka-Malen S, Quintillani Jr R and Courvalin P (1996) Mechanisms of glycopeptide resistance in enterococci. *J. Infect*. 32, 11–16.

Azucena E and Mobashery S (2001) Aminoglycoside-modifying enzymes: mechanisms of catalytic processes and inhibition. *Drug Res. Updates*. 4, 106–117.

Baldry, P. (1976). The battle against bacteria – a fresh look. Cambridge University Press; pp 156.

Barbosa TM and Levy SB (2000) Differential expression of over 60 chromosomal genes in *Escherichia coli* by constitutive expression of MarA. *J. Bacteriol*. 182, 3467–3474.

Bjedov I, Tenaillon O, Gerard B, Souza V, Denamur E, Radman M, Taddei F and Matic I (2003) Stress-induced mutagenesis in bacteria. *Science*. 300, 1404–1409.

Blazquez J (2003) Hypermutation as a factor contributing to the acquisition of antimicrobial resistance, *Clin. Infect. Dis*. 37, 1201–1209.

Bonnet R (2004) Growing group of extended spectrum β-lactamases: the CTX-M enzymes. *Antimicrob. Agents Chemother*. 48, 1–14.

Boucher Y, Labbate M, Koenig JE and Stokes HW (2007) Integrons: Mobilizable platforms that promote genetic diversity in bacteria. *Trends Microbiol*. 15, 301–309.

Bradford PA (2001) Extended spectrum β-lactamases (ESBL) in the 21st century: Characterisation, epidemiology and detection of this important resistance threat. *Clin. Microbiol. Rev*. 48, 933–951.

Bush K, Jacoby GA and Medeiros AA (1995) A functional classification of β-lactamases and its correlation with molecular structure. *Antimicrob. Agents Chemother*. 39, 1211–1233.

Canton R and Coque TM (2006) The CTX-M β-lactamase pandemic. *Curr. Opin. Microbiol*. 9, 466–475.

Chopra I, O'Neill AJ and Miller K (2003) The role of mutators in the emergence of antibiotic-resistant bacteria. *Drug Resist. Update*. 6, 137–145.

Courvalin P (2006) Vancomycin resistance in Gram-positive cocci. *Clin. Infect. Dis*. (*Suppl. 1*). 42, 25–34

Decousser JW, Poirel L and Nordman P (2001) Characterisation of chromosomally encoded, extended spectrum class 4, β-lactamase from *Kluyvera cryocrescens*. *Antimicrob. Agents Chemother*. 45, 3595–3598.

Denamur E, Bonacorsi S, Giraud A, Duriez P, Hilali F, Amorin C, Bingen E, Andremont A, Picard B, Taddei F and Matic I (2002) High frequency of mutator strains among human uropathogenic *Escherichia coli* isolates. *J. Bacteriol*. 184, 605–609

Depardieu F, Podglajen I, Leclercq R, Collatz E and Courvalin P (2007) Modes and modulations of antibiotic resistance gene expression. *Clin. Microbiol. Rev*. 20, 79–114.

Doi Y and Arakawa Y (2007) 16S ribosomal RNA methylation: emerging resistance mechanism against amino glycosides. *Clin. Infect. Dis.* 45, 88–94.

Dzidic S, Bacun-Druzina V and Petranovic M (2003) The role of mismatch repair in bacterial evolution. *Food Technol. Biotechnol.* 41, 177–182.

Dzidic S and Bedekovic V (2003) Horizontal gene transfer-emerging multidrug resistance in hospital bacteria. *Acta Pharmacol. Sin.* 24, 519–226.

Giraud A, Matic I, Radman M, Fons M and Taddei F (2002) Mutator bacteria as a risk factor in treatment of infectious diseases. *Antimicrob. Agents Chemother.* 46, 863–865

Hansman, D., Devitt, L., Miles, H. Riley, J. (1974). Pneumococci relatively unsusceptible to penicillin in Australia and New Guniea. *Medical Journal of Australia*; 2: 353 – 356.

Hart, C.A. and Kariuki, S. (1998). Antimicrobial resistance in developing countries. *British Medical Journal*; 317: 647 – 650.

Hawkey, P.M. (1998). The origins and the molecular basis of antibiotic resistance. *British Medical Journal*; 317: 657 – 660.

Hoge, C.W., Gambel, J.M., Srijan, A *et al.* (19980. Trends in antibiotic resistance among diarrheal pathogens isolated in Tailand over 15 years. *Clin. Infect. Disease,* 26: 341 – 345.

Hooper DC (1999) Mechanisms of fluoroquinolone resistance. *Drug Resist. Update.,* 2, 38–55.

Humeniuk C, Arlet G and Gautier V (2002) β-Lactamases of *Kluyvera ascorbita*, probable progenitors of some plasmid-encoded CTX-M types. *Antimicrob. Agents Chemother.* 46, 3045–3049.

Jayaraman R. (2009) Antibiotic resitance: an overview of mechanisms and a paradigm shift. *Current Science,* 96(11): 1475 – 1484.

Jin D and Gross C (1988) Mapping and sequencing of mutations in the *Escherichia coli rpo* B gene that lead to rifampicin resistance. *J. Mol. Biol.* 202, 45–58.

Komolafe, O.O. (2003) Antibiotic resistance in bacteria- an emerging public health problem. *Malawi Medical Journal,* 15(2): 63 – 67.

Kraig, E. (1998) Facing the microbial threat. *British Medical Journal,* 317 – 620.

Krasovec R and Jerman I (2003) Bacterial multicellularity as a possible source of antibiotic resistance. *Med. Hypotheses.* 60, 484–488.

Kumar AN and Jayaraman R (1991) Molecular cloning, characterization and expression of nitrofuran reductase gene of *Escherichia coli*. *J. Biosci.* 16, 145–159.

Kumarasamy KK, Toleman MA, Walsh TR, Bagaria J, Butt F, Balakrishnan R *et al.* (2010). Emergence of a new antibiotic resistance mechanism in India, Pakistan and the UK: a molecular, biological and epidemiological study. *Lancet;*

Kunin, C.M. (1993) Resistance to antimicrobial drugs - a worldwide calamity. *Annals of Internal Medicine,*118: 557 – 561.

LeClerc JE, Li B, Payne WL and Cebula TA (1996) High mutation frequencies among *Escherichia coli* and *Salmonella* pathogens. *Science.* 274, 1208–1211.

Li X and Nikaido H (2004) Efflux-mediated drug resistance in bacteria. *Drugs.* 64, 159–204.

Livermore DM and Woodford N (2000) Carbapenemases: a problem in waiting? *Curr. Opin. Microbiol.* 3, 489–495

Macia MD, Blanquer D, Togores B, Sauleda J, Perez JL and Oliver A (2005) Hypermutation is a key factor in development of multiple-antimicrobial resistance in *Pseudomonas aeruginosa* strains causing chronic lung infections. *Antimicrob. Agents Chemother.* 49, 3382–3386.

Martinez JL and Baquero F (2000) Mutation frequencies and antibiotic resistance. *Antimicrob. Agents Chemother.* 44, 1771–1777.

Matic I (2003) Stress-induced mutagenesis in bacteria. *Science.* 300, 1404–1409.

Michel M, Guttmann L (1997). Methicillin-resistant *Staphylococcus aureus* and vancomycin resistant enterococci: therapeutic realties and possibilities. *Lancet,* 349: 1901 – 1906

Mirza, S.H., Beeching, N.J., Hart, C.A. (1996) Multi-drug resistant typhoid: a global problem. *Journal of Medical Microbiology,* 44: 317 – 319.

Mosher RH, Camp DJ, Yang K, Brown MP, Shaw WV and Vining LC (1995) Inactivation of chloramphenicol by Ophosphorylation: A novel mechanism of chloramphenicol resistance in *Streptomyces venezuelae* ISP 5230, a CAM producer. *J. Biol. Chem.* 270, 27000–27006.

Mukhtar TA, Koteva KP, Hughes DW and Wright GD (2001) Vgb from *Staphylococcus aureus* inactivates streptogramin B antibiotics by an elimination mechanism, not hydrolysis. *Biochem.* 40, 8877–8886.

Nikaido, H. (1989) Outer membrane barrier as a mechanism of antimicrobial resistance. *Antimicrobial Agents and Chemotherapy,* 33: 1831 – 1836.

Nikaido H (1996) Multidrug efflux pumps of Gram-negative bacteria. *J. Bacteriol.* 178, 5853–5869.

Nordman P and Poirel L (2002) Emerging carbapenemases in Gramnegative aerobes. *Clin. Microbiol. Infect.* 8, 321–331.

Normark BH and Normark S (2002) Evolution and spread of antibiotic resistance. *J. Intern. Med.* 252, 91–106.

Oyamada Y, Ito H, Inoue M and Yamagashi J (2006) Topoisomerase mutations and efflux are associated with fluoroquinolone resistance in *Enterococcus faecalis*. *J. Med. Microbiol.* 55, 1395–1401.

Padayachee T and Klugman KP (1999) Molecular basis of rifampicin resistance in *Staphylococcus aureus*. *Antimicrob. Agents Chemother.* 43, 2361–2365.

Park CH, Robiscek A, Jacoby GA, Sahm D and Hooper DC (2006) Prevalence in the United States of a aac (6')-Ib-Cr encoding a ciprofloxacine modifying enzyme. *Antimicrob. Agents Chemother.* 50, 3953–3955.

Piddock LJ and Wise R (1987) Induction of the SOS response in *Escherichia coli* by 4-quinolone antimicrobial agents. *FEMS Microbiol. Lett.* 41, 289–294.

Ploy MC, Lambert T, Couty JP and Denis F (2000) Integrons: An antibiotic resistance gene capture and expression system. *Clin. Chem. Lab. Med.* 38, 483–487.

Poirel L, Kampfer P and Nordman P (2002) Chromosome encoded ambler class A β-lactamase of *Kluyvera georgiana*, a probable progenitor of a sub-group of extended spectrum β-lactamases. *Antimicrob. Agents Chemother.* 46, 4038–4040.

Pos KM (2009) Drug transport mechanism of the AcrB efflux pump. *Biochim Biophys Acta* 1794, 782-793.

Queenan AM and Bush K (2007) Carbapenemases: the versatile β-lactamases. *Clin. Microbiol. Rev.* 20, 440–458.

Rahal, K., Wang, F., Schindler, J *et al.* (1997). Reports on surveillance of antimicrobial resistance on individual countries. *Clin Infect. Disease,* 24(1): S69 – S 75.

Rasmussen, B.A., Bush, K., Tally, F.P. 1997. Antimicrobial resistance in anaerobes. *Clin Infect. Disease*; 24: S110- S120.

Rayssiguier C, Thaler DS and Radman M (1989) The barrier to recombination between *Escherichia coli* and *Salmonella typhimurium* is disrupted in mismatch-repair mutants. *Nature*. 342, 396–401.

Robiscek A *et al.* (2006) Fluoroquinolone-modifying enzyme: a new adaptation of a common aminoglycoside acetyl transferase. *Nature Med*. 12, 83–88.

Rosche WA and Foster P (2000) Mutation under stress: Adaptive mutation in *Escherichia coli*. In: *Bacterial stress responses*, G. Storz, R. Hengge-Aronis (Eds.), ASM press, Washington DC, USA.

Rowe-Magnus DA and Mazel D (1999) Resistance gene capture. *Curr. Opin. Microbiol.* 2, 483–488.

Ruiz J (2003) Mechanisms of resistance to quinolones: Target alteration, decrease accumulation and gyrase protection. *J. Antimicrob. Chemother.* 51, 1109–1117.

Sack, R.B., Rahman, M., Yunus, M., Khan, E.H. 1997. Antimicrobial resistance in organisms casuing diarrhoeal disease. *Clin. Infect. Disease*; 24(1): S102- S105.

Schwarz, S., Werckenthin, C., Pinter, L. *et al.* (1995) Chloramphenicol resistance in *Staphylococcus intermedius* from a single veterinary centre: Evidence for plasmid and chromosomal location of the resistance genes. *Veterinary Microbiology,,* 43: 151- 159.

Schwarz S, Kehrenberg C, Doublet B and Clockaart A (2004) Molecular basis of bacterial resistance to chloramphenicol and florphenicol. *FEMS Microbiol. Rev.* 28, 519–542.

Seoane A and Garcia-Lobo JM (2000) Identification of a streptogramin A acetyl transferase gene in the chromosome of *Yersinia enterocolitica*. *Antimicrob. Agents Chemother.* 45, 905–909.

Simjee S and Gill MJ (1997) Gene transfer, gentamicin resistance and *enterococci*. *J. Hosp. Infect.* 36, 249–259.

Somoskovi A, Parsons LM and Salfinger M (2001) The molecular basis of resistance to isoniazid, rifampin and pyrazinamide in *Mycobacterium tuberculosis*. *Respir. Res.* 2, 164–168.

Suganito M and Roderick SL (2002) Crystal structure of Vat D: an acetyl transferase that inactivates streptogramin A group of antibiotics. *Biochem.* 41, 2209–2216.

Sutton MD, Smith BT, Godoy VG and Walker GC (2000) The SOS response: Recent insights into *umuDC*-dependent mutagenesis and DNA damage tolerance, *Annu. Rev. Genet.* 34, 479–497.

Taddei F, Radman M, Maynard-Smith J, Toupance B, Gouyon PH, Godelle B (1997) Role of mutator alleles in adaptive evolution. *Nature*. 387, 700–702.

Tomasz, A., Munaz, R. 1995. ß-lactam antibiotic resistance in Gram-positive bacteria pathogens of upper respiratory tract: a brief overview of mechanism. *Microbial Drug Resistance*; 1:103 - 109

Viveiros M, Dupont M, Rodrigues L, Davin-Regli A, Martin M, Pages J and Amaral J (2007) Antibiotic stress, genetic response and altered permeability of *E. coli*. *PLoS One*. 2, e365.

Vulic M, Dionisio F, Taddei F and Radman M (1997) Molecular keys to speciation: DNA polymorphism and the control of genetic exchange in enterobacteria. *Proc. Natl. Acad. Sci. USA*. 94 (1997) 9763–9767.

Walsh CT, Fisher SL, Park IS, Proholad M and Wu Z (1996) Bacterial resistance to vancomycin: five genes and one missing hydrogen bond tell the story. *Chem. Biol.* 3, 21–26.

Walther-Ramussen J and Hoiby N (2004) Cefotaximases (CTXMases), an extended family of extended spectrum β-lactamases. *Can. J. Microbiol.* 50, 137–165.

Whiteway J, Koziraz P, Veall J, Sandhu N, Kumar P and Hoecher B (1998) Oxygen insensitive nitroreductases: analysis of the roles of *nfs* A and *nfs* B in development of resistance to 5- nitrofuran derivatives in *Escherichia coli*. *J. Bacteriol.* 180, 5529–5539.

WHO fact sheet, Antimicrobial resistance, 1998; No. 194.

Wise, R. 1998. Antimicrobial resistance is a major threat to public health (Editorial). *British Medical Journal,*;

Wright GD (2007) The antibiotic resistome: the nexus of chemical and genetic diversity. *Nature Rev. Microbiol.* 5, 175–186.

Woodford N and Ellington MJ (2007) The emergence of antibiotic resistance by mutation. *Clin. Microbiol. Infect.* 13, 5–18.

Zapun A, Conters-Martel C and Vernet T (2008) Penicillin-binding proteins and β-lactam resistance. *FEMS Micribiol. Rev.* 32, 361–385.

Zenno S, Koike H, Kumar AN, Jayaraman R, Tanokura M and Saigo K (1996) Biochemical characterisation of Nfs A, the *Escherichia coli* major nitroreductase exhibiting a high amino acid sequence homology to Frp, a *Vibrio harveyi* flavin oxidoreductase. *J. Bacteriol.* 178, 4508–4514.

2

The Natural Antibiotic Resistances of the Enterobacteriaceae *Rahnella* and *Ewingella*

Wilfried Rozhon, Mamoona Khan and Brigitte Poppenberger
Max F. Perutz Laboratories, University of Vienna,
Austria

1. Introduction

The antibiotic resistance genes present in clinical isolates are usually acquired and located on mobile elements allowing their horizontal transfer to other strains or even across bacterial species. Consequently, resistance genes with 100% sequence identity may be found in otherwise unrelated genera while the occurrence of such an acquired resistance within a certain species is highly variable.

In contrast, a number of bacteria are naturally resistant against some antibiotics. The molecular basis for natural resistance may be a general factor like the lack of the targeted pathway, a variant of the targeted molecule that is not inhibited by the antibiotic or a membrane limiting entry of the antibiotic into the cell. In addition natural resistance may also be mediated by a resistance gene belonging to the cell's core genes. Such resistance genes are vertically inherited, shared by (nearly) all isolates of a species and co-evolve with their hosts. They are often encoded by the chromosome, are usually immobile and their expression level is tightly regulated or very low. The establishment of such a resistance requires a long lasting, usually mild selection pressure as it may be present in the soil, which contains many microorganisms producing antibiotics. Examples for this type of natural resistance are the chromosomally encoded β-lactamases found in several species of the Enterobacteriaceae (Naas et al., 2008), many of them colonising plants and soil.

Although these environmental microorganisms pose a low risk to human health, concerns about the spread of their antibiotic resistance genes to pathogens have arisen. Their resistance genes are usually non-mobile, but inclusion into mobile genetic elements may allow the spread to unrelated bacteria. In the last two decades the CTX-M type enzymes have become the most prevalent extended-spectrum β-lactamases (EBSLs) in pathogenic Enterobacteriaceae (Canton & Coque, 2006). The CTX-M enzymes are believed to originate from *Klyvera ascorbata* and *Klyvera georgiana* chromosomal β-lactamases (Olson et al., 2005; Rodriguez et al., 2004). The inclusion of these genes in integrons located on large conjugative plasmids has likely facilitated their spread among the Enterobacteriaceae. Such plasmids contain frequently multiple resistance genes, which might have further enhanced spread of the CTX-M genes in microbial communities by co-selection (Canton & Coque, 2006). Once established in pathogens the spectrum of the resistance genes may be increased by point mutations further impeding treatment of infections with antibiotics. Thus improved understanding of natural resistance, conditions favouring transfer of resistance genes to pathogens and the underlying molecular mechanisms are important areas of research.

Rahnella and *Ewingella*, two closely related genera of the Enterobacteriaceae, are naturally resistant to several β-lactam antibiotics. *Rahnella* is widespread in nature and routinely present in the daily human diet but also *Ewingella* may be present at high titers in some kinds of food. Both microorganisms have been infrequently isolated from clinical specimens. Here the biology, natural habitats, clinical significance and antibiotic susceptibility patterns of *Ewingella* and *Rahnella* will be addressed. Novel results about their resistance genes will be presented and the evolution of these genes and the potential for their transfer to other bacteria will be discussed.

2. Biology, clinical significance and antibiotic resistances of *Rahnella* and *Ewingella*

In 1976 a new class of Enterobacteriaceae was defined during a numerical taxonomy study and provisionally named 'group H2' (Gavini et al., 1976). Based on DNA relatedness studies this group was later proposed as a new species, *Rahnella aquatilis* (Izard et al., 1979). In the following years strains belonging to this novel genus were infrequently isolated from water and clinical specimens and *Rahnella* was thought to be a rare microorganism (Farmer et al., 1985) until it was found to be frequent in plant and soil specimens. Also *Ewingella* was recognised as a separate group of the Enterobacteriaceae in a phenotypical study, which was subsequently confirmed by DNA-DNA hybridisation experiments (Grimont et al., 1983). Based on current reports *Ewingella* is believed to be a rare member of the Enterobacteriaceae (Brenner & Farmer 2005) but some studies indicate that it might be common in some ecological niches. Investigations of clinical isolates revealed that *Rahnella* and *Ewingella* are resistant to several antibiotics, mainly β–lactams. The susceptibility patterns suggested the presence of an extended spectrum Ambler class A β-lactamase (ESBL) in *Rahnella* (Stock et al., 2000), which could be confirmed by cloning and sequencing of the resistance gene (Bellais et al., 2001). The susceptibility pattern and detection of the enzyme by SDS-PAGE/nitrocefin staining suggested an Ambler class C β-lactamase (AmpC) for *Ewingella* (Stock et al., 2003). Here we report for the first time a DNA sequence-based phylogenetic analysis confirming that the *Ewingella* β-lactamase belongs to the AmpC class.

2.1 Biology, habitat and possible applications of *Rahnella* and *Ewingella*

The genus *Rahnella* comprises three genomospecies, *Rahnella aquatilis* (= genomospecies 1), *Rahnella* genomospecies 2 and *Rahnella* genomospecies 3 (Brenner et al., 1998), while the genus *Ewingella* consists of only one species: *Ewingella americana*. Based on phenotypical tests two biogroups of *Ewingella americana* have been defined, which show differences in L-rhamnose and D-xylose fermentation (Grimont et al., 1983). Strains belonging to *Rahnella* and *Ewingella* have no special nutritional requirements and can use a number of carbon sources. They are able to grow in the temperature range from close to 0°C to approximately 40°C, although many strains show a reduced biochemical activity at elevated temperatures (Brenner & Farmer 2005; Brenner et al., 1998; Davis & Eyles, 1992; Jensen et al., 2001; McNeil et al., 1987).

Rahnella is widely distributed and has been isolated from many types of samples. It is frequently found in the rhizosphere and tightly associated with roots and tubers of plants (Berge et al., 1991; Heulin et al., 1994; Jafra et al., 2009; Rozhon et al., 2010) but is also present on other parts of plants including leaves (Hamilton-Miller & Shah, 2001; Hashidoko et al., 2002), fruits (Lindow et al., 1998) and seeds (Cankar et al., 2005; Iimura & Hosono, 1996). Other sources are water (Brenner et al., 1998; Gavini et al., 1976; Niemi et al., 2001), soil (Martinez et al., 2007) and the intestine of snails, slugs (Brenner et al., 1998) and even American mastodon remains (Rhodes et al., 1998). Recently, *Rahnella* was also found at a high frequency in the gut of ghost moths (Yu et al., 2008) and to be associated with larvae and adults of the mountain pine beetle (Winder et al., 2010). *Rahnella* is frequently present in the human diet and has been isolated from different types of food including vegetables (Hamilton-Miller & Shah, 2001; Raphael et al., 2011; Rozhon et al., 2010; Ruimy et al., 2010a), sprouts (Cobo Molinos et al., 2009), fruits (Rozhon et al., 2006), meat (Brightwell et al., 2007; Lindberg et al., 1998) and beverages (Hamze et al., 1991; Jensen et al., 2001). In contrast to its wide distribution in nature *Rahnella* is rarely isolated from clinical specimens.

Ewingella has also been isolated from vegetables (Hamilton-Miller & Shah, 2001) and vacuum-packaged meat (Brightwell et al., 2007), but seems to be significantly less frequent than *Rahnella* in such samples. In contrast, *Ewingella* is very common on mushrooms including button mushroom, shiitake and oyster mushroom (Reyes et al., 2004). Importantly, *Ewingella* is the causative agent of a browning disorder of button mushroom called 'internal stipe necrosis' (Inglis & Peberdy, 1996), which causes significant economic loss. In addition, *Ewingella* has also been isolated from molluscs (Müller et al., 1995). Clinical specimens tested positive for *Ewingella* were mainly blood and swabs from the respiratory tract and wounds.

Rahnella and *Ewingella* have some interesting properties for agronomic and industrial applications. Both seem to promote plant growth and *Rahnella* may be useful as antagonist for controlling plant pathogens including *Erwinia amylovora*, causing fire blight of pear and apple trees (Laux et al., 2002), and *Xanthomonas campestris*, the causative agent of black rot (El-Hendawy et al., 2005). In addition, *Rahnella* might improve the supply of plants with nutrients like phosphate (Kim et al., 1997) and it is able to fix nitrogen (Heulin et al., 1994). The polysaccharides levan and lactan produced by different strains of *Rahnella* have interesting properties for industrial processes (Kim et al., 2003; Matsuyama et al., 1999; Pintado et al., 1999; Seo et al., 2002). The high uranium(VI) resistance of *Rahnella* and its ability to bind this toxic heavy metal is currently intensively investigated and its potential for bioremediation is studied (Beazley et al., 2007; Geissler et al., 2009; Martinez et al., 2007). Because of the increasing interest a project for sequencing of the *Rahnella* genome was launched and recently finished. The sequence of environmental strain *Rahnella aquatilis* Y9602 is available from the genbank database (www.ncbi.nlm.nih.gov) under accession number NC_015061.

2.2 Clinical significance

Rahnella and *Ewingella* are only occasionally isolated from clinical specimens and the clinical significance of both microorganisms is still under debate. Both are believed to be opportunistic pathogens. The pathogenic potential of *Rahnella* seems to be relatively low while a few fatal outcomes of infections caused by *Ewingella* have been reported.

2.2.1 Clinical significance of *Rahnella*

Several reports describe the isolation of *Rahnella* in a clinical context (Table 1). However, in some cases the clinical significance is difficult to assess particularly because many patients had some underlying conditions including haematologic and solid organ malignancy, diabetes and AIDS or had undergone surgery. The age of the patients ranged from 11 months to 78 years and an, although statistically insignificant, male predominance has been recognised among them (Gaitán & Bronze, 2010). Typical sites of isolation were blood, wounds and urine. Interestingly, a significant number of patients developed symptoms during hospitalisation suggesting nosocomial infections.

The first description of *Rahnella* in a clinical context dates back to 1985, where it was isolated from a burn wound (Farmer et al., 1985). In another case *Rahnella* was isolated from a surgical wound that had persisted for more than eight months and was repeatedly tested negative for bacteria before a purulent exudate appeared. At that time pure cultures of *Rahnella* could be isolated from the wound exudate (Maraki et al., 1994). Since *Rahnella* is easy to cultivate and previous efforts to detect bacteria in the wound were negative it seems most likely that the wound was infected recently before the exudate appeared, for instance during the daily wound cleansing procedure. In a further case *Rahnella* was isolated from a diabetes mellitus associated foot wound. Although the infection reacted well to treatment with ampicillin-sublactam the toe and the second digit of the foot had to be amputated because of severe necrosis. This course of disease belongs to the most severe described for an infection with *Rahnella*. However, the ulceration of the wound had begun two month before any medical treatment was started and a co-infection with *Candida sp.* was diagnosed.

While, in a clinical context, *Rahnella* was first isolated from a wound swab, its most frequent site of isolation was blood. *Rahnella* bacteraemia was associated with fever and in two cases with septic shock (Chang et al., 1999; Gaitán & Bronze, 2010). Most patients showed *Rahnella* bacteraemia during hospitalisation (9 of 15 cases) and venous catheters, surgery and drug abuse seem to pose risk factors for infection with this bacterium (Funke & Rosner, 1995; Gaitán & Bronze, 2010; Hoppe et al., 1993; Oh & Tay, 1995). In two epidemiologically related cases a parenteral nutrition fluid was identified as the most probable source of *Rahnella* (Caroff et al., 1998). Both cases appeared in the same hospital within three days and the bacterial strains isolated from the blood of both patients showed identical biochemical profiles and antibiograms and shared the same macrorestriction and ribotyping profiles. Also other patients who had received the same batch of the parenteral nutrition fluid experienced episodes of shivers but blood cultures were not taken impeding further analysis (Caroff et al., 1998). In one very unusual case a contaminated intravenous infusion fluid that a patient had self-administrated could be identified as the source of *Rahnella* (Chang et al., 1999). Thus in a number of cases *Rahnella* cells were directly introduced into the blood circulation. Under certain circumstances *Rahnella* may also be able to spread from the urinary tract to the blood system. Blood cultures of a febrile 76-year old man complaining of nausea and vomiting grew *Rahnella*. The patient had a history of a benign prostatic hypertrophy and the analysis of his urine revealed "many" bacteria. Because of these results and the underlying conditions pyelonephritis was suggested as a possible source of the patient's bacteraemia (Tash, 2005). Since the bacteria isolated from blood and urine of this patient were not compared by biochemical and molecular methods a causal link between the urinary tract infection and bacteraemia remains speculative. With respect to that it is important to note that *Rahnella* was isolated from urine in some other cases but no signs for bacteraemia were reported (Alballaa et al., 1992; Domann et al., 2003; O'Hara et al., 1998).

Case	Year, country	Age, sex	Signs and symptoms	Site	Underlying condition(s)	Treatment	Outcome	Reference
1	1985ª, USA	NA	NA	Burn wound	Burn	NA	NA	(Farmer et al., 1985)
2	1986, USA	37 y, M	Cough, fever, night sweats, diarrhoea	Bronchial washings	AIDS; co-infection with Cryptococcus neoformans	Ampicillin, gentamycin	Cure	(Harrell et al., 1989)
3	1987, Belgium	79 y, M	Fever, expectoration	Sputum, bronchial aspirate	Chronic lymphocytic leukaemia emphysema, bronchopulmonary infection with Pneumococcus	Trimethoprim-sulfamethoxazole	Cure	(Christiaens et al., 1987)
4	1988, France	42 y, F	Septicaemia, leukaemic relapse	Blood	Acute lymphocytic leukaemia, diabetes mellitus, bronchial asthma, Hickman catheter	Vancomycin, ceftazidime	NA	(Goubau et al., 1988)
5	1991, Saudi Arabia	40 y, M	Dysuria	Urine	Renal transplant (status post)	Amoxicillin; ciprofloxacin	Cure	(Alballaa et al., 1992)
6	1992, Greece	63 y, F	Purulent exudate	Surgical wound	Osteoporosis, alcoholism, operation at the left knee	Trimethoprim-sulfamethoxazole	Cure	(Maraki et al., 1994)
7	1992, Germany	7 y, M	Fever (39.5°C)	Blood	Bone marrow transplant recipient; Hickman catheter	Gentamycin, azlocillin, flucloxacillin; amikacin, ceftriaxone, vancomycin	Cure	(Hoppe et al., 1993)
8	1994ª, Italy	59 y, F	Fever	Blood	Chronic renal failure, parenteral nutrition via a Hickman catheter	Ciprofloxacin	Cure	(Caraccio et al., 1994)
9	1994, Switzerland	21 y, M	Fever (39°C)	Blood	AIDS, positive for HBV, HCV and HDV antibodies, recent infection with Staphylococcus aureus, intravenous drug abuse	Ciprofloxacin	Cure	(Funke & Rosner, 1995)
10	1995ª, Singapore	48 y, M	Fever (38.2°C)	Blood	Diabetes mellitus (for 2 y), pulmonary tuberculosis, appendicular abscess	Ampicillin, gentamycin, amoxicillin–clavulanate, gentamycin	Cure	(Oh & Tay, 1995)
11	1995ª, Singapore	57 y, M	Fever	Blood	Laryngeal carcinoma, total laryngectomy	Metronidazole, ceftriaxone; gentamycin	Cure	(Oh & Tay, 1995)
12	1996ª, Spain	2 y, F	Acute gastroenteritis	Faeces	None	None	Cure	(Reina & Lopez, 1996)
13	1996ª, Spain	2 y, M	Acute gastroenteritis	Faeces	AIDS	None	Cure	(Reina & Lopez, 1996)

Case	Year, country	Age, sex	Signs and symptoms	Site	Underlying condition(s)	Treatment	Outcome	Reference
14	1996[c], Japan	11 m, F	Fever (39.7°C), cough	Blood	Congenital heart disease	Cefpodoxime-proxetil; cefotaxime; cefazolin, netilmicin, ceftazidime	Cure	(Matsukura et al., 1996)
15	1997, France	32 y, F	Fever (>38°C)	Blood	Ingestion of a caustic product, parenteral nutrition via a catheter	Removal of the catheter	Cure	(Caroff et al., 1998)
16	1997, France	61 y, M	Fever (40°C)	Blood	Relapse from a renal carcinoma (status post), parenteral nutrition via a catheter	Ticarcillin-clavulanate, vancomycine	Cure	(Caroff et al., 1998)
17	1998[a,b], Japan	NA	NA	Urine	Chronic urinary tract infection	NA	NA	(O'Hara et al., 1998)
18	1999, Korea	26 y, M	Fever (38.2°C), septic shock	Blood	Contaminated intravenous fluid; healthy individual	Ceftriaxone, imipenem	Cure	(Chang et al., 1999)
19	1999, Tunisia	65 y, F	Fever (38.5°C), ketosis	Blood	Diabetes mellitus for 5 y	Cefotaxime, trimethoprim-sulfamethoxazole	Cure	(Boukadida et al., 1999)
20	2000, USA	46 y, M	Fever	Blood	B-cell lymphoblastic leukaemia, immunosuppressive medication, Hickman catheter	Piperacillin-tazobactam, gentamycin	Cure	(Carinder et al., 2001)
21	2000, Spain	63 y, M	Fever (37.8°C), excessive exudate	Trache-ostomy exudate	Laryngeal carcinoma (status post)	Amoxicillin-clavulanic acid; cefotaxime, amikacin	Cure	(Fajardo & Bueno, 2000)
22	2003[a], NA	NA, F	NA	Urine	Co-infection with Candida albicans	None	NA	(Domann et al., 2003)
23	2004[a], USA	76 y, M	Fever (39.8°C)	Blood	Benign prostatic hypertrophy, bacteria in urine	Tracheostomy tube Levofloxacin	Cure	(Tash, 2005)
24	2009, Turkey	57 y, F	Ulcerated foot wound	Wound	Diabetes mellitus for 20 years, co-infection with Candida sp.	Ampicillin-sublactam; Amputation of a toe	Cure	(Aktaş et al., 2009)
25	2009, Italy	78 y, M	Fever, sepsis	Blood	hospitalised at an intensive care unit, co-infection with Candida famata and Pantoea agglomerans[c]	Meropenem	NA	(Liberto et al., 2009)
26	2011, USA	27 y, F	Septic shock, fever (38.1°C)	Blood	Sickle cell disease, central venous catheter	Ciprofloxacin, removal of the catheter	Cure	(Gaitán & Bronze, 2010)

Table 1. Infections caused by *Rahnella*. All cases we could find in the literature are included. [a] Year of report (the year of isolation is not available); [b] The isolates were obtained in the 1990s; [c] *Pantoea agglomerans* is considered as the reason for the sepsis.

Rahnella was also isolated from the faeces of two children with acute diarrhoea. In both cases typical enteropathogenic bacteria, parasites and viruses could not be detected. However, the detection of *Rahnella* in the faeces of patients with diarrhoea is not a sufficient reason for the conclusion that this microorganism is the true cause of the infectious process (Reina & Lopez, 1996). It seems indeed unlikely that *Rahnella* is an enteropathogen since this organism is frequently present in food, particularly vegetables which are frequently eaten raw, while the isolation of *Rahnella* from faeces from patients suffering acute gastroenteritis seems to be a rare exception.

Infections with *Rahnella* reacted very well to treatment with antibiotics and most patients recovered rapidly, though even many of them were immunocompromised. Some patients recovered even without antibiotic treatment (Caroff et al., 1998; Reina & Lopez, 1996). Importantly, no deaths were reported as outcome of an infection with *Rahnella*. These data and the fact that *Rahnella* is a frequent microorganism routinely present in the human diet suggest that it has only a slight pathogenic capacity and its ability to infect humans may be highly dependent on their immunological status.

Currently few data about the pathogenic capacities of the three genomospecies of *Rahnella* are available. The routinely used phenotypic tests allow identification of *Rahnella* only at the genus level. Thus the genomospecies of the isolates of the cases summarised in Table 1 is unknown. A study using DNA-DNA hybridisation revealed that three clinical isolates belonged to *Rahnella aquatilis* (= genomospecies 1) and three were identified as *Rahnella* genomospecies 2 (Brenner et al., 1998) indicating that both genomospecies may act as opportunistic pathogens. However, a study including more strains is highly demanded to assess any potential differences of the pathogenic potential of the *Rahnella* genomospecies.

2.2.2 Clinical significance of *Ewingella americana*

Ewingella americana has been isolated from a variety of clinical specimens, particularly blood and wound swabs and less frequently from sputum (Brenner & Farmer 2005). Typical underlying conditions were surgeries, injuries from accidents, drug abuse and renal failure (Table 2). Some patients had diabetes, received immunosuppressive therapy, were HIV positive or suffered from other chronic infections. However, in contrast to infections with *Rahnella*, a significant number of patients were fully immunocompetent.

Most patients had undergone surgery prior development of bacteraemia, suggesting nosocomial infections. Pien and Bruce (1986) described a nosocomial outbreak of *Ewingella* bacteraemia. Six cases of *Ewingella* bacteraemia appeared in an intensive care unit of a hospital within six weeks. All infected patients had high fever or leukocytosis and had undergone either cardiovascular or peripheral vascular surgery. A careful environmental culturing study identified a contaminated ice bath used to cool syringes for cardiac output determinations as most likely source for the bacteria. *Ewingella americana* was cultured from the bath and its removal from the intensive care unit terminated the outbreak (Pien & Bruce, 1986). In another hospital *Ewingella americana* was diagnosed in blood drawn from 20 patients (Gardner et al., 1985). None of the patients had symptoms typical for *Ewingella americana* sepsis. An environmental investigation revealed that the bacteria were present in a citric buffer anticoagulant used to fill coagulation tubes. Review of blood drawing procedures showed that the non-sterile coagulation tubes were frequently filled first

Case	Year, country	Age, sex	Signs and symptoms	Site	Underlying condition(s)	Treatment	Outcome	Reference
1	1982–1983, USA	55 y, F	Postoperative fever, sepsis	Blood	Aortoiliac graft bypass, aorta occlusion, diabetes	Ampicillin, carbenicillin, gentamicin	Cure	(Pien & Bruce, 1986)
2	1982–1983, USA	57 y, M	Postoperative fever	Blood	Ventricular aneurysmetomy, lower extremity thrombectomy	Cefotaxime, gentamicin, mezlocillin	Cure	(Pien & Bruce, 1986)
3	1982–1983, USA	58 y, M	Postoperative fever	Blood	Coronary artery bypass surgery	Gentamicin, mezlocillin, trimethoprim-sulfamethoxazole	Cure	(Pien & Bruce, 1986)
4	1982–1983, USA	54 y, F	Postoperative fever	Blood	Aorta-iliac artery bypass	Gentamicin, trimethoprim-sulfamethoxazole, doxycycline	Cure	(Pien & Bruce, 1986)
5	1983ᵃ, USA	41 y, M	Postoperative fever (39.2°C)	Blood	Bypass surgery; atherosclerosis, diabetes mellitus; intravascular catheters; co-infection with Pseudomonas sp.	Gentamicin, trimethoprim-sulfamethoxazole	Cure	(Pien et al., 1983)
6	1985, South Africa	46 y, M	Wound (traffic accident)	Wound swab	Wounds originating from a traffic accident; co-infection with Staphylococcus aureus	None	Cure	(Bear et al., 1986)
7	1989, Germany	30 y, F	adhesive eyelids, itching	Conjunctivae (swab)	None	Amoxicillin–clavulanate	Cure	(Heizmann & Michel, 1991)
8	1991, Belgium	75 y, M	Cholecystis, fever (39.4°C)	Blood	Surgery of the gallbladder; also Pseudomonas aeruginosa, Candida albicans and Serratia marcescens were isolated from the patient	Temocillin	Cure	(DeVreese et al., 1992)
9	1991ᵃ, Spain	31 y, M	Balanitis	Penile exudate	HIV, intravenous drug abuse, several opportunistic infections	Tobramycin	Cure	(Sanmartin Jimenez et al., 1991)
10	1995ᵃ, Spain	18 m, M	Acute gastroenteritis	Faeces	None	None	Cure	(Reina et al., 1995)
11	1999ᵃ, Greece	70 y, F	Peritonitis, fever (37.4°C)	Peritoneal dialysate	End-stage renal disease , ambulatory dialysis for 5 years	Amikacin, vancomycin	Cure	(Kati et al., 1999)

Case	Year, country	Age, sex	Signs and symptoms	Site	Underlying condition(s)	Treatment	Outcome	Reference
12	1999, France	38 y, M	Fever (39°C)	Blood	AIDS, intravenous drug abuse (a syringe used was rinsed with water from a fountain), co-infection with *Candida sp.*	Ceftriaxone, amikacin	Cure	(Le Gall et al., 2000)
13	2000, Belgium	57 y, F	Fever (38.8°C)	Blood	Peripheral blood progenitor cell transplantation, treatment with cyclosporine A; Hickman catheter	Removal of the catheter	Cure	(Maertens et al., 2001)
14	2000[a], Brasilia	38 y, F	Kerato-conjunctivitis	Conjuncti-vae (swab)	Soft contact lens	Ciprofloxacin	Cure	(Da Costa et al., 2000)
15	2003[a], Germany	74 y, F	Waterhouse-Friderichsen syndrome	Blood from heart and spleen	Pain in the left leg; otherwise healthy	Tramadol (for treatment of pain)	Death	(Tsokos, 2003)
16	2004[a], Greece	72 y, M	Fever (38.5°C), diffuse abdominal pain	Peritoneal effluent	end-stage renal failure, dialysis for 3 years	Ceftazidime, tobramycin	Cure	(Papaefstathiou et al., 2004)
17	2003[a], Korea	35 y, M	Pneumonia, fever (38.2°C)	Sputum	Chronic renal failure for 7 y; rejection of the transplanted kidney; coinfection with alpha-haemolytic streptococci	Ceftriaxone, isepamicin	Cure	(Ryoo et al., 2005)
19	2007[a], USA	77 y, F	Shortness in breath	Sputum	Infection with *Mycobacterium tuberculosis* and *M. avium* (status post); Cohen's disease	Trimethoprime-sulfamethoxazole	Cure	(Pound et al., 2007)
20	2007, Saudi Arabia	30 y, M	Pneumonia	Tracheal aspirate	Multiple severe injuries from a traffic accident, coma, contusion on the right upper lung, multiple organ failure	No treatment with antibiotics is described	Death	(Bukhari et al., 2008)

Table 2. Infections caused by *Ewingella*. All cases we could find in the literature are included. [a] Year of report (the year of isolation is not available).

allowing contamination of the subsequently filled culture tubes (McNeil et al., 1985). At least some of the patients received inappropriate, unnecessary antimicrobial therapy, incurring the risk of adverse drug reactions and the selection of drug-resistant bacteria (McNeil et al., 1987).

A fatal case of Waterhouse–Friderichsen syndrome was associated with an *Ewingella* infection of a previously healthy 74-year-old women (Tsokos, 2003). She experienced dragging pain in her left leg. Since the physical examination was unremarkable except for restricted mobility caused by the painful leg and her temperature was normal, just an analgetic was administered and bed rest ordered. On the next morning she was found dead in her bed. An autopsy revealed intraparenchymal haemorrhages in both adrenal glands, the heart showed granulocytic infiltration, clots were present in the larger arterial vessels and her brain and lungs were oedematous. *Ewingella americana* could be isolated from heart and spleen blood obtained during autopsy. In agreement with a suspected sepsis a highly increased level of procalcitonin was measured. Death was attributed to acute adrenal insufficiency due to Waterhouse–Friderichsen syndrome caused by *Ewingella americana* (Tsokos, 2003). In a second case the death of a 30-year-old man was associated with pneumonia caused by *Ewingella americana* (Bukhari et al., 2008). In this case the patient was admitted deeply comatose with multiple severe injuries caused by a road traffic accident to hospital. His brain showed oedema, intercerebral haemorrhage in basal ganglia to the right thalamus and subarachnoid haemorrhage along with the fracture of the frontal bone. The upper part of his right lung showed contusion. *Ewingella americana* was identified in his tracheal aspirate but not from any other sample of the patient. The isolated strain exhibited multiple antibiotic resistances but it was not reported whether the patient received any antibiotic treatment. On the eighth day of admission he went to a stage of multiple organ failure and died. It was hypothesised that the cause of death may be pneumonia associated with brain damage (Bukhari et al., 2008). However, because of the underlying conditions it is difficult to rate whether the infection with *Ewingella* was indeed the cause of death. Only two other cases of respiratory infection caused by *Ewingella* have been reported. In both cases the patients recovered quickly after treatment with antibiotics. However, it is important to note that in one of these cases the isolated strain was multidrug resistant (Pound et al., 2007).

In two cases *Ewingella* was associated with eye infection (Da Costa et al., 2000; Heizmann & Michel, 1991). Swabs of the conjunctivae grew the microorganism. Symptoms were keratoconjunctivitis, adhesive eyelids, itching and impaired secretion of tears. In both cases the infection reacted well to antibiotic treatment and the symptoms were relieved in a few days. One report describes also the isolation of *Ewingella* from faeces of a patient with diarrhoea. However, like in the cases of isolation of *Rahnella* from faeces, the clinical significance of this finding is unclear. Since *Ewingella* may be present on some kinds of food, isolated bacteria may originate from the ingested food and be unrelated to diarrhoea. Studies on the frequency of *Ewingella* in the human diet and additional case reports are necessary to rate the enteropathogenic potential of this microorganism.

Taken together these reports suggest that *Ewingella* has a higher pathogenic capacity than *Rahnella*. Several cases of infection in immunocompetent patients were reported. *Ewingella* may also cause infections with fatal outcome. Furthermore, while all *Rahnella* strains isolated so far are susceptible to most antibiotics, two multiple drug resistant isolates of *Ewingella* have been reported. The origin of these resistances, their molecular basis and capacity to spread to other genera are intriguing questions to be addressed in the future.

2.3 Identification of *Rahnella* and *Ewingella*

Reliable identification of strains is crucial for determining appropriate treatments of infections, hygiene monitoring in medical centres and industry and for basic research studies investigating the biology and ecology of microorganisms. In the past *Rahnella* strains were often identified as *Enterobacter agglomerans*, which may also explain that *Rahnella* was thought to be a rare genus while it is now considered as a relatively frequent bacterium.

Rahnella and *Ewingella* can be isolated using media not inhibitory for Enterobacteriaceae such as MacConkey agar or Bromothymol blue lactose agar. Levine EMB agar is especially suitable for *Rahnella*, which forms dark colonies on this medium (Rozhon et al., 2010). *Ewingella* was successfully isolated from mushrooms using VRBG agar (Reyes et al., 2004) or LB agar plates. The latter were anaerobically incubated to suppress growth of *Pseudomonas* (Inglis & Peberdy, 1996). Since a single phenotypic test allowing identification of *Rahnella* or *Ewingella* is lacking, a complete set of biochemical tests is necessary for identification. *Rahnella* is often described to be phenylalanine deaminase positive, which is a very rare characteristic among the Enterobacteriaceae, and to be motile at 25°C but not at 37°C. However, it must be emphasised that *Rahnella* shows only a very weak positive reaction for phenylalanine deaminase and some isolates react negative. Similarly, some strains are also immotile at 25°C. Thus the results of these two tests should be interpreted with care. It is important to note that the three *Rahnella* genomospecies can not be differentiated by biochemical tests (Brenner et al., 1998). Nevertheless, in many reports strains are claimed to be identified as '*Rahnella aquatilis*' although only phenotypic tests were performed. Such classifications should be evaluated very critically. The three *Rahnella* genomospecies were originally identified by DNA-DNA hybridisation experiments (Brenner et al., 1998). With the rapid development of molecular techniques in the last decades DNA sequencing of housekeeping genes is now the method of choice for identification of *Rahnella* at the genomospecies level and for confirmation of the identification of *Ewingella*. For sequencing

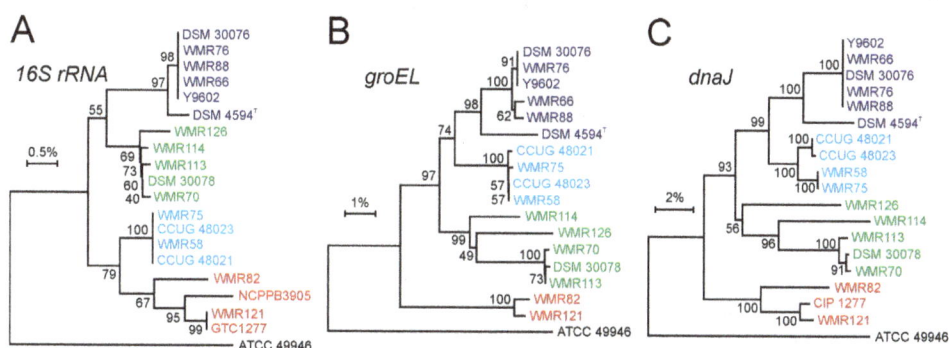

Fig. 1. Neighbour-joining trees based on partial *16S rRNA* (A), *groEL* (B) and *dnaJ* (C) gene sequences of *Rahnella* and *Ewingella*. The trees were constructed with MEGA4 (Tamura et al., 2007) using the p-distance model. Percentage bootstrap values of 1000 replicates are indicated at the corresponding nodes. The scale bars represents the indicated sequence difference. *Erwinia amylovora* ATCC 49946 was used as outgroup. Strains belonging to *Rahnella aquatilis*, *Rahnella* genomospecies 2, *Rahnella* genomospecies 3 and *Ewingella americana* are shown dark blue, light blue, green and red, respectively.

of the (partial) *16S rRNA* gene the primer pair 16S-3/16S-5 can be employed (sequences: 5'-ATATTGCACAATGGGCGC-3' and 5'-GCCATTGTAGCACGTGTGTAG-3', respectively; amplicon: 881 bp) (Rozhon et al., 2011). For verification a part of the *groEL* gene can be sequenced using the primer pair groEL-fwd/groEL-rev (sequences: 5'-ATGGCAGCTAAAGACGTAAAATT-3' and 5'- TTACGACGRTCGCCRAAGC-3', respectively; amplicon: 857 bp) (Rozhon et al., 2011). In addition a part of the *dnaJ* gene can be sequenced using the primer pair dnaJ-fwd/dnaJ-rev (sequences: 5'-CAGTATGGTCATGCAGCCTTTGAACA-3' and 5'-TCAAAGAACTTTTTCACGCCGTC-3', respectively; amplicon: 917 bp). Neihgbour-joining trees constructed with such sequences are shown in Figure 1. The genbank database contains numerous *Rahnella* and *Ewingella* *16S rRNA* and several *groEL* and *dnaJ* gene sequences. Since little is known about the identification of most of these strains only sequences of strains deposited to strain collections should be used for analysis of the obtained data (Table 3).

Strain	Synonyms	*16S rRNA*	*groEL*	*dnaJ*
Rahnella aquatilis DSM 4594[T]	CCUG 14185[T]	FM876214	FM877005	HE577308
Rahnella aquatilis DSM 30076		FM876215	FM877006	HE577309
Rahnella genomospecies 2 CCUG 48021 [a]		U88434	FM877008	HE577311
Rahnella genomospecies 2 CCUG 48023		U88438	FM877009	HE577312
Rahnella genomospecies 2 CCUG 21213		FM876216	FM877007	NA
Rahnella genomospecies 3 DSM 30078 [b]	LMG 2640	U90758	FM877012	HE577310
Ewingella americana GTC 1277	DSM 4560, CCUG 14506	AB273745	NA	AB272652
Ewingella americana NCPPB 3905		X88848	NA	NA

Table 3. Accession numbers of *16S rRNA*, *groEL* and *dnaJ* gene sequences of *Rahnella* and *Ewingella* strains. Abbreviations: CCUG: Culture Collection, University of Göteborg (www.ccug.se); DSM: Deutsche Sammlung von Mikroorganismen (www.dsmz.de); GTC: Gifu Type Culture Collection; LMG: BCC/LMG Belgian Co-ordinated Collection of Microorganisms (bccm.belspo.be); NCPPB: National Collection of Plant Pathogenic Bacteria (www.ncppb.com); NA: not available. [a] Reference strain for genomospecies 2. [b] Reference strain for genomospecies 3.

2.4 Antibiotic resistance of *Rahnella* and *Ewingella*

2.4.1 Susceptibility patterns

The susceptibility patterns of more than 180 *Rahnella* strains have been described in the literature (Table 4). Many of these strains were isolated from clinical specimens but more than 75 originate from environmental samples (most of them were obtained in the study of Ruimy et al. (2010b) and in this study). *Rahnella* was found to be resistant to narrow spectrum penicillins, aminopenicillins, carboxypenicillins and most strains showed a low-level resistance to ureidopenicillins with MICs below 16 mg/l (Stock et al., 2000). Resistance was also observed for 1st and 2nd generation cephalosporins while most strains were sensitive or at least intermediate for 3rd and all strains were sensitive to 4th generation cephalosporins and carbapenems. Addition of β-lactamase inhibitors including clavulanic acid, sublactam and tazobactam decreased the MICs of all β-lactams tested. This pattern suggests the presence of a cavulainc acid-sensitive extended spectrum Ambler class A β-lactamase (Ambler, 1980) resembling the chromosomally encoded class A β-lactamase of *Klebsiella* sp. (Labia et al., 1979; Sykes & Matthew, 1976), *Escherichia hermanii* (Stock &

Antibiotic [a]	Class [b]	(Christiaens et al., 1987)	(Freney et al., 1988)	(Goubau et al., 1988)	(Harrell et al., 1989)	(Hohl et al., 1990)	(Alballaa et al., 1992)	(Hoppe et al., 1993)	(Maraki et al., 1994)	(Oh & Tay, 1995)	(Funke & Rosner, 1995)	(Matsukura et al., 1996)	(Caroff et al., 1998)	(O'Hara et al., 1998)	(Chang et al., 1999)	(Stock et al., 2000)	(Fajardo & Bueno, 2000)	(Bellais et al., 2001)	(Carinder et al., 2001)	(Tash, 2005)	(Aktaş et al., 2009)	(Ruimy et al., 2010b)	(Gaitán & Bronze, 2010)	This study
No. of strains tested		1	12	1	1	6	1	1	1	2	1	1	2	1	1	72	1	2	1	1	1	55	1	20
Amikacin	AMG						S	S	S		S					S				S	S			
Amoxicillin	APEN	R						R			R			R		R	R	R				R		R
Amoxicillin + In	APEN	S	S		SIR		S	R			S			S		S	R	S		S	S	S		S
Ampicillin	APEN	R	R	I	R		R				R	R	R	I		R			R	R	R	R		IR
Ampicillin + In	APEN															R				S	S			
Azlocillin	UPEN									S						IR								
Aztreonam	MOB								S	S								S		S	S	S	S	
Benzylpenicillin	NPEN															R								R
Carbenicillin	CPEN														S									R
Cefaclor	CEF2																	SIR						IR
Cefamandole	CEF2	S							S															
Cefazolin	CEF1			R	R		R	R				S						SIR		R	S	R		S
Cefepime	CEF4															S			S		S	S		
Cefotaxime	CEF3								S		S			S	S	I				S	S	SI		SI
Cefoxitin	CEF2		S					R				S		S		SIR		S		S	S			
Ceftazidime	CEF3								S	S		S				S		S	S	S	S	S		
Ceftriaxone	CEF3					S	S	S	S	I								SIR	S	S	S		S	
Cefoperazone	CEF3														S			SIR		S				
Cefuroxime	CEF2	S		R				R			I		I					IR	R	S				
Cephalothin	CEF1	S	R		R			R	R	R		R		R				R	R	S				IR
Chloramphenicol	O	S		S				R			S	S			S			SI			S			
Ciprofloxacin	FQU				S	S		S	S	S						S				S	S	S	S	
Fosfomycin	O							R							R	R								
Gentamycin	AMG	S		S		S	S	S	S	S	S			S	S	S				S	S	S		S
Imipenem	CARB								S	S	S	S	S	S	S	S	S	S	S	S	S	S	S	
Meropenem	CARB															S		S						S
Netilmicin	AMG								S	S		S				S								
Piperacillin	UPEN								S		S			S		SIR			I	S	S	R	R	S
Piperacillin + In	UPEN															S			S		S	S		
Tetracycline	TET			S	S			S	S	S						SIR					S			
Ticarcillin	CPEN	R								S			R			R		R				R	R	
Ticarcillin + In	CPEN															S			S			S		
TMP/SMX	SUL		S	S	S	R	S	S	S			S			S	S				S	S	S		S
Tobramycin	AMG								S	S		S				S						S		

Table 4. Susceptibility pattern of *Rahnella*. [a] In: β-lactamase inhibitor (clavulanic acid, sublactam or tazobactam); TMP/SMX: trimethoprim/sulfamethoxazole. [b] Classes of antibiotics: AMG: aminoglucosides; APEN: aminopenicillins; CARB: carbapenems; CEF1-4: 1st to 4th generation cephalosporins; CPEN: carboxybenicillins; FQU: flouroquinolons; MOB: monobactams; NPEN: narrow spectrum penicillins; O: other; SUL: sulfonamides; TET: tetracyclines; UPEN, ureidopenicillins. S: susceptible; I: intermediate; R: resistant.

Antibiotic [a]	Class [b]	(Pien et al., 1983)	(Bear et al., 1986)	(Pien & Bruce, 1986)	(Freney et al., 1988)	(Hohl et al., 1990)	(Heizmann & Michel, 1991)	(DeVreese et al., 1992)	(Reina et al., 1995) [c]	(Kati et al., 1999)	(Da Costa et al., 2000) [c]	(Maertens et al., 2001)	(Stock et al., 2003)	(Papaefstathiou et al., 2004)	(Ryoo et al., 2005)	(Pound et al., 2007)	(Bukhari et al., 2008)	This study
No. of strains tested		1	1	4	8	3	1	1	1	1	1	1	20	1	1	1	1	2
Amikacin	AMG	R	S	S						S			S			S	R	R
Amoxicillin	APEN												SIR					R
Amoxicillin + In	APEN		R		SIR	IR			R	S		S	SIR	S			I	R
Ampicillin	APEN	S		S	SIR		S	S	R	S	R	S		S	S	R		R
Ampicillin + In	APEN						S					R	SI		S	R	R	
Aztreonam	MOB							S					S	S	S	R	R	
Benzylpenicillin	PEN									R	R		R					R
Carbenicillin	CPEN	S		S				S		S								R
Cefaclor	CEF2												R					R
Cefamandole	CEF2	S		S														
Cefazolin	CEF1											R	SIR			R	R	
Cefepime	CEF4									S			S		S	R	R	
Cefotaxime	CEF3	S	S	S	SI		S			S		S	S		S	I	R	S
Cefoxitin	CEF2	S	S	R	R								SIR		S	R		
Ceftazidime	CEF3		S					S		S			S			I	R	
Ceftriaxone	CEF3					S				S			S			R	R	
Cefuroxime	CEF2							S		I		I	SR			R	R	
Cephalothin	CEF1	S		R	R				R	R					R	R		R	R
Cephradine	CEF1		R															
Chloramphenicol	O	S	S	S									S	S				
Ciprofloxacin	FQU					S							S	S	S	R		
Ertapenem	CARB															R		
Fosfomycin	O												SIR					
Gentamycin	AMG	R					S			S		S				R	R	
Imipenem	CARB			S				S					S	S	S	R	R	
Levofloxacin	FQU															R		
Meropenem	CARB												S					S
Netilmicin	AMG		S					S										
Ofloxacin	FQU									S		S	S					
Piperacillin	UPEN	S		S								S	S	S	S			
Piperacillin + In	UPEN		S				S	S					S		S	I	R	
Tetracycline	TET	S	S	S							R		SI	R	S	R	R	R
Ticarcillin	CPEN				R								S					R
Ticarcillin + In	CPEN														S	R		
TMP/SMX	SUL	S		S		S		S					S	S	S	R		
Tobramycin	AMG	R	S					S				S				R	R	

Table 5. Susceptibility pattern of *E. americana*. [a, b] For codes see Table 4. [c] Only resistance information was published.

Wiedemann, 1999) and *Serratia fonticola* (Peduzzi et al., 1997). In contrast to *Rahnella*, *Escherichia hermanii* and the *Klebsiella* isolates were sensitive to 1st and 2nd generation cephalosporins while the *Serratia fonticola* β-lactamase showed activity even against 3rd generation cephalosoprins. The unique susceptibility pattern of *Rahnella* indicates an enzyme distant from the other Ambler class A β-lactamases.

Also most *Ewingella* strains are resistant to several β-lactamases, mainly 1st and 2nd generation cephalosporins, while they were sensitive to 3rd and 4th class cephalosporins. In contrast to *Rahnella* only a low or medium-level resistance for penicillins could be observed. The distribution of the MICs of these antibiotics showed a peak at the concentration range clinically defined as 'intermediate' resulting in strains that were sensitive, intermediate or resistant (Stock et al., 2003). This overlap is likely the reason that the phenotypes of ampicillin and amoxicillin resistance seem to be inconsistent in the literature (see Table 4). The β-lactamase of *Ewingella* is insensitive to inhibitors, which is typical for class C β-lactamases.

Apart from β-lactams the most remarkable resistance of *Rahnella* and *Ewingella* was for fosfomycin. The MICs of most strains exceeded 64 mg/l and often reached 512 mg/l (Stock et al., 2000; Stock et al., 2003). Also one highly resistant *Rahnella* isolate with a MIC exceeding 1600 mg/l was reported (O'Hara et al., 1998). Other resistances shared by most strains included only such to which other species of the Enterobacteriaceae are also intrinsically resistant, for instance macrolides, lincosamides and glycopeptides.

Remarkably, two multidrug resistant strains of *Ewingella* were reported. Based on an antibiogram a successful treatment with cefotetan and trimethoprim/sulfamethoxazole was initiated in one case (Pound et al., 2007), while no information about antibiotic therapy was reported in the second case (Bukhari et al., 2008). Further reports of strains with unusual susceptibility patterns are rare and usually only one or two additional resistances were observed (Table 4 and 5). Thus treatment of infections is usually simple. In several cases trimethoprim/sulfamethoxazole, ciprofloxacin, gentamycin and 3rd generation cephalosporins were successfully used. For *Rahnella* also combinations of penicillins with β-lactamase inhibitors may be an option, while this is inappropriate for *Ewingella* infections.

2.4.2 Antibiotic resistance genes and their evolution

Cloning and sequencing of the *Rahnella* β-lactamase (bla_{RAHN-1}) confirmed that it belongs to the Ambler group C (Bellais et al., 2001). The bla_{RAHN-1} gene comprises 888 bp and its translated amino acid sequence shows 75%, 71% and 67% identity to the chromosomally encoded β-lactamases of *Serratia fonticola*, *Kluyvera cryocrescens* and *Citrobacter sedlakii* and approximately 70% identity to plasmid encoded CTX-M type ESLBs found in isolates of *Klebsiella pneumoniae*, *Escherichia coli*, *Acinetobacter baumanii* and other species (Figure 2B). Currently the sequences of the complete bla_{RAHN} loci of four different strains are available. They show a similar pattern: bla_{RAHN} and its surrounding genes have the same transcriptional orientation. An upstream transcriptional regulator that may regulate bla_{RAHN} expression is lacking (Figure 2A). The expression of many chromosomally encoded class A β-lactamases including that of *Citrobacter diversus* (Jones & Bennett, 1995) and *Proteus vulgaris* (Ishiguro & Sugimoto, 1996) is regulated by LysR-type transcription factors but also some examples lacking such a control system, for instance bla_{KLUC-1} of *Kluyvera cryocrescens* (Decousser et al., 2001), are known. A recent phylogenetic study using partial β-lactamase gene sequences of *Rahnella* strains isolated from different vegetables and fruits revealed two

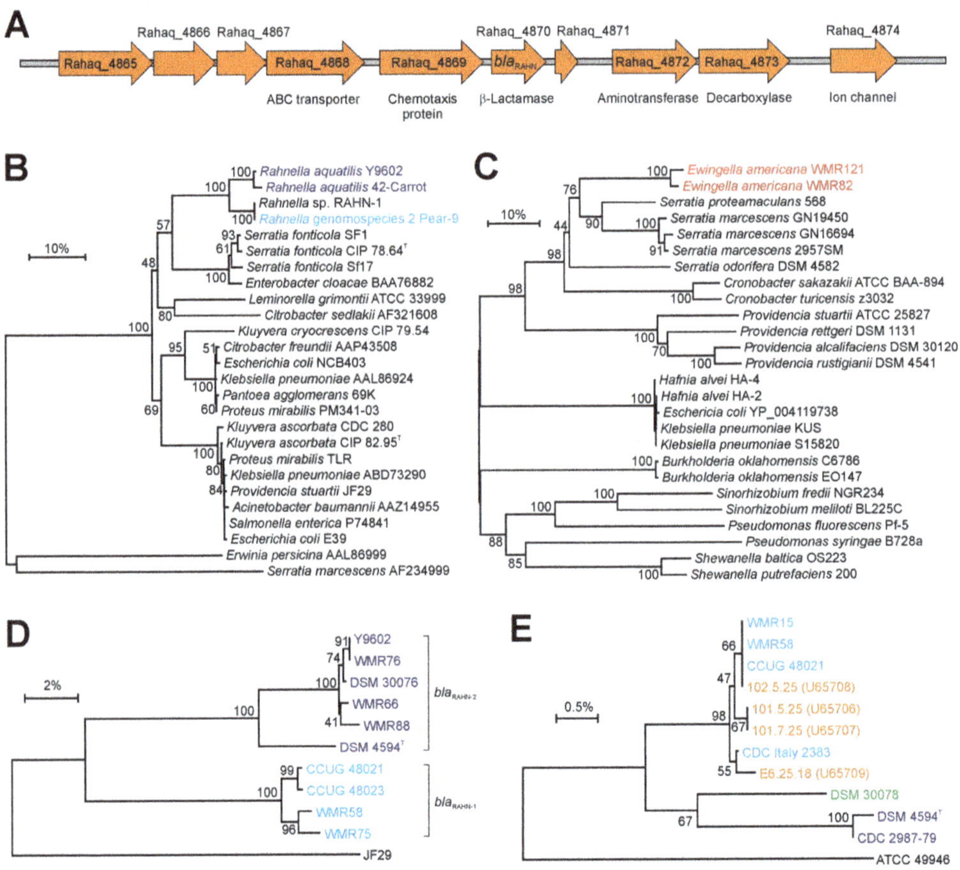

Fig. 2. The antibiotic resistance genes of *Rahnella* and *Ewingella*. (A) The bla$_{RAHN}$ locus and its surrounding genes from strain *Rahnella aquatilis* Y9602 are shown. (B) Phylogentic trees of class A β-lactamases related to *bla*$_{RHAN}$ and (C) class C enzymes related to AmpC of *Ewingella americana*. (D) β-lactamases of *Rahnella aquatilis* and *Rahnella* genomospecies 2 cluster in two different clades. *Providencia stuartii* JF29 was used as outgroup. (E) *Rahnella* isolates obtained from 12,000 year old mastodon remains (shown in orange; the accession numbers are given in brackets) cluster with recent strains belonging to *Rahnella* genomospecies 2. The tree shown is based on partial *16S rRNA* gene sequences. The same methods and colour codes like in Figure 1 were used.

clusters (Ruimy et al., 2010b). A similar dichotomy was also observed for a phlyogenetic tree based on partial *16S rRNA* and *rpoB* sequences (Ruimy et al., 2010a). The originally described *bla*$_{RHAN-1}$ gene (Bellais et al., 2001) clustered with the sequences obtained from *Rahnella* genomospecies 2. The variant found in *Rahnella aquatilis* was named *bla*$_{RHAN-2}$ (Ruimy et al., 2010b). Here we provide data confirming the results of these studies: we sequenced the (partial) *bla* gene of a number of reference strains and environmental isolates. The obtained phylogenetic tree (Figure 2D) is in agreement with that obtained for the *16S rRNA*, *groEL* or *dnaJ* gene (Figure 1). These data clearly suggest that *bla*$_{RHAN}$ was present in the ancestor before the divergence in genomospecies. Previously the isolation of *Rahnella* strains from 12,000 year old American mastodon remains was reported. We used the partial *16S rRNA* gene sequence of these isolates and of recent reference strains to construct a phlyogenetic tree (Figure 2E). The four prehistoric strains cluster clearly with genomospecies 2. This indicates that divergence in genomospecies occured significantly more than 12,000 years ago. Thus the bla_{RHAN} seems to be present in *Rahnella* for a long time and thus represents a natural resistance of this microorganism.

However, we were unable to obtain any PCR product for strains belonging to *Rahnella* genomospecies 3 although these strains were intermediate or resistant to amoxicillin and cephalothin. Thus *Rahnella* genomospecies 3 may either possess a β-lactamase resistance gene unrelated to bla_{RAHN-1} and bla_{RAHN-2} or the primer binding sites may be different. Since the β-lactam susceptibility pattern of the three *Rahnella* genomospecies is very similar, the latter explanation seems more plausible.

Based on the susceptibility pattern an Abler class C β-lactamase was suggested for *Ewingella americana* (Stock et al., 2003). Using different primer combinations we could amplify and sequence the (partial) *ampC* gene of the strains WMR82 and WMR121. The amino acid sequence shows 72% identity to AmpC of *Serratia proteamaculans* and approximately 67% and 59% to AmpC of other *Serratia* species and to the *Providencia* cluster, respectively (Figure 2C). It is interesting to note that the AmpC sequences of the two *Ewingella* isolates share only 96.3% sequence identity. In contrast the plasmid encoded mobile β-lactamases found in some *Klebsiella pneumoniae* and *Escherichia coli* isolates exceed 98% identity (Figure 2C). It is believed that they originate from the chromosomally encoded *ampC* gene of *Hafnia alvei* (Girlich et al., 2000). This result and the observation that the vast majority of *Ewingella americana* strains have a similar susceptibility pattern suggest natural rather than acquired β-lactam resistance for this microorganism.

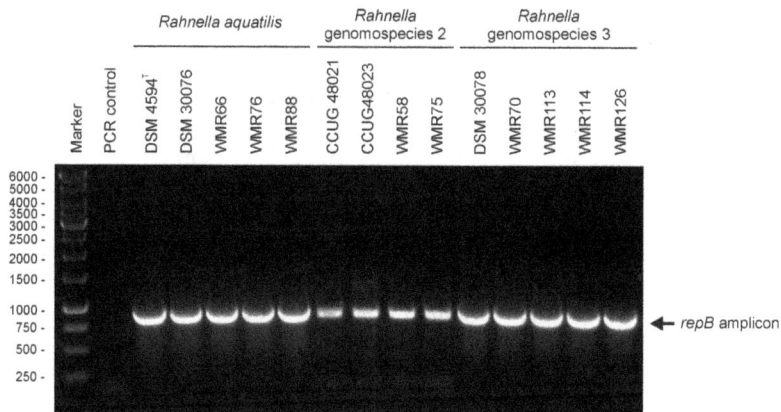

Fig. 3. The plasmid pRAHAQ01 is ubiquitously present in *Rahnella*. The (putative) replication gene *repB* of plasmid pRAHAQ01 could be detected by PCR in all strains tested.

While the molecular basis of β-lactam resistance is well known, the genotype of the fosfomycin resistance remains elusive. The high level of fosfomycin resistance observed in several strains and the report of successful transfer of the fosfomycin resistance to *Serratia marcescens* (O'Hara et al., 1998) rather suggest the presence of a specific fosfomycin:glutation-S-transferase than mutations in the GlpT, a transporter necessary for entry of fosfomycin into the cell.

2.4.3 The plasmid complement of *Rahnella*

Originally bla_{RAHN-1} was thought to be chromosomally encoded, since transfer experiments to *Escherichia coli* failed (Bellais et al., 2001). The recently completed *Rahnella* genome sequencing project showed unambiguously that the β-lactamase gene of strain Y9602 is located on a 617 kb megaplasmid, pRAHAQ01. The bla_{RAHN-2} locus and the surrounding genes of pRAHAQ01 share striking homology to three previously reported bla_{RAHN-1} and bla_{RAHN-2} sequences (Bellais et al., 2001; Ruimy et al., 2010b), indicating that they may also be plasmid born. To investigate this in more detail we analysed the sequence of pRAHAQ01 for putative plasmid replication genes and found only one candidate: Rahaq_4731 or *repB*. RepB shares 82% amino acid sequence identity with the replication protein of pEA29, a large plasmid of the plant pathogen *Erwinia amylovora* (McGhee & Jones, 2000). PCR analysis using primers for a conserved part of the *repB* gene showed a positive result for all strains tested (Figure 3). Moreover, in a previous study the presence of 400 kb to 700 kb megaplasmids in *Rahnella* soil isolates has been described (Evguenieva-Hackenberg & Selenska-Pobell, 1995). This substantiates that bla_{RAHN} may be commonly plasmid encoded. pRAHAQ01 and a second large plasmid found in strain Y9602 seem to be immobile since no known transfer system could be found on their backbones. Furthermore, no evidence could be found that bla_{RAHN} is located on a transposon or an integron.

A number of *Rahnella* strains possess also small plasmids. The majority of them were found to belong to the ColE1 family but also some ColE2 and rolling circle plasmids were isolated. Interestingly, the *Rahnella* ColE1 plasmids formed a distinct cluster in the ColE1 family and lacked any mobilisation system, suggesting that they rarely spread by horizontal gene transfer events. The ColE2 and the rolling circle plasmids possessed mobilisation systems but, like the ColE1 plasmids, were cryptic and did not encode any resistance gene (Rozhon et al., 2010).

Taken together these results suggest that the *Rahnella* β-lactamase, although plasmid encoded, is hardly mobilised to other microorganisms. Indeed, any evidence for its spread to human pathogens is currently lacking (Ruimy et al., 2010b). Similarly, also the *ampC* gene of *Ewingella* has so far remained restricted to its natural host but further experiments are necessary to rate its ability for mobilisation. Such studies would be important because previous reports provide evidence that *Ewingella americana* may be present in clinical environments (McNeil et al., 1987; Pien & Bruce, 1986) and the appearance of multiple drug resistant *Ewingella americana* strains (Bukhari et al., 2008; Pound et al., 2007) indicates that this micoorganism may exchange genetic information with human pathogens.

3. Conclusion

Rahnella is commonly associated with plants and *Ewingella* has been found at high titers in cultured mushrooms. Thus these two Enterobacteriaceae may be frequent in some types of food. Both may appear as infrequent human opportunistic pathogens. Infections are easy to treat if the specific antibiotic resistance patterns of these bacteria are considered. *Rahnella* and *Ewingella* are naturally resistant to several β-lactams, which is mediated by an Ambler class A and an Ambler class C β–lactamase, respectively. The β-lactam resistance gene of *Rahnella*, bla_{RAHN}, is located on the large non-mobile plasmid pRAHAQ01. This plasmid belongs to the pEA29 family, which is commonly found in plant associated bacteria. *Rahnella* acquired bla_{RAHN} presumably in prehistoric times before the divergence into genomospecies. Since then bla_{RAHN} has co-evolved with its host and diverged to bla_{RAHN-1} and bla_{RAHN-2} found in *Rahnella* genomospecies 2 and in *Rahnella aquatilis*, respectively. The variant present in *Rahnella* genomospecies 3 remains to be identified. Although bla_{RAHN} is located on a plasmid it is not per se mobile and so far no hint for its mobilisation to other species has been found. However, since several examples of chromosomal resistance genes that were transferred into pathogens have been documented, it can not be excluded that also bla_{RAHN} may spread to other bacteria in the future. Based on the suceptibility pattern it was previously hypothesised that the β-lactamase of *Ewingella americana* is an Ambler class C enzyme. Here we have provided compelling data confirming this assumption. However, further studies are necessary to assess whether the *Ewingella ampC* gene is chromosome or plasmid born and its potential for transfer needs to be investigated. *Rahnella* and *Ewingella* are also naturally resistant to fosfomycin. The molecular basis of this resistance remains elusive. Other resistances were rarely reported for *Rahnella*, while recently two multidrug resistant strains of *Ewingella* were described. These characteristics should be considered for treatment of infections and for potential applications of *Rahnella* and *Ewingella*.

4. Acknowledgment

We would like to thank Harald Preßlmayer for translation of French, Spanish and Italian manuscripts. This work was supported by the Austrian Science Fund.

5. References

Aktaş, E.; Külah, C.; Cömert, F.; Bektaş, Z. & Kargi, E. (2009). Isolation of *Rahnella aquatilis* from bone and soft tissue of a foot of a patient with diabetes (case report). *Türk Mikrobiyoloji Cemiyeti Dergisi*, Vol.39, No.1-2, (January 2009), pp. 54-57, ISBN 0258-2171

Alballaa, S.R.; Qadri, S.M.; al-Furayh, O. & al-Qatary, K. (1992). Urinary tract infection due to *Rahnella aquatilis* in a renal transplant patient. *Journal of clinical microbiology*, Vol.30, No.11, (November 1992), pp. 2948-2950, ISBN 0095-1137

Ambler, R.P. (1980). The structure of beta-lactamases. *Philosophical transactions of the Royal Society of London, Series B*, Vol.289, No.1036, (May 1980), pp. 321-331, ISBN 0962-8436

Bear, N.; Klugman, K.P.; Tobiansky, L. & Koornhof, H.J. (1986). Wound colonization by *Ewingella americana*. *Journal of clinical microbiology*, Vol.23, No.3, (March 1986), pp. 650-651, ISBN 0095-1137

Beazley, M.J.; Martinez, R.J.; Sobecky, P.A.; Webb, S.M. & Teillefert, M. (2007). Uranium biomineralization as a result of bacterial phosphatase activity: Insights from bacterial isolates from a contaminated subsurface. *Environmental science and technology*, Vol.41, No.16, (August 2007), pp. 5701-5707, ISBN 0013-936X

Bellais, S.; Poirel, L.; Fortineau, N.; Decousser, J.W. & Nordmann, P. (2001). Biochemical-genetic characterization of the chromosomally encoded extended-spectrum class A beta-lactamase from *Rahnella aquatilis*. *Antimicrobial agents and chemotherapy*, Vol.45, No.10, (October 2001), pp. 2965-2968, ISBN 0066-4804

Berge, O.; Heulin, T.; Achouak, W.; Richard, C.; Bally, R. & Balandreau, J. (1991). *Rahnella aquatilis*, a nitrogen-fixing enteric bacterium associated with the rhizosphere of wheat and maize. *Canadian journal of microbiology*, Vol.37, No.3, (March 1991), pp. 195-203, ISBN 0008-4166

Boukadida, J.; Maaroufi, A. & Chaib, A. (1999). Septidmie à *Rahnella aquatilis*. *Médecine et maladies infectieuses*, Vol.29, No.11, (November 1999), pp. 718-720, ISBN 0399-077X

Brenner, D.J. & Farmer , J.J. (2005). Order XIII. "Enterobacteriales", In: *Bergey's Manual of Systematic Bacteriology, Volume 2, Part B*, D.J. Brenner, N.R. Krieg, J.T. Staley, (Eds.). *Springer*, pp. 587-850, ISBN 978-0387-24144-9, New York, USA

Brenner, D.J.; Muller, H.E.; Steigerwalt, A.G.; Whitney, A.M.; O'Hara, C.M. & Kampfer, P. (1998). Two new *Rahnella* genomospecies that cannot be phenotypically differentiated from *Rahnella aquatilis*. *International journal of systematic bacteriology*, Vol.48, No.1, (January 1998), pp. 141-149, ISBN 0020-7713

Brightwell, G.; Clemens, R.; Urlich, S. & Boerema, J. (2007). Possible involvement of psychrotolerant Enterobacteriaceae in blown pack spoilage of vacuum-packaged raw meats. *International journal of food microbiology*, Vol.119, No.3, (November 2007), pp. 334-339, ISBN 0168-1605

Bukhari, S.Z.; Hussain, W.M.; Fatani, M.I. & Ashshi, A.M. (2008). Multi-drug resistant *Ewingella americana*. *Saudi medical journal*, Vol.29, No.7, (July 2008), pp. 1051-1053, ISBN 0379-5284

Cankar, K.; Kraigher, H.; Ravnikar, M. & Rupnik, M. (2005). Bacterial endophytes from seeds of Norway spruce (*Picea abies* L. Karst). *FEMS microbiology letters*, Vol.244, No.2, (March 2005), pp. 341-345, ISBN 0378-1097

Canton, R. & Coque, T.M. (2006). The CTX-M beta-lactamase pandemic. *Current opinion in microbiology*, Vol.9, No.5, (October 2006), pp. 466-475, ISBN 1369-5274

Caraccio, V.; Rocchetti, A. & Garavelli, P. (1994). *Rahnella aquatilis* bacteremia in a patient with chronic renal failure. *Giornale di malattie infettive e parassitarie*, Vol.46, No.5, (May 1994), pp. 330-331, ISBN 0017-0321

Carinder, J.E.; Chua, J.D.; Corales, R.B.; Taege, A.J. & Procop, G.W. (2001). *Rahnella aquatilis* bacteremia in a patient with relapsed acute lymphoblastic leukemia. *Scandinavian journal of infectious diseases*, Vol.33, No.6, (June 2001), pp. 471-473, ISBN 0036-5548

Caroff, N.; Chamoux, C.; Le Gallou, F.; Espaze, E.; Gavini, F.; Gautreau, D.; Richet, H. & Reynaud, A. (1998). Two epidemiologically related cases of *Rahnella aquatilis* bacteremia. *European Journal of Clinical Microbiology and Infection Diseases*, Vol.17, No.5, (May 1998), pp. 349-352, ISBN 0934-9723

Chang, C.L.; Jeong, J.; Shin, J.H.; Lee, E.Y. & Son, H.C. (1999). *Rahnella aquatilis* sepsis in an immunocompetent adult. *Journal of clinical microbiology*, Vol.37, No.12, (December 1999), pp. 4161-4162, ISBN 0095-1137

Christiaens, E.; Hansen, W. & J., M. (1987). Isolement des expectorations d'un patient atteint de leucemie lymphoide chronique et de broncho-emphyseme d'une

Enterobacteriaceae nouvellement decrite: *Rahnella aquatilis*. *Médecine et maladies infectieuses*, Vol.17, No.12, (December 1987), pp. 732-734, ISBN 0399-077X

Cobo Molinos, A.; Abriouel, H.; Ben Omar, N.; Lopez, R.L. & Galvez, A. (2009). Microbial diversity changes in soybean sprouts treated with enterocin AS-48. *Food microbiology*, Vol.26, No.8, (December 2009), pp. 922-926, ISBN 1095-9998

Da Costa, P.S.; Tostes, M.M. & de Carvalho Valle, L.M. (2000). A case of keratoconjunctivitis due to *Ewingella americana* and a review of unusual organisms causing external eye infections. *Braz J Infect Dis*, Vol.4, No.5, (October 2000), pp. 262-267, ISBN 1413-8670

Davis, J.A. & Eyles, M.J. (1992). Discolouration of cottage cheese caused by *Rahnella aquatilis* in the presence of gluco delta-lactone. *Australian journal of diary technology*, Vol.47, No.1, (January 1992), pp. 62-63, ISBN 0004-9433

Decousser, J.W.; Poirel, L. & Nordmann, P. (2001). Characterization of a chromosomally encoded extended-spectrum class A beta-lactamase from *Kluyvera cryocrescens*. *Antimicrobial agents and chemotherapy*, Vol.45, No.12, (December 2001), pp. 3595-3598, ISBN 0066-4804

DeVreese, K.; Claeys, G. & Verschraegen, G. (1992). Septicemia with *Ewingella americana*. *Journal of clinical microbiology*, Vol.30, No.10, (October 1992), pp. 2746-2747, ISBN 0095-1137

Domann, E.; Hong, G.; Imirzalioglu, C.; Turschner, S.; Kuhle, J.; Watzel, C.; Hain, T.; Hossain, H. & Chakraborty, T. (2003). Culture-independent identification of pathogenic bacteria and polymicrobial infections in the genitourinary tract of renal transplant recipients. *Journal of clinical microbiology*, Vol.41, No.12, (December 2003), pp. 5500-5510, ISBN 0095-1137

El-Hendawy, H.H.; Osman, M.E. & Sorour, N.M. (2005). Biological control of bacterial spot of tomato caused by *Xanthomonas campestris* pv. *vesicatoria* by *Rahnella aquatilis*. *Microbiological research*, Vol.160, No.4, pp. 343-352, ISBN 0944-5013

Evguenieva-Hackenberg, E. & Selenska-Pobell, S. (1995). Genome analysis of five soil bacterial isolates named formerly *Enterobacter agglomerans*. *Journal of Applied Bacteriology*, Vol.79, No.1, (July 1995), pp. 49-60, ISBN 1365-2672

Fajardo, M. & Bueno, M.J. (2000). Isolation of *Rahnella aquatilis* in the tracheostomy exudate from a patient with laryngeal cancer. *Enfermedades infecciosas y microbiologia clinica*, Vol.18, No.5, (May 2000), pp. 251, ISBN 0213-005X

Farmer, J.J.; R., D.B.; Hickman-Brenner, F.W.; McWhorter, A.; Huntleycarter, G.P.; Asbury, M.A.; Riddle, C.; Wathen-Grady, H.G.; Elias, C.; Fanning, G.R.; Steigerwalt, A.G.; O'Hara, C.M.; Morris, G.K.; Smith, P.B. & Brenner, D.J. (1985). Biochemical identification of new species and biogroups of Enterobacteriaceae isolated from clinical specimens. *J Cin Microb*, Vol.21, No.1, (January 1985), pp. 46-76, ISBN 0095-1137

Freney, J.; Husson, M.O.; Gavini, F.; Madier, S.; Martra, A.; Izard, D.; Leclerc, D. & Fleurette, D. (1988). Susceptibilities to antibiotics and antiseptics of new species of the family Enterobacteriaceae. *Antimicrobial agents and chemotherapy*, Vol.62, No.6, (June 1988), pp. 873-876, ISBN 0066-4804

Funke, G. & Rosner, H. (1995). *Rahnella aquatilis* bacteremia in an HIV-infected intravenous drug abuser. *Diagnostic microbiology and infectious disease*, Vol.22, No.3, (July 1995), pp. 293-296, ISBN 0732-8893

Gaitán, J.I. & Bronze, M.S. (2010). Infection caused by *Rahnella aquatilis*. *The American journal of the medical sciences*, Vol.339, No.6, (June 2010), pp. 577-579, ISBN 1538-2990

Gardner, S.; Kabat, K. & Shulman, S.T. (1985). An outbreak of pseudobacteremia caused by *Ewingella americana*. *Pediatric Research*, Vol.19, No.4/2, (April 1985), pp. 200, ISBN 0031-3998

Gavini, F.; Ferragut, C.; Lefebvre, B. & Leclerc, H. (1976). Étude taxonomique d'entérobactéries appartenant ou apparentés au genre Enterobacter. *Annales de microbiologie*, Vol.127, No.B, (February 1976), pp. 317-335, ISBN 0300-5410

Geissler, A.; Merroun, M.; Geipel, G.; Reuther, H. & Selenska-Pobell, S. (2009). Biogeochemical changes induced in uranium mining waste pile samples by uranyl nitrate treatments under anaerobic conditions. *Geobiology*, Vol.7, No.3, (June 2009), pp. 282-294, ISBN 1472-4669

Girlich, D.; Naas, T.; Bellais, S.; Poirel, L.; Karim, A. & Nordmann, P. (2000). Biochemical-genetic characterization and regulation of expression of an ACC-1-like chromosome-borne cephalosporinase from *Hafnia alvei*. *Antimicrobial agents and chemotherapy*, Vol.44, No.6, (June 2000), pp. 1470-1478., ISBN 0066-4804

Goubau, P.; Van Aelst, F.; Verhaegen, J. & Boogaerts, M. (1988). Septicaemia caused by *Rahnella aquatilis* in an immunocompromised patient. *European Journal of Clinical Microbiology Infection Diseases*, Vol.7, No.5, (October 1988), pp. 697-699, ISBN 0934-9723

Grimont, P.A.; Farmer, J.J.; Grimont, F.; Asbury, M.A.; Brenner, D.J. & Deval, C. (1983). *Ewingella americana* gen.nov., sp.nov., a new Enterobacteriaceae isolated from clinical specimens. *Annales de microbiologie*, Vol.134A, No.1, (January 1983), pp. 39-52, ISBN 0300-5410

Hamilton-Miller, J.M. & Shah, S. (2001). Identity and antibiotic susceptibility of enterobacterial flora of salad vegetables. *International journal of antimicrobial agents*, Vol.18, No.1, (July 2001), pp. 81-83, ISBN 0924-8579

Hamze, M.; Mergaert, J.; van Vuuren, H.J.; Gavini, F.; Beji, A.; Izard, D. & Kersters, K. (1991). *Rahnella aquatilis*, a potential contaminant in lager beer breweries. *International journal of food microbiology*, Vol.13, No.1, (May 1991), pp. 63-68, ISBN 0168-1605

Harrell, L.J.; Cameron, M.L. & O'Hara, C.M. (1989). *Rahnella aquatilis*, an unusual gram-negative rod isolated from the bronchial washing of a patient with acquired immunodeficiency syndrome. *Journal of clinical microbiology*, Vol.27, No.7, (July 1989), pp. 1671-1672, ISBN 0095-1137

Hashidoko, Y.; Itoh, E.; Yokota, K.; Yoshida, T. & Tahara, S. (2002). Characterization of five phyllosphere bacteria isolated from *Rosa rugosa* leaves, and their phenotypic and metabolic properties. *Bioscience, biotechnology, and biochemistry*, Vol.66, No.11, (November 2002), pp. 2474-2478, ISBN 0916-8451

Heizmann, W.R. & Michel, R. (1991). Isolation of *Ewingella americana* from a patient with conjunctivitis. *European Journal of Clinical Microbiology and Infection Diseases*, Vol.10, No.11, (November 1991), pp. 957-959, ISBN 0934-9723

Heulin, T.; Berge, O.; Mavingui, P.; Gouzou, L.; Hebbar, K.P. & Balandreau, J. (1994). *Bacillus polymyxa* and *Rahnella aquatilis*, the dominant N$_2$-fixing bacteria associated with wheat rhizosphere in French soils. *European Journal of Soil Biology*, Vol.30, No.1, (January 1994), pp. 35-42, ISBN 1164-5563

Hohl, P.; Lüthy-Hottenstein, J.; Zollinger-Iten, J. & Altwegg, M. (1990). *In vitro* activities of fleroxacin, cefetamet, ciprofloxacin, ceftriaxone, trimethoprim-sulfamethoxazole, and amoxicillin-clavulanic acid against rare members of the family Enterobacteriaceae primarily of human (clinical) origin. *Antimicrobial agents and chemotherapy*, Vol.34, No.8, (August 1990), pp. 1605-1608, ISBN 0066-4804

Hoppe, J.E.; Herter, M.; Aleksic, S.; Klingebiel, T. & Niethammer, D. (1993). Catheter-related *Rahnella aquatilis* bacteremia in a pediatric bone marrow transplant recipient. *Journal of clinical microbiology*, Vol.31, No.7, (July 1993), pp. 1911-1912, ISBN 0095-1137

Iimura, K. & Hosono, A. (1996). Biochemical characteristics of *Enterobacter agglomerans* and related strains found in buckwheat seeds. *International journal of food microbiology*, Vol.30, No.3, (July 1996), pp. 243-253, ISBN 0168-1605

Inglis, P.W. & Peberdy, J.F. (1996). Isolation of *Ewingella americana* from the cultivated mushroom, *Agaricus bisporus*. *Current microbiology*, Vol.33, No.5, (November 1996), pp. 334-337, ISBN 0343-8651

Ishiguro, K. & Sugimoto, K. (1996). Purification and characterization of the *Proteus vulgaris* BlaA protein, the activator of the beta-lactamase gene. *Journal of biochemistry*, Vol.120, No.1, (July 1996), pp. 98-103, ISBN 0021-924X

Izard, D.; Gavini, F.; Trinel, P.A. & Leclere, H. (1979). *Rahnella aquatilis*, nouveau membre de la famille des Enterobacteriaceae. *Annales de microbiologie*, Vol.130, No.2, (February 1979), pp. 163-177, ISBN 0300-5410

Jafra, S.; Przysowa, J.; Gwizdek-Wisniewska, A. & van der Wolf, J.M. (2009). Potential of bulb-associated bacteria for biocontrol of hyacinth soft rot caused by *Dickeya zeae*. *Journal of applied microbiology*, Vol.106, No.1, (January 2009), pp. 268-277, ISBN 1365-2672

Jensen, N.; Varelis, P. & Whitfield, F.B. (2001). Formation of guaiacol in chocolate milk by the psychrotrophic bacterium *Rahnella aquatilis*. *Letters in applied microbiology*, Vol.33, No.5, (November 2001), pp. 339-343, ISBN 0266-8254

Jones, M.E. & Bennett, P.M. (1995). Inducible expression of the chromosomal *cdiA* from *Citrobacter diversus* NF85, encoding an ambler class A beta-lactamase, is under similar genetic control to the chromosomal *ampC*, encoding an Ambler class C enzyme, from *Citrobacter freundii* OS60. *Microbial drug resistance*, Vol.1, No.4, (Winter 1995), pp. 285-291, ISBN 1076-6294

Kati, C.; Bibashi, E.; Kokolina, E. & Sofianou, D. (1999). Case of peritonitis caused by *Ewingella americana* in a patient undergoing continuous ambulatory peritoneal dialysis. *Journal of clinical microbiology*, Vol.37, No.11, (November 1999), pp. 3733-3734, ISBN 0095-1137

Kim, H.; Park, H.-E.; Kim, M.-J.; Lee, H.G.; Yang, J.-Y. & Cha, J. (2003). Enzymatic characterization of a recombinant levansucrase from *Rahnella aquatilis* ATCC 15552.

Journal of microbiology and biotechnology, Vol.13, No.2, (February 2003), pp. ISBN 1738-8872

Kim, K.Y.; Jordan, D. & Krishnan, H.B. (1997). *Rahnella aquatilis*, a bacterium isolated from soybean rhizosphere, can solubilize hydroxyapatite. *FEMS microbiology letters*, Vol.153, No.2, (August 1997), pp. 273-277, ISBN 0378-1097

Labia, R.; Fabre, C.; Masson, J.M.; Barthelemy, M.; Heitz, M. & Pitton, J.S. (1979). *Klebsiella pneumonia* strains moderately resistant to ampicillin and carbenicillin: characterization of a new beta-lactamase. *The Journal of antimicrobial chemotherapy*, Vol.5, No.4, (July 1979), pp. 375-382, ISBN 0305-7453

Laux, P.; Baysal, Ö. & Zeller, W. (2002). Biological control of fire blight by using *Rahnella aquatilis* Ra39 and *Pseudomonas spec.* R1. *Acta Hortiulturae*, Vol.590, (November 2002), pp. 225-229, ISBN 978-90-66058-06-4

Le Gall, S.; Pellissier, L.; Delmas, P.; Esterni, J.P. & Roblin, X. (2000). Septicémie à *Ewingella americana* chez un patient toxicomane, au stade sida. *Médecine et maladies infectieuses*, Vol.30, No.7, (July 2000), pp. 484, ISBN 0399-077X

Liberto, M.C.; Matera, G.; Puccio, R.; Lo Russo, T.; Colosimo, E. & Foca, E. (2009). Six cases of sepsis caused by *Pantoea agglomerans* in a teaching hospital. *The new microbiologica*, Vol.32, No.1, (January 2009), pp. 119-123, ISBN 1121-7138

Lindberg, A.M.; Ljungh, A.; Ahrne, S.; Lofdahl, S. & Molin, G. (1998). Enterobacteriaceae found in high numbers in fish, minced meat and pasteurised milk or cream and the presence of toxin encoding genes. *International journal of food microbiology*, Vol.39, No.1-2, (January 1998), pp. 11-17, ISBN 0168-1605

Lindow, S.E.; Desurmont, C.; Elkins, R.; McGourty, G.; Clark, E. & Brandl, M.T. (1998). Occurrence of indole-3-acetic acid-producing bacteria on pear trees and their association with fruit russet. *Phytopathology*, Vol.88, No.11, (November 1998), pp. 1149-1157, ISBN 0031-949X

Maertens, J.; Delforge, M.; Vandenberghe, P.; Boogaerts, M. & Verhaegen, J. (2001). Catheter-related bacteremia due to *Ewingella americana*. *Clin Microbiol Infect*, Vol.7, No.2, (Febuary 2001), pp. 103-104, ISBN 1198-743X

Maraki, S.; Samonis, G.; Marnelakis, E. & Tselentis, Y. (1994). Surgical wound infection caused by *Rahnella aquatilis*. *Journal of clinical microbiology*, Vol.32, No.11, (November 1994), pp. 2706-2708, ISBN 0095-1137

Martinez, R.J.; Beazley, M.J.; Taillefert, M.; Arakaki, A.K.; Skolnick, J. & Sobecky, P.A. (2007). Aerobic uranium(VI) bioprecipitation by metal-resistant bacteria isolated from radionuclide- and metal-contaminated subsurface soils. *Environmental microbiology*, Vol.9, No.12, (December 2007), pp. 3122-3133, ISBN 1462-2912

Matsukura, H.; Katayama, K.; Kitano, N.; Kobayashi, K.; Kanegane, C.; Higuchi, A. & Kyotani, S. (1996). Infective endocarditis caused by an unusual gram-negative rod, *Rahnella aquatilis*. *Pediatric cardiology*, Vol.17, No.2, (April 1996), pp. 108-111, ISBN 0172-0643

Matsuyama, H.; Sasaki, R.; Kawasaki, K. & Yumoto, I. (1999). Production of a novel exopolysaccharide by *Rahnella aquatilis*. *Journal of bioscience and bioengineering*, Vol.87, No.2, (July 1999), pp. 180-183, ISBN 1389-1723

McGhee, G.C. & Jones, A.L. (2000). Complete nucleotide sequence of ubiquitous plasmid pEA29 from *Erwinia amylovora* strain Ea88: gene organization and intraspecies variation. *Applied and environmental microbiology*, Vol.66, No.11, (November 2000), pp. 4897-4907, ISBN 0099-2240

McNeil, M.M.; Davis, B.J.; Anderson, R.L.; Martone, W.J. & Solomon, S.L. (1985). Mechanism of cross-contamination of blood culture bottles in outbreaks of pseudobacteremia associated with nonsterile blood collection tubes. *Journal of clinical microbiology*, Vol.22, No.1, (July 1985), pp. 23-25, ISBN 0095-1137

McNeil, M.M.; Davis, B.J.; Solomon, S.L.; Anderson, R.L.; Shulman, S.T.; Gardner, S.; Kabat, K. & Martone, W.J. (1987). *Ewingella americana*: recurrent pseudobacteremia from a persistent environmental reservoir. *Journal of clinical microbiology*, Vol.25, No.3, (March 1987), pp. 498-500, ISBN 0095-1137

Müller, H.E.; Fanning, G.R. & Brenner, D.J. (1995). Isolation of *Ewingella americana* from mollusks. *Current microbiology*, Vol.31, No.5, (November 1995), pp. 287-290, ISBN 0343-8651

Naas, T.; Poirel, L. & Nordmann, P. (2008). Minor extended-spectrum beta-lactamases. *Clin Microbiol Infect*, Vol.14, No.1, (January 2008), pp. 42-52, ISBN 1198-743X

Niemi, R.M.; Heikkila, M.P.; Lahti, K.; Kalso, S. & Niemela, S.I. (2001). Comparison of methods for determining the numbers and species distribution of coliform bacteria in well water samples. *Journal of applied microbiology*, Vol.90, No.6, (June 2001), pp. 850-858, ISBN 1364-5072

O'Hara, K.; Chen, J.; Shigenobu, F.; Nakamura, A.; Taniguchi, K.; Shimojima, M.; Ida, H.; Yoshikawa, E.; Tsuboi, I.; Mizuoka, K. & Sawai, T. (1998). Appearance of fosfomycin resistant *Rahnella aquatilis* clinically isolated in Japan. *Microbios*, Vol.95, No.381, (May 1998), pp. 109-115, ISBN 0026-2633

Oh, H.M. & Tay, L. (1995). Bacteraemia caused by *Rahnella aquatilis*: report of two cases and review. *Scandinavian journal of infectious diseases*, Vol.27, No.1, (January 1995), pp. 79-80, ISBN 0036-5548

Olson, A.B.; Silverman, M.; Boyd, D.A.; McGeer, A.; Willey, B.M.; Pong-Porter, V.; Daneman, N. & Mulvey, M.R. (2005). Identification of a progenitor of the CTX-M-9 group of extended-spectrum beta-lactamases from *Kluyvera georgiana* isolated in Guyana. *Antimicrobial agents and chemotherapy*, Vol.49, No.5, (May 2005), pp. 2112-2115, ISBN 0066-4804

Papaefstathiou, C.; Vlassopoulos, D.; Zoumberi, M.; Mangana, P.; Hadjiconstantinou, V. & Kouppari, G. (2004). *Ewingella americana* peritonitis in an adult patient on continuous ambulatory peritoneal dialysis. *Clinical Microbiology Newsletter*, Vol.26, (December 2004), pp. 184-185, ISBN 0196-4399

Peduzzi, J.; Farzaneh, S.; Reynaud, A.; Barthelemy, M. & Labia, R. (1997). Characterization and amino acid sequence analysis of a new oxyimino cephalosporin-hydrolyzing class A beta-lactamase from *Serratia fonticola* CUV. *Biochimica et biophysica acta*, Vol.1341, No.1, (August 1997), pp. 58-70, ISBN 0006-3002

Pien, F.D. & Bruce, A.E. (1986). Nosocomial *Ewingella americana* bacteremia in an intensive care unit. *Archives of internal medicine*, Vol.146, No.1, (January 1986), pp. 111-112, ISBN 0003-9926

Pien, F.D.; Farmer, J.J., 3rd & Weaver, R.E. (1983). Polymicrobial bacteremia caused by *Ewingella americana* (family Enterobacteriaceae) and an unusual *Pseudomonas* species. *Journal of clinical microbiology*, Vol.18, No.3, (Sepember 1983), pp. 727-729, ISBN 0095-1137

Pintado, M.E.; Pintado, I.E. & Malcata, F.X. (1999). Production of polysaccharide by *Rahnella aquatilis* with whey feedstock. *Journal of food science*, Vol.64, No.2, (February 1999), pp. 348-352, ISBN 0022-1147

Pound, M.W.; Tart, S.B. & Okoye, O. (2007). Multidrug-resistant *Ewingella americana*: a case report and review of the literature. *The Annals of pharmacotherapy*, Vol.41, No.12, (December 2007), pp. 2066-2070, ISBN 1542-6270

Raphael, E.; Wong, L.K. & Riley, L.W. (2011). Extended-spectrum beta-lactamase gene sequences in gram-negative saprophytes on retail organic and nonorganic spinach. *Applied and environmental microbiology*, Vol.77, No.5, (March 2011), pp. 1601-1607, ISBN 1098-5336

Reina, J. & Lopez, A. (1996). Clinical and microbiological characteristics of *Rahnella aquatilis* strains isolated from children. *The Journal of infection*, Vol.33, No.2, (September 1996), pp. 135-137, ISBN 0163-4453

Reina, J.; López, A.; Fernández-Baca, V. & Ros, M.J. (1995). Aislamiento de *Ewingella americana* en las heces de un paciente con diarrea scretora. *Revista espanola de pediatria*, Vol.51, No.4, (April 1995), pp. 393-395, ISBN 0034-947X

Reyes, J.E.; Venturini, M.E.; Oria, R. & Blanco, D. (2004). Prevalence of *Ewingella americana* in retail fresh cultivated mushrooms (*Agaricus bisporus*, *Lentinula edodes* and *Pleurotus ostreatus*) in Zaragoza (Spain). *FEMS microbiology ecology*, Vol.47, No.3, (March 2004), pp. 291-296, ISBN 1574-6941

Rhodes, A.N.; Urbance, J.W.; Youga, H.; Corlew-Newman, H.; Reddy, C.A.; Klug, M.J.; Tiedje, J.M. & Fisher, D.C. (1998). Identification of bacterial isolates obtained from intestinal contents associated with 12,000-year-old mastodon remains. *Applied and environmental microbiology*, Vol.64, No.2, (February 1998), pp. 651-658, ISBN 0099-2240

Rodriguez, M.M.; Power, P.; Radice, M.; Vay, C.; Famiglietti, A.; Galleni, M.; Ayala, J.A. & Gutkind, G. (2004). Chromosome-encoded CTX-M-3 from *Kluyvera ascorbata*: a possible origin of plasmid-borne CTX-M-1-derived cefotaximases. *Antimicrobial agents and chemotherapy*, Vol.48, No.12, (December 2004), pp. 4895-4897, ISBN 0066-4804

Rozhon, W.; Khan, M.; Petutschnig, E. & Poppenberger, B. (2011). Identification of *cis*- and *trans*-acting elements in pHW126, a representative of a novel group of rolling circle plasmids. *Plasmid*, Vol.65, No.1, (January 2011), pp. 70-76, ISBN 1095-9890

Rozhon, W.; Petutschnig, E.; Khan, M.; Summers, D.K. & Poppenberger, B. (2010). Frequency and diversity of small cryptic plasmids in the genus *Rahnella*. *BMC microbiology*, Vol.10, (February 2010), pp. 56, ISBN 1471-2180

Rozhon, W.M.; Petutschnig, E.K. & Jonak, C. (2006). Isolation and characterization of pHW15, a small cryptic plasmid from *Rahnella* genomospecies 2. *Plasmid*, Vol.56, No.3, (November 2006), pp. 202-215, ISBN 0147-619X

Ruimy, R.; Brisabois, A.; Bernede, C.; Skurnik, D.; Barnat, S.; Arlet, G.; Momcilovic, S.; Elbaz, S.; Moury, F.; Vibet, M.A.; Courvalin, P.; Guillemot, D. & Andremont, A. (2010a). Organic and conventional fruits and vegetables contain equivalent counts of Gram-negative bacteria expressing resistance to antibacterial agents. *Environmental microbiology*, Vol.12, No.3, (March 2010), pp. 608-615, ISBN 1462-2920

Ruimy, R.; Meziane-Cherif, D.; Momcilovic, S.; Arlet, G.; Andremont, A. & Courvalin, P. (2010b). RAHN-2, a chromosomal extended-spectrum class A beta-lactamase from *Rahnella aquatilis*. *The Journal of antimicrobial chemotherapy*, Vol.65, No.8, (August 2010), pp. 1619-1623, ISBN 1460-2091

Ryoo, N.H.; Ha, J.S.; Jeon, D.S.; Kim, J.R. & Kim, H.C. (2005). A case of pneumonia caused by *Ewingella americana* in a patient with chronic renal failure. *Journal of Korean medical science*, Vol.20, No.1, (Febuary 2005), pp. 143-145, ISBN 1011-8934

Sanmartin Jimenez, O.; Botella Estrada, R.; Roig Rubino, P.; Febrer Bosch, I.; Nieto Hernandez, A. & Navarro Ibanez, V. (1991). Balanitis por *Ewingella americana* en un paciente inmunodeprimido. *Actas dermo-sifiliograficas*, Vol.82, No.3, (March 1991), pp. 125-126, ISBN 1138-8196

Seo, J.W.; Jang, K.H.; Kang, S.A.; Song, K.B.; Jang, E.K.; Park, B.S.; Kim, C.H. & Rhee, S.K. (2002). Molecular characterization of the growth phase-dependent expression of the *lsrA* gene, encoding levansucrase of *Rahnella aquatilis*. *Journal of bacteriology*, Vol.184, No.21, (November 2002), pp. 5862-5870, ISBN 0021-9193

Stock, I.; Gruger, T. & Wiedemann, B. (2000). Natural antibiotic susceptibility of *Rahnella aquatilis* and *R. aquatilis*-related strains. *Journal of chemotherapy (Florence, Italy)*, Vol.12, No.1, (Feburay 2000), pp. 30-39, ISBN 1120-009X

Stock, I.; Sherwood, K.J. & Wiedemann, B. (2003). Natural antibiotic susceptibility of *Ewingella americana* strains. *Journal of chemotherapy (Florence, Italy)*, Vol.15, No.5, (October 2003), pp. 428-441, ISBN 1120-009X

Stock, I. & Wiedemann, B. (1999). Natural antibiotic susceptibility of *Escherichia coli, Shigella, E. vulneris*, and *E. hermannii* strains. *Diagnostic microbiology and infectious disease*, Vol.33, No.3, (March 1999), pp. 187-199, ISBN 0732-8893

Sykes, R.B. & Matthew, M. (1976). The beta-lactamases of gram-negative bacteria and their role in resistance to beta-lactam antibiotics. *The Journal of antimicrobial chemotherapy*, Vol.2, No.2, (June 1976), pp. 115-157, ISBN 0305-7453

Tamura, K.; Dudley, J.; Nei, M. & Kumar, S. (2007). MEGA4: Molecular Evolutionary Genetics Analysis (MEGA) software version 4.0. *Molecular biology and evolution*, Vol.24, No.8, (August 2007), pp. 1596-1599, ISBN 0737-4038

Tash, K. (2005). *Rahnella aquatilis* bacteremia from a suspected urinary source. *Journal of clinical microbiology*, Vol.43, No.5, (May 2005), pp. 2526-2528, ISBN 0095-1137

Tsokos, M. (2003). Fatal Waterhouse-Friderichsen syndrome due to *Ewingella americana* infection. *The American journal of forensic medicine and pathology*, Vol.24, No.1, (March 2003), pp. 41-44, ISBN 0195-7910

Winder, R.S.; Macey, D.E. & Cortese, J. (2010). Dominant bacteria associated with broods of mountain pine beetle, *Dendroctonus ponderosae* (Colepotera: Curculionidae, Scolytinae). *Journal of the entomological society of Britisch Columbia*, Vol.107, (December 2010), pp. ISBN 0071-0733

Yu, H.; Wang, Z.; Liu, L.; Xia, Y.; Cao, Y. & Yin, Y. (2008). Analysis of the intestinal microflora in *Hepialus gonggaensis* larvae using *16S rRNA* sequences. *Current microbiology*, Vol.56, No.4, (April 2008), pp. 391-396, ISBN 0343-8651

3

Antibiotic Resistance in Nursing Homes

Giorgio Ricci[1], Lucia Maria Barrionuevo[1], Paola Cosso[1],
Patrizia Pagliari[1] and Aladar Bruno Ianes[2]
*[1]Residenza Sanitaria Assistenziale Villa San Clemente,
Segesta Group Korian, Villasanta (MB)
[2]Medical Direction, Segesta Group Korian, Milan
Italy*

1. Introduction

Until early 20th century, infectious diseases were primarily responsible for mortality in the United States; the average life expectancy were 47 years (US Department of Health and Human Services [DHHS], 1985).

The advent of antiseptic techniques, vaccinations, antibiotics and other public health measures, raised life expectancy. In the early 21st century life expectancy has risen to 76 to 80 years in most developed nations (Center for Diseases Control and Prevention, 2003). Therefore, it is estimated that, by the year 2030, in the United States, 70 million persons will be over 65 years old. (National Nursing Home Week, 2005)

This epidemiologic transition has shifted the burden of morbidity from infections and acute illness to chronic diseases and degenerative illness. (Centers for Diseases Control and Prevention, 2003)

Therefore, with multiple comorbid diseases, many older persons develop functional decline and dependency requiring institutionalization in nursing homes (Juthani-Mehta & Quagliariello, 2010). Nowadays there are over 16000 nursing homes in United States and approximately 1.5 million Americans reside in nursing homes. By 2050 the number of Americans requiring long-term care is expected to double, and this trend is expected in all developed nations (Jones AL & Al, 2009).

The patient population and environment of the nursing home, provide a milieu that permits the development of infections and promote transmission of infectious agents (Nicolle LE & Al, 2001; Juthani-Mehta M & Quagliariello VJ, 2010). This is because nursing home residents have a number of risk factors, including age-associated immunological changes (High K, 2007; van Duin D 2007a, 2007b), organ systems changes, multiple comorbid diseases (e.g dementias, diabetes mellitus, cardio-vascular diseases, chronic obstructive pulmonary disease, impaired dentition) (Bettelli G, 2011), and degenerative disease requiring the insertion of prosthetic devices (e.g. joint prostheses, implantable cardiac devices) that lead to frailty and disability with a high impact on development of infections (Jackson ML & Al, 2004; Curns AT & Al, 2005; Fry AM & Al, 2005).

1.1 Immunosenescence

A functional immune system is considered vital for the host's continued survival against onslaught of pathogens. In humans, as well as in many other species, it is becoming recognized that the immune system declines with age (immunosenescence), which leads to a higher incidence of infections, cancers and autoimmune diseases (Pawelec G, 1999). Immunosenescence involves both the host's capacity to respond to infections and the development of long-term immune memory, especially by vaccination (Muszkat M & Al, 2003; Aspinall R & Al, 2007; Jackson MI & Al, 2008; Boog CJP, 2009), therefore it is considered a major contributory factor to the increased frequency of morbidity and mortality among the elderly (Ginaldi, L & Al, 2001)

Immunosenescence is a multifactorial condition leading to many pathologically significant health problems in the aged population. Some of the age-dependent biological changes that contribute to the onset of immunosenescence are listed in Table 1.

Cells	Biological Changes	References
Hematopoietic stem cells	↓ Self-renewal capacity	Ito K & Al, 2004
Phagocytes	↓ Total number, ↓ Bactericidal activity	Lord JM & Al, 2001; Strout, R.D & Suttles J, 2005
Natural Killer (NK)	↓ Cytotoxicity	Bruunsgaard H & Al, 2001; Mocchegiani E & Malavolta M, 2004
Dendritic Cells	↓ Antigen-Presenting function	Uyemura K, 2002
B- lymphocytes	↓ Antibodies production ↑ AutoAntibodies	Han S & Al, 2003
Naïve lymphocytes	↓ Production	Hakim FT & Gress RE, 2007
Memory cells	↓ Functional competence	Ginaldi L & Al, 2001
Macrophages	Disregulation	Cambier J, 2005
Thymus	↓ Epithelial volume	Aspinall R & Andrew D, 2000
Thymocytes (i.e. premature T-cells)	Reduction/Exhausion on the number	Min H & Al, 2004
Lymphokines	↓ Production (e.g. IL-2)	Murciano C & Al, 2006; Voehringer D & Al, 2002; Ouyang Q & Al, 2003
T-cell receptor (TcR)	Shrinkage of antigen-recognition repertoire diversity	Naylor K & Al, 2005; Weng NP, 2006
Response to Antigenic stimulation	Impaired proliferation of T-cells	Murciano C & Al, 2006; Naylor K & Al, 2005; Weng NP, 2006; Voehringer DM & Al, 2006
Memory & Effector T-cells	Accumulation and Clonal expansion	Franceschi C & Al, 1999; Voehringer DM & Al, 2006
Changes in cytokine profile	e.g. ↑ Pro-inflammatory cytokines milieu	Suderkotter C & Kalden H, 1997

Table 1. Age-dependent biological changes of immunosenescence

At a glance, Hematopoietic stem cells (HSC), which provide the regulated lifelong supply of leukocyte progenitors that are in turn able to differentiate into a diversity of specialized immune cells (including lymphocytes, antigen-presenting dendritic cells and phagocytes) diminish in their self-renewal capacity. This is due to the accumulation of oxidative damage to DNA by aging and cellular metabolic activity and the shortening of telomeric terminals of chromosomes (Ito K & Al, 2004). There is a decline in the total number of phagocytes in aged hosts, coupled with an intrinsic reduction of their bactericidal activity (Lord JM & Al, 2001; Strout, R.D & Suttles J, 2005).

The cytotoxicity of Natural Killer (NK) cells and the antigen-presenting function of dendritic cells is known to diminish with old age (Bruunsgaard H & Al, 2001; Mocchegiani E & Malavolta M, 2004); the age-associated impairment of dendritic Antigen Presenting Cells (APCs) has profound implications as this translates into a deficiency in cell-mediated immunity and thus, the inability for effector T-lymphocytes to modulate an adaptive immune response (Uyemura K, 2002). There is a decline in humoral immunity caused by a reduction in the population of antibody producing B-cells along with a smaller immunoglobulin diversity and affinity (Han S & Al, 2003)

As age advances, there is a decline in both the production of new naive lymphocytes (Hakim FT & Gress RE, 2007), and the functional competence of memory cell populations, with increased frequency and severity of diseases such as cancer, chronic inflammatory disorders and autoimmunity (Ginaldi L & Al, 2001) .

A problem of infections in the elderly is that they frequently present with non-specific signs and symptoms, and clues of focal infection are often absent or obscured by underlying chronic conditions (Ginaldi L & Al, 2001). Ultimately, this provides problems in diagnosis and subsequently, treatment. In addition to changes in immune responses, the beneficial effects of inflammation devoted to the neutralisation of dangerous and harmful agents, early in life and in adulthood, become detrimental late in life in a period largely not foreseen by evolution, according to the antagonistic pleiotropy theory of aging (Franceschi C & Al, 2000a). It should be further noted that changes in the lymphoid compartment is not solely responsible for the malfunctioning of the immune system in the elderly. Although myeloid cell production does not seem to decline with age, macrophages become dysregulated as a consequence of environmental changes (Cambier J, 2005). The functional capacity of T-cells is most influenced by the effects of aging: the age-related alterations are evident in all stages of T-cell development, making them a significant factor in the development of immunosenescence (Linton P & Al, 2006). After birth, the decline of T-cell function begins with the progressive involution of the thymus, which is the organ essential for T-cell maturation following the migration of precursor cells from the bone marrow. This age-associated decrease of thymic epithelial volume results in a reduction/exhaustion on the number of thymocytes (i.e. pre-mature T-cells), thus reducing output of peripheral naïve T-cells (Aspinall R & Andrew D, 2000; Min H & Al, 2004).

Once matured and circulating throughout the peripheral system, T-cells still undergo deleterious age-dependent changes. Together with the age-related thymic involution and the consequent age-related decrease of thymic output of new T cells, this situation leaves the body practically devoid of virgin T cells, which makes the body more prone to a variety of infectious and non-infectious diseases. (Franceschi C & Al 2000b)

T-cell components associated with immunosenescence include: deregulation of intracellular signal transduction capabilities (Fulop T & Al, 1999), diminished capacity to produce effector lymphokines (Murciano C & Al, 2006; Voehringer D & Al, 2002; Ouyang Q & Al, 2003), shrinkage of antigen-recognition repertoire of T-cell receptor (TcR) diversity (Naylor K & Al, 2005; Weng NP, 2006), cytotoxic activity of Natural Killer T-cells (NKTs) decreases (Mocchegiani E & Malavolta M, 2004), impaired proliferation in response to antigenic stimulation (Murciano C & Al, 2006; Naylor K & Al, 2005; Weng NP, 2006; Voehringer DM & Al, 2006), the accumulation and the clonal expansion of memory and effector T-cells (Franceschi C & Al, 1999; Voehringer DM & Al, 2006), hampered immune defenses against viral pathogens, especially by cytotoxic CD8+ T cells (Ouyang, Q & Al, 2003) and changes in cytokine profile e.g. increased pro-inflammatory cytokines milieu present in the elderly (Suderkotter C & Kalden H, 1997).

1.2 Organ system and aging

Alterations in organ systems occur with normal aging, and many of these physiologic alterations contribute to the development of infections (Vergese A & Berk S, 1990; Smith PW, 1994) (Table 2)

System	Aging changes
Skin	Epidermal thinning (Ghadially R & Al, 1995), ↓ elasticity, ↓ subcutaneous tissue, ↓ vascularity (Norman RA, 2003; Gilchrest BA, 1999)
Respiratory	↓ cough reflex, ↓ mucociliary transport, ↓ elastic tissue (Mittman C & Al, 1965), ↑ IgA/IgM in bronchoalveolar lavage and ↑ CD4+/CD8* lymphocytes (Meyer KC & Al, 1996) , ↓ antioxidant levels in epithelial lining fluid (Kelly FJ & Al, 2003)
Gastrointestinal	↓ motility, ↓ gastric acidity (Hall KE & Wiley JW, 1998)
Urinary	↓ urine osmolarity, ↑ perineal-vaginal colonization (women) (Farage MA & Maibach HI, 2011) ↑ prostate size and ↓ prostate secretion (men) (Nickel JC, 2003)

Table 2. Physiologic organ systems changes in the elderly

Although generally efficient defenses against infections are associated with the immune systems, many other elements have an important role.

Epithelia from skin, bladder, the bronchial and the digestive system, for a physical barrier and thereby play a key part in preventing bacteria from invading the human body (Ben-Yehuda A & Weksler ME, 1992). In particular, the skin changes, associated with aging lead to delayed wound healing (Ghadially R & Al, 1995).

Changes in respiratory tract function increase the likehood of aspiration and pneumonia. Apart for a decrease in immune function, various mechanisms are likely to contribute to the pneumonia risk of the elderly: blunting of protective reflexes in the airway, seen after stroke but also a part of normal ageing (Yamaya M & Al, 1991), decreased in mucociliary clearance (Incalzi RA & Al, 1989), loss of local immunity (decreased T-cell subsets and immunoglobulin in respiratory secretions) (Meyer KC, 2001).

Alterations in gastrointestinal tract physiology (e.g. decreased mobility and gastric acidity, decreased intestinal mobility, modifications of resident intestinal flora and intestinal mucus) increase the likelihood of infection after ingestion of a potential pathogen (Ben-Yehuda A & Weksler ME, 1992; Klontz KC & Al, 1997)

Moreover, the urinary tract is more vulnerable to infections in both elderly men and women even in absence of other diseases. Factors contributing to this vulnerability include mechanical changes (reduction in bladder capacity, uninhibited contractions, decreased urinary flow rate and post-void residual urine), urothelial change (enhanced bacterial adherence), prostatic hypertrophy in men (Ben-Yehuda A & Weksler ME, 1992) and hormonal changes (lack of estrogen in post menopausal women) (Yoshikawa TT & Al, 1996)

1.3 Chronic diseases and comorbility

The nursing home population has a high frequency if chronic diseases, many of which increase the likelihood of infections. These chronic diseases are often the major factor necessitating institutional care (Ouslander J, 1989; Hing F & Bloom B, 1990; Van Rensbergen G & Nawrot T, 2010). The most frequent diagnosed underlying chronic diseases include

dementia and neurologic diseases (Banaszak-Koll & Al, 2004; Bowman C & Al, 2004; Van Rensbergen G & Nawrot T, 2010), peripheral diseases (Chong WF & Al, 2011), cerebrovascular diseases (Bowman C & Al, 2004; Van Rensbergen G & Nawrot T, 2010; Chong WF & Al, 2011), chronic pulmonary conditions (Mc Nabney MK & Al, 2007; Van Rensbergen G & Nawrot T, 2010), hearth diseases (Chan KM & Al, 1998; Van Rensbergen G & Nawrot T, 2010; Chong WF & Al, 2011). The prevalence of diabetes mellitus varies from 10 to 30 per cent in the nursing home population (Garibaldi RA & Al, 1981; Nicolle LE & Al, 1984; Ahmed A & Al, 2003; Valiyeva E & Al, 2006; Mc Nabney MK & Al, 2007; IKED Report, 2007; Van Rensbergen G & Nawrot T, 2010).

Comorbidities contribute to the high frequency of infections in nursing homes because the high risk profile of nursing homes residents (Jette AM & Al, 1992): demented residents often have neurogenic bladder and inability to empty the bladder that results in an increased frequency of urinary tract infections (Nicolle LE, 2000; 2002). Patients with peripheral vascular disease have an high risk for skin and soft tissue infections because the impaired vascular supply to extremities and peripheral edema (Sieggreen MY & Kline RA, 2004; Ely JW & Al; 2006). Patients with chronic obstructive pulmonary disease are likely to have bacterial colonization of tracheobronchial tree and recurrent bronchopulmonary infections (Marin A & Al, 2010). Moreover, patients with diabetes mellitus, have increased prevalence of infections (Shah BR & Hux JE, 2003; Bertoni AG & Al, 2001): pneumonia (Valdez R & Al, 1999; Tan JS, 2000), lower urinary tract infections and pyelonephritis (Zhanel GG & Al, 1995; Stamm WE & Hooton TM, 1993), soft tissue infections, including the "diabetic foot", necrotizing fasciitis and mucocutaneous Candida infections (Votey SR & Peters Al, 2005; Fridkin SK & Al, 2005; Miller LG & Al, 2005). Others infections such as invasive (malignant) otitis externa, rhinocerebral mucormycosis (Durand M & Joseph M, 2005; Earhart KC, Baugh WP, 2005) and emphysematous infections (cholecystitis and pyelonephritis) (Votey SR & Al, 2005) occur almost exclusively in diabetics. The optimal management of infections in nursing homes residents includes ensuring optimal therapy of these associated diseases.

1.4 Functional impairment

Disability, functional dependence and deteriorating cognitive performance are strong predictors of nursing home admission among older adults (Jette AM & Al, 1992; Pourat N, 1995; Krauss NA & Altmann, 2004; Miller SC & Al, 1998; Gaugler JE & Al, 2007). On the other hand the chronic diseases affecting the elderly nursing home residents, lead to functional impairment and dependency in activity of daily living (Bajekal M , 2002; Flacker JM & Kiely DK, 2003; Sutcliffe C & Al, 2007; Andresen M & Puggaard L, 2009; Jones AL & Al, 2009).

Poor functional status in nursing home residents has been reported to be associated with increased occurrence of infections and high mortality rate (Curns AT & Al 2005; Jackson ML & Al, 2008; Juthani-Mehta M & Quagliariello VJ, 2010). Chair and bed-bound residents are at risk of pressure ulcers (Galvin J, 2002; Henoch I & Gustaffson M, 2003; Pressure Ulcer Advisory Panel/European Pressure Ulcer Advisory Panel Pressure Ulcer Prevention and Treatment Clinical Practice Guideline, 2009; Jankowski IM; 2010). Urinary incontinence is common, affecting as many as 50% of residents in nursing home and approaches to the management of incontinence (including indwelling bladder catheters and external collecting devices for elderly men), increase the incidence of urinary infections (Gammack JK, 2003; Richards CL. 2004; Eriksen HM & Al, 2007; Ricci G & Al, 2010). Fecal incontinence is also associated with an higher risk of urinary infection (Topinkovà E & Al, 1997;) and both urinary and fecal incontinence may contribute to extensive environmental contamination with pathogens and antimicrobial agent-resistant bacteria (Schnelle JF & Al, 1997; Leung FW & Schnelle JF, 2008; Pagliari P & Al, 2011).

1.5 Nutrition and malnutrition

There are a number of studies that document that 10 to 50% of nursing home residents are malnourished (Donini LM & Al, 2000; Saletti A & Al, 2000; Omran ML & Morley JE, 2000; Nakamura H & Al, 2006; Pauly L & Al, 2007). Over 50% of nursing home residents have reported to suffer from protein caloric malnutrition (Nakamura H & Al, 2006; Ordòñez J & Al, 2010). Vitamin, zinc and micronutrients deficiencies are also reported (Mandal SK & Ray AK, 1987; Girodon F & Al, 1997; Bates CJ & Al, 1999a; 1999b; Gosney MA & Al, 2008). The reasons for this high frequency of malnutrition might be comorbidities (Bostrőm AM & Al, 2011; Shahin ES & Al, 2010), feeding difficulties (Hildebrandt GH & Al, 1997; Lamy M & Al, 1999; Lelovics Z, 2009; Chang CC & Roberts BL, 2011), impaired cognition (Blandford G & Al, 1998; Magri et Al, 2003; Bartholomeyczik S & Al, 2010; Bostrőm AM & Al, 2011), bacterial overgrowth of the small bowel (e.g. Escherichia coli or anaerobic organisms) leading to malabsorption (Mc Evoy AJ & Al, 1983; Elphick HL & Al, 2006; Ziegler TR & Cole R, 2011) and poorer clinical outcomes (Kaganski N & Al, 2005; Stratton RJ & Al, 2006) .

1.6 Invasive devices

Because of multiple comorbidities and disabilities, nursing home residents are more likely to require invasive medical devices (e.g. indwelling urinary catheter, percutaneous and naso-gastric feeding tube, tracheostomy, intravenous catheter and cardiac device). Feeding tubes are present from 7 to 41% of cognitive impaired nursing homes residents and urinary catheterization rate range from 11 to 12%. (Warren JI & Al, 1989; Juthani-Mehta M & Quagliariello VJ, 2010)

Moreover the use of some devices, including tracheostomies and intravenous catheters, is increasing in the nursing homes, reflecting the increasing level of impairment among elderly patients admitted to these facilities.

Device use has been associated with both colonization and infection with antibiotic resistant organisms in nursing home residents (Mody L & Al, 2007; 2008; Rogers MA & Al, 2008; L, & Al, 2008; 2010): from 5 to 10% of nursing home residents have long-term indwelling urinary catheters with associated persistent polymicrobial bacteriuria, urinary tract infections (Warren JW & Al, 1982; Beck-Sague C & Al, 1993; Garibaldi RA, 1999; Ha US & Cho YH,

2006; Regal RE & Al, 2006;) and their complications (Ouslander J & Al, 1987; Warren JW & Al 1987; 1988), while enteral feeding solution given to patients with nasogastric and percutaneous feeding tubes, may be contaminated with bacteria of the family of Enterobacteriaceae, including Serratia spp and Enterobacter spp. (Freedland CP & Al, 1989; Greenow JE & Al, 1989). Moreover, nasogastric tubes have been reported to be associated with a greater occurrence of aspiration pneumonia (Fay DE & Al, 1991) which is one of factor promoting the use of percutaneous gastric or jejunal feeding tubes with subsequent complication of stomal site infections, peritonitis (Luman W & Al, 2001) and risk of developing Clostridium difficile antibiotic-associated diarrhea (AAD) (Asha NJ & Al, 2006).

Finally, intravenous peripheral line, peripherally inserted central catheter, tracheostomy and suprapubic urinary catheter are other commonly used devices in nursing home with an increasingly risk of developing sepsis, pneumonia, skin infections, soft tissue infections (Tsan L & Al, 2008). Device use has therefore associated with repeated courses of antimicrobial therapy foster the emergence of resistant pathogens. (Rogers MA & Al, 2008)

1.7 Drugs use in elderly nursing homes residents

Residents in nursing homes often have a complex and complicated illness profile ranging from simultaneous occurrence of several chronic diseases, depression, pain, sleep problems and dementia with the psychiatric and behavioral symptoms (Selbaek G & Al, 2007; Ricci G & Al, 2009) . Thus "polypharmacy" is the norm in nursing home population. The average nursing home resident receives from 5 to 10 different medications at any time (Beers MH & Al, 1992; Furniss L & Al, 1998; Doshi JA & Al, 2005; Kersten H & Al, 2009). Some of these medications may increase the likelihood of infections: atypical antipsychotics may impair consciousness and increase the frequency of aspiration (Knol W & Al, 2008; Gau JT & Al, 2010); H2 blockers and protonic pump inhibitors (PPI) lead to decreased gastric acidity and may contribute to increased gastrointestinal infections (Laheij RI & Al; 2004; Gulmez SE & Al, 2007;Eom CS & Al 2011; Laria A & Al, 2011). Oral and inhaled glucocorticoid therapy are associated with an increased dose-dependent risk of infections (Ernst P & Al, 2007; Calverley PM & Al, 2007; Kardos P & Al, 2007; Drummond MB & Al, 2008; Singh S & Al, 2009; Smitten AL, & Al 2008; Dixon WG & Al, 2011).

2. Management of infections in nursing homes

Clinical criteria used in the diagnosis and surveillance for infections in nursing homes, have generally been developed from observations in younger population with limited comorbidities. It was not until 2000 that the multifaceted nature of the evaluation of patients in long-term care facilities has led the Society for Healthcare Epidemiology of America and the American Geriatric Society to participation, review and support the Guidelines concerning the multidimensional assessment as part of the infectious disease evaluation in an older adult. (Bentley DW & Al, 2000; Kinsella K & Velkoff, VA , 2001; High KP & Al, 2005; Centre for Diseases Control and Prevention, 2003)

These guidelines are specifically intended to apply to older adult nursing home residents of the potential heterogeneity of conditions present in these facilities residents, suggests that the recommendations are intended to assist with the management of the majority of residents: older adults with multiple comorbidities and functional disabilities.

2.1 Clinical presentation of infections

Presentation of infections in nursing home residents are sometimes atypical (McGeer A & Al, 1991; Norman D & Toledo S, 1992; High K & Al, 2009). Several factors contribute to the difficulty of establishing a clinical diagnosis in these patients. Hearing and cognition are often impaired in nursing home patients: symptoms may not be expressed or correctly interpreted by caregivers. Chronic clinical conditions may obscure the sign of infection leading to misinterpretation or overlooking symptoms. For instance, urinary incontinence may mask symptoms of urinary infection, or congestive heart failure may mask symptoms of pulmonary infection. The presence of coexisting diseases such as chronic bronchitis, which may mask acute pneumonia, or rheumatoid arthritis, which can confound the presence of septic arthritis, may compound difficulties in making the diagnosis of infection. (Cantrell M & Norman DC, 2010)

Altered physiologic responses to infection, or for the manner to any acute illness, are due to man factors including the decremental biologic changes of normal aging, which may be exacerbated by lifestyle. For example, age-related changes in chest wall expansion and lung tissue elasticity, which may be made worse by smoking, contribute to a diminished cough reflex. A weakened cough has the double negative effect of contributing to a decline in pulmonary host defenses and making the diagnosis of respiratory infection more difficult.

Another example of an altered physiologic response to infection in older persons that deserves special mention is the often-observed blunted fever response (Harper C & Newton P, 1989; Wasserman M & Al, 1989; Norman D & Toledo S, 1992; Norman D & Yoshikawa TT, 1996) and increased frequency of afebrile infection (Gleckman B & Hibert D, 1982; Meyers B & Al, 1989)

Although fever is the cardinal sign of infection, the traditional definition of fever (oral temperature of 38° to 38.3°C) may not be sensitive enough to diagnose infection in elderly patients. Castle SC & Al (1991) found that, in a nursing home population, baseline body temperatures are approximately 0.5°C below those of a normal young person and that with infection, despite a rise in temperature comparable to that seen in the young, the maximum temperature may be below the traditional definition of fever. However, a temperature of 37.8°C coupled with a decline in functional status is highly indicative of infection in this population. (Castle SC & Al, 1991)

The presence or absence of fever — aside from facilitating or inhibiting the diagnosis of infection — has other implications. The presence of fever (as defined by an oral temperature of 38.3°C) is highly specific for the presence of a serious, usually bacterial, infection (Keating MJ III, & Al, 1984; Wasserman M & Al, 1989). Moreover, when the syndrome of fever of unknown origin (FUO) occurs in elderly persons, it typically signifies a treatable condition such as intra-abdominal infection, infective endocarditis, temporal arteritis, or other rheumatologic condition. (Knockaert DC & Al, 1993; Berland B & Gleckman RA, 1992).

A blunted fever response to infection frequently portends a poor prognosis (Weinstein MP & Al, 1983).

This may be relevant to the mounting evidence that fever may play an important role in host defenses (Kluger MJ & Al, 1996; Norman D & Yoshikawa TT, 1996). The peripheral leukocyte count in bacterial infection is not as high as that observed for younger population and leukocytosis is often absent. (Werner H & Kuntsche J, 2000). So, the elevation of acute phase protein may be a more reliable marker of infection than elevation of erythrocyte sedimentation rate.

In summary, an acute infection in the elderly may present with either typical clinical manifestations or subtle findings.

Signs and symptoms pointing to a specific organ system infection may be lacking. Thus, an infection should be sought in any elderly person with an unexplained acute to subacute (days to weeks) decline in functional status, falls, delirium, anorexia, weakness, disorientation (Gavazzi G, Krause KH, 2002)

2.2 Antimicrobial agent use in nursing homes

Antimicrobials agents are among the most frequently prescribed pharmaceutical agents in nursing homes; the account for approximately 40% of all systemic drugs used (Crossley K & Al, 1987; Wayne SJ & Al, 1992). It is estimated that two to four million courses of antibiotics are prescribed for residents of US nursing homes annually (Strausbaugh LJ & Joseph CL, 2000) . As a result, from 50 to 70% of residents receive at least one systemic antimicrobial agent during 1 year (Montgomery P & Al, 1995) and the prevalence of systemic antibiotic use is reported to be 8% (Crossley K & Al, 1987; Jacobson C & Strausbaugh LJ, 1990; Warren JW & Al, 1991; Montgomery P & Al, 1995; Lee YL & Al, 1996; Mylotte JM, 1996; Loeb M & Al, 2001a). In a 9-month surveillance study in a nursing home care unit (Jacobson C & Strausbaugh LJ, 1990), 51% of the 321 study patients received antimicrobial agents at some time during their stay. More than one agent was prescribed for 30% of these patients. In addition as many as 30% of nursing home residents receive at least one prescription for a topical antimicrobial agent each year (Yakabowich MR & Al, 1994; Montgomery P & Al, 1995).

A substantial proportion of antimicrobial treatment in nursing homes is considered inappropriate: from 30 to 75% of systemic antimicrobial agents (Zimmer JG & Al, 1986; Crossley K & Al 1987; Jones SR & Al, 1987; Katz PR & Al, 1990; Warren JW & Al, 1991; Yakabowich MR & Al, 1994; Pickering TD & Al, 1994; Montgomery P & Al, 1995) and up to 60% of topical antimicrobial agents (Montgomery P & Al, 1995) are inappropriately used.

The inappropriate use of antibiotics, especially in frail elderly nursing home residents, can be burdensome and harmful (Morrison RR & Al, 1998). From a broader public health perspective, antimicrobial use is the primary factor leading to the emergence of antimicrobial-resistant bacteria. Antibiotic resistance among bacteria implicated in the most common infections is rising exponentially throughout the word (D'Agata E & Mitchell SL, 2008). Infections caused by antimicrobial-resistant bacteria are associated with up to 5 times higher mortality rates and lead to more frequent and prolonged hospitalization compared with infections caused by antimicrobial-susceptible bacteria (Carmeli Y & Al, 2002; Cosgrove SE & Al, 2002; 2005). These issues are relevant for older patients who arbor relatively high of antimicrobial-resistant bacteria, and in nursing homes, where antimicrobials are the most frequently prescribed pharmaceutical agents (Crossley K & Al 1987; Warren JW & Al, 1991; Flamm RK & Al, 2004)

3. Infections in nursing homes

Infections are a frequent occurrence in nursing homes. The most important aspects are represented by endemic infections, epidemics and infections with resistant organisms

3.1 Endemic infections

The most frequent endemic infections are respiratory tract, urinary tract, skin and soft tissue, and gastrointestinal infections (primarily manifesting as diarrhea) (Strausbaugh LJ & Joseph CJ, 1999).

3.1.1 Occurrence of endemic infections

In United States nursing homes, 1.6 to 3,8 million infections occur (Strausbaugh LJ & Al, 2000). These infections are largely endemic and have an overall infection rate that ranges from 1,8 to 13,5 infections per 1000 resident care days (Strausbaugh LJ & Al, 2000). The variability of prevalence (Cohen E & Al, 1979; Garibaldi R & Al, 1981; Standfast SJ & Al, 1984; Setia U & Al, 1985; Scheckler W & Peterson P, 1986; Alvarez S & Al, 1988; Magaziner J & Al, 1991; Steinmiller A & Al, 1991; Eikelenboom-Boskamp A & Al, 2011) and incidence (Magnussen M & Robb S, 1980; Farber BF & Al, 1984; Nicolle LE & Al, 1984; Franson T & Al, 1986; Scheckler W & Peterson P, 1986; Viahov D & Al, 1987; Alvarez S & Al, 1988; Schicker JM & Al, 1988; Hoffman N & Al, 1990; Jacobson C & Strausbaugh LJ, 1990; Darnowsky S & Al, 1991; Jackson M & Al, 1992) rate of infections, reflects differences in patients populations in different study institutions, as well as differing surveillance definitions and methods for case ascertainment .

Many of these reports are from Veteran Administration facilities, where over 90% of the population are male and, thus, non representative of the general nursing home population, in which only 20 to 30% are male. The most frequent infections identified are usually respiratory tract infections, varying in rate from 0.46 to 4.4 per 1000 resident days. In most reports, this includes both upper and lower respiratory infections, because the difficulties in distinguishing the two diagnoses on the basis of clinical criteria alone (Cohen E & Al, 1979; Garibaldi R & Al, 1981; Standfast SJ & Al, 1984; Scheckler W & Peterson P, 1986; Magaziner J & Al, 1991). (Table 3)

The reported incidence of symptomatic urinary infections varies from 0,1 to 2,4 per 1000 resident days. (Nicolle LE, 2000)

The influence of different surveillance definition is notable in reports of incidence of febrile urinary infections. Symptomatic urinary infection may be defined permissively as a positive urine culture in a patient with fever and no other apparent source or, restrictively as a positive urine culture in a patient with fever and acute symptoms referable to the urinary tract (Schaeffer AJ & Schaeffer EM, 2007; High K & Al, 2009). Report using the permissive definition overestimate the occurrence of febrile urinary infection, while those using the restrictive definition certainly underestimate the incidence.

The clinical and economic impact of endemic infections in the nursing home residents is difficult to define, because these patients are highly chronic impaired, and additional morbidity from intercurrent infection is difficult to measure. Moreover, in case of fully dependent, non communicative, demented resident, mortality may not be considered an undesiderable outcome. Similarly, the prolongation of institutionalization may also not be meaningful as a measure of morbidity or cost in these permanently institutionalized elderly residents.

Reference	Incidence per 1000 resident days				
	All infections	Respiratory	Urinary	Skin & soft tissue	Gastrointest inal tract
Magnussen M & Robb S, 1980	3.4	0.46	2.4	0.3	0
Alvarez S & Al, 1988	2.7	0.7	1.2	0.5	Not stated
Nicolle LE & Al, 1984	4.1	1.8	0.1	1.0	0.9
Farber BF & Al, 1984	6.7	3.2	1.8	0.1	0
Franson T & Al, 1986	4.6	1.0	2.3	1.0	Not stated
Scheckler W & Peterson P, 1986	3.6	1.3	1.6	0.5	0.04
Vlahov D & Al, 1987	3.6	1.1	1.2	0.2	0.7
Schicker JM & Al, 1988	5.4	2.0	1.9	0.7	0.24
Jacobson C & Strausbaugh L, 1990	2.6	0.9	1.0	0.45	0.15
Hoffman N & Al, 1990	4.6	1.0	1.9	0.09	0
Darnowski S & Al, 1991	9.5	4.4	1.5	2.1	Not stated
Jackson M & Al, 1992	7.1	3.3	1.3	1.8	0.09
Brusaferro S & Moro ML, 2005	4.8	1.8	1.5	0.7	Not stated

Table 3. Incidence of infections in nursing homes (described in published studies)

Indices that may be used as measures of the impact of endemic infections include the volume of antimicrobial agent use (Warren JW & Al, 1982; Crossley K & Al, 1987; Montgomery P & Al, 1995), frequency of transfer to acute-care facilities for management of infection and infection-related mortality. Reports summarizing antimicrobial agent use consistently identify urinary infection as the most frequent diagnosis for which treatment is prescribed, with respiratory infections second in frequency (Zimmer JG & Al, 1986; Crossley K & Al, 1987; Warren JW & Al, 1991; Waine SJ & Al, 1992; Montgomery P & Al, 1995; Bentley DW & Al, 2000).

From 7 to 30% of elderly residents transferred from nursing homes to acute-care institutions, are transferred for management of infections (Irvine P & Al, 1984; Gordon WZ & Al, 1985; Jacobson C & Strausbaugh LJ, 1990; Kerr H & Byrd J, 1991); respiratory and urinary infections are the diagnoses that most commonly require transfer (Irvine P & Al, 1984; Gordon WZ & Al, 1985). One prospective study reported that 6,3% of all infectious episodes in nursing homes were associated with death, or 10,3 deaths per 100 residents per year (Nicolle LE & Al, 1984). However, overall mortality is reported to be similar in residents with and without infection (Jacobson C & Strausbaugh LJ, 1990). The only common infection with a high case/fatality ratio is pneumonia (Ahlbrecht H & Al, 1999). Autopsy series of elderly nursing home residents consistently fail to identify an infection other than pneumonia as an immediate cause of death (Nicolle LE & Al, 1987a; Gross JS & Al, 1988)

3.1.2 Respiratory tract infections

3.1.2.1 Upper respiratory tract infections

Upper respiratory infections in nursing home patients include sinusitis, otitis media, otitis externa and pharyngitis. Generally, the incidence of upper respiratory tract infections is reported to be less than that of lower respiratory tract infections: Scheckler and Peterson (1986) reported 1,1 upper respiratory tract infections per 100 resident months, compared with 1,9 pneumonia and bronchitis. The different clinical syndromes included as upper respiratory tract infections are usually reported as a single group, and the incidence of infection at each side is not known for nursing home residents. Group A streptococcus may cause pharyngitis, but most reports of streptococcal pharyngitis describe relatively uncommon episodes of epidemic infections (Schwartz B & Ussery X, 1992). Overall, these infections seem to have limited impact in the nursing home population.

3.1.2.2 Lower respiratory tract infections

Lower respiratory tract infections, including both pneumonia and bronchitis, are the most important infections occurring in nursing homes in both frequency and clinical consequences (Jackson M & Al, 1992; Beck-Sague C & Al, 1994). Increased aspiration of oropharyngeal contents and impairment pulmonary clearance mechanism resulting from physiologic aging changes, as well chronic pulmonary, cardiovascular and neurologic disease, contribute to the high incidence of pneumonia.

Pneumonia is the only infection that is an important contributor to mortality, in this population, with a reported case/fatality rate of 6 to 23% (Nicolle LE & Al, 1984; Scheckler W & Peterson P, 1986; Jackson M & Al, 1992; Jacobson C & Strausbaugh LJ, 1990).

Studies of the etiologies of nursing home-acquired pneumonia are generally flawed because they rely on expectorated sputum specimens to define bacteriology, and sputum specimens cannot differentiate oropharyngeal colonization from pulmonary infection.

Invasive methods to estabilish an etiologic cause (transtracheal or transthoracic aspiration, bronchoscopy) are infrequently performed in nursing home population. Bacteriemia occurs in less than 25% of cases, even if it would allow the identification of the causative agent.

With this limitations, streptococcus pneumoniae, remains the most important pathogen (Phair J & Al, 1978; Bentley DW, 1984; Farber BF & Al, 1984; Marrie TJ & Al, 1986; Peterson PK & Al, 1988). (Table 4)

Patients with chronic obstructive pulmonary disease have an increased frequency of bronchopneumonia, associated with Haemophilus influenzae and Moraxella catarrhalis. There is an increased occurrence of Gram-negative organism such Klebsiella pneumonia in the nursing home relative to other populations.

In at least one study in which specimen for culture were obtained through transtracheal aspiration, 37% of episodes were reported to have mixed respiratory flora (Bentley DW, 1984). Atypical pathogens such as Chlamydia pneumonia, Mycoplasma pneumonia and Legionella pneumophila may cause pneumonia in nursing home residents, but appear to be relatively infrequent.

Bacteria (percentage of total isolates)	Garb J & Al, 1978 (n=47)	Marrie TJ & Al, 1986 (n=12)	Peterson PK & Al, 1988 (n=129)	Bentley DW, 1984 (n=115)	Phillips SL & Brahaman-Phillips MA, 1993 (n=92)	Lim WS & Macfarlane JT, 2001 (n=22)	El-Sohl AA & Al, 2002 (n=21)	El-Sohl AA & Al, 2004 (n=93)	Carratala J & Al, 2007 (n=126)	Kothe H & Al, 2008 (n=1349)	Shindo Y & Al, 2009 (n=141)
Streptococcus pneumoniae	19	17	30	32	34	55	0.04	25	27.8	43.3	13.5
Klebsiella pneumoniae	30	25	7.5	-	2.2	-	0.04	-	-	-	7.1
Hemophilus influentiae	4.3	-	23	5.2	23	-	-	-	11.9	3.4	-
Enterobacter spp	11	8.3	-	-	1.1	-	24	28	-	-	-
Escherichia coli	6.4	17	13	-	6.5	-	-	-	2.4	-	3.5
Serratia marcescens	4.3	-	-	-	-	-	-	-	-	-	-
Pseudomonas aeruginosa	4.3	-	2.5	-	6.5	-	14	-	1.6	-	5.7
Citrobacter spp	2.1	-	2.5	-	2.2	-	-	-	-	-	-
Proteus spp	-	-	2.5	-	2.2	-	-	-	-	-	2.8
Branhamella catarrhalis	-	-	13	-	4.3	-	-	-	-	-	-
Other Gram-	-	-	-	17	6.5	22	-	-	6.4	7.1	2.8
Staphylococcus aureus	19	8.3	7.5	1.7	12	-	33	31	2.4	2.2	9.9
Mixed	-	25	-	43	-	-	38	5	-	20.9	20.3

Table 4. Bacteria reported in published studies as a etiologic agents in subjects with nursing home-acquired pneumonia

3.1.2.3 Tuberculosis

The occurrence of Mycobacterium tuberculosis is variable among different institutions, although it is an important cause of infection in some nursing homes (Stead W, 1981; Stead W & Al, 1985; Brennen C & Al, 1988; Bentley DW, 1990a).

The prevalence of positive tuberculin skin test in nursing home residents has been reported to vary from 21 to 35% (Stead W & Al, 1985; Welty C & Al, 1985; Perez-Stable EJ & Al, 1988).

While active tuberculosis in nursing home residents is usually due to reactivation of latent infection, primary infection or reinfection may occur following exposure to an infectious case (Bentley DW, 1990a). Stead W (1985) reported that residents with negative skin test on admission to nursing homes, had a 5% year conversion rate in a home with a known infectious case, while the rate was 3,5% year in a home without a known case.

About 10% of skin test convertors who did not receive prophylactic isoniazid therapy developed active infection.

When an infectious case occurs, delay in diagnosis due to preexisting chronic pulmonary symptoms, or delay in obtaining a chest radiography, may lead to prolonged, extensive exposure of other residents and staff.

3.1.3 Urinary tract infections

3.1.3.1 Symptomatic urinary infections

In most survey the leading infection in nursing homes and in long-term care facilities is urinary tract infection (Bentley DW & Al, 2000; Philip W & Al, 2008) although with restrictive clinical definitions, symptomatic urinary infection is less frequent than respiratory infection (Stevenson KB & Al, 2005). Bacteriuria is very common in nursing home residents but, by itself, is not associated with adverse outcomes and does not affect survival (Eberle CM & Al 1993; Smith PW, 1985; Nicolle LE & Al, 2005a), therefore practitioners must distinguish symptomatic UTI from asymptomatic bacteriuria in making therapeutic decisions.

Diagnosing urinary tract infection in nursing home residents is problematic. Given the high incidence of asymptomatic bacteriuria and pyuria, a positive urine culture and pyuria on urinalysis are non-diagnostic (Nicolle LE, 2000). Practitioners utilize clinical criteria to differentiate symptomatic urinary tract infection from asymptomatic bacteriuria, but existing clinical criteria were developed by expert consensus (McGeer A & Al, 1991; Philip W & Al, 2008) . The McGeer consensus criteria for urinary tract infection are widely accepted as surveillance and treatment standards (Centers for Medicare and Medicaid (CMS) Manual System, 2005).

For residents without an indwelling catheter, three of the following criteria must be met to identify urinary tract infection : (1) fever ≥38°C; (2) new or increased burning on urination, frequency, or urgency; (3) new flank or suprapubic pain or tenderness; (4) change in character of urine; (5) worsening of mental or functional status (McGeer A & Al, 1991) The Loeb consensus criteria for urinary tract infection are minimum criteria necessary for empiric antibiotic therapy. For residents without an indwelling catheter, criteria include acute dysuria alone or fever (>37.9° or 1.5°C increase above baseline temperature) plus at least one of the following: new or worsening urgency, frequency, supra-pubic pain, gross hematuria, costovertebral angle tenderness, or urinary incontinence. (Loeb M & Al, 2001) The reliability, specifically inter-observer variability, for elements of these consensus criteria has not been determined.

If the typical symptoms of urinary tract infection are dysuria and frequency (cystitis) or fever and flank pain (pyelonephritis), the elderly may present with atypical or non-localizing symptoms. Chronic genitourinary symptoms are also common but are not attributable to bacteriuria (Nicolle LE & Al, 2005a; Ouslander JG & Schnelle JF, 2005). Because the prevalence of bacteriuria is high, a positive urine culture, with or without pyuria, is not sufficient to diagnose urinary infection (Nicolle LE & Al, 2005a). Clinical findings for diagnosis of urinary tract infection in non-catheterized residents must include some localization to the genitourinary tract (Mc Geer & Al, 1991). The diagnosis also requires a positive quantitative urine culture obtained by the clean-catch voided technique, by in and out catheterization, or by aspiration through a catheter system sampling port. A negative test for pyuria or a negative urine culture obtained prior to initiation of antimicrobial therapy, excludes urinary infection, while a positive urine culture is not helpful in defining a urinary source for symptoms. Given these provisos, rates of symptomatic urinary infection of 0,11 to 0,15 per bacteriuric year have been reported in studies with restrictive clinical definition, that require the presence of localizing genitourinary symptoms or signs (Nicolle LE, 1983; 1987). Moreover, symptomatic urinary infection is reported as the diagnosis necessitating transfer from a nursing home to an acute-care facility in 1 to 8% of such transfers (Irvine P, 1984; Gordon WZ, & Al, 1985). The urinary tract is the most common source of bacteriemia in the institutionalized elderly, contributing to over 50% of episodes (Setia U & Al, 1984; Rudman D & Al, 1988; Muder RR & Al, 1992; Nicolle LE & Al, 1994a) with a case/fatality ratio of 16 to 23% (Setia U & Al, 1985; Muder RR & Al, 1992; Nicolle LE & Al, 1994a). The prevalence of indwelling urethral catheters in the nursing homes is 7 to 10% (Ribeiro BJ & Smith SR, 1985; Warren JW & Al, 1989; Kunin CM & Al, 1992). Catheterization predisposes to clinical urinary tract infection and the catheterized urinary tract is the most common source of bacteriemia in nursing homes (Smith PW, 1985; Nicolle LE & Al, 1996). Bacteriemia occurs significantly more frequently in subjects with indwelling urinary catheters (Rudman D & Al, 1988; Muder RR & Al, 1992). Residents with long-time catheters often present with fever alone.

Nursing home residents with indwelling urinary catheters, are uniformly colonized with bacteria, largely attributable to biofilm oñ the catheter (Warren JW & Al, 1982). These organisms are often more resistant to oral antibiotics than bacteria isolated from elderly persons in the community (Gambert SR & Al, 1982; Daly PB & Al, 1991). Specimen collected through the catheter present for more than few days, reflect biofilm microbiology. For residents with chronic indwelling catheters and symptomatic infections, changing the catheter immediately prior to instituting antimicrobial therapy, allows collection of a bladder specimen, which is a more accurate reflection of infecting organisms (Raz R & Al, 2000). Catheter replacement immediately prior therapy is also associated with more rapid defervescence and lower risk of early symptomatic relapse post-therapy (Raz R & Al, 2000).

Guidelines for prevention of catheter-associated urinary tract infections in hospitalized patients (Wong ES & Hooden TM, 1981), are generally applicable to catheterized nursing home residents (Philip W & Al, 2008). Recommended measures include limiting use of catheters, insertion of catheters aseptically by trained personnel, use of as small diameter a catheter as possible, handwashing before and after catheter manipulation, maintenance of a closed catheter system, avoiding irrigation unless the catheter is obstructed, keeping the collecting bag below the bladder and maintaining good hydration in residents. Urinary catheters coated with antimicrobial materials have the potential to decrease urinary tract infections, but have not been studied in the nursing home setting (Ha US & Cho YH, 2006; Schumm K & Lam TB, 2008). For some residents with impaired voiding, intermittent catheterization is an option, and clean technique is as safe as sterile technique (Duffy LM & Al, 1995). External catheter are also a risk factor for urinary tract infections in male residents (Smith PW & Al, 1991), but are significantly more comfortable and associated with fewer adverse effects, including symptomatic urinary infection, than indwelling catheter (Saint S & Al, 2006). Local external care is required.

The reported microbiology of symptomatic urinary tract infections in nursing homes shows that E. coli in women, and Proteus Mirabilis in men are the most frequently isolated infecting organisms (Nicolle LE & Al, 1987; 1996; Ricci G & Al, 2010). Gram-negative organisms of increased antimicrobial resistance, including Klebsiella pneumoniae, Providencia spp, Morganella morganii, Enterobacter spp, Citrobacter spp and Pseudomonas aeruginosa are frequently isolated (Nicolle LE & Al, 1987; 1996; Ricci G & Al, 2010). Gram-positive organisms, including Enterococcus spp, coagulase-negative Staphylococci, and less frequently, Staphylococcus aureus, are also identified (Ricci G & Al, 2010). (Table 5)

Bacteria (percentage of total isolates)	Grude N & Al, 2001	Mathai D & Al, 2001	Nicolle LE, 2005	Das & Al, 2009	Ricci & Al, 2010
Escherichia coli	56.7%	46.9%	15%	53.6%	55,5%
Proteus Mirabilis	72%	5.0%	42%	14.6%	12.4%
Klebsiella pneumoniae	-	11%	8.2%	13.9%	11.8%
Providencia spp	-	-	22%	3.7%	0.26%
Morganella Morganii	-	-	-	1.5%	0.52%
Enterobacter cloacae	0.9%	-	7.1%	-	3.52%
Citrobacter spp	0.2%	-	-	-	0.26%
Pseudomonas aeruginosa	1.3%	7.5%	27%	2.6%	7.64%
Enterococcus faecalis	7.9%	12.8%	-	4.5%	2.35%
Coagulase-negative Staphylococci	12.5%	3.4%	2.4%	-	-
Staphylococcus aureus	2.2%	-	-	4.1%	-

Table 5. Bacteria reported in published studies as etiologic agents in urinary tract infections

Providentia stuartii, is an organism with a unique proclivity for causing infections in nursing homes (Flerer J & Ekstrom M, 1981; Muder RR & Al, 1992). The major site of isolation of the organism is the urinary tract of patients with long-term indwelling urinary catheters or external urine-collecting devices (Flerer J & Ekstrom M, 1981; Warren JW & Al, 1982). The occurrence of Providencia stuartii is highly variable among different facilities. When present, it is often identified in urine cultures from virtually all patients with long-term indwelling urinary catheters: this observation suggest that cross-infection either through the environment or on the hands of staff members is the major determinant of Providencia stuartii urinary infections in the nursing home setting (Nicolle LE & Al, 1983)

3.1.3.2 Asymptomatic bacteriuria

If the prevalence and the incidence of symptomatic urinary infection is high, the prevalence and the incidence of asymptomatic bacteriuria are also high (Table 6). In a male population from whom monthly urine cultures were obtained, the incidence of new episodes of bacteriuria was 45 per 100 patients/years (Nicolle LE & Al, 1983). In a female population, 1,2 infections per resident/year were identified (Nicolle LE & Al, 1987) and in a 58 month follow up of an Italian nursing home population, the rate of positive urine samples in asymptomatic subjects was higher than 45% (Ricci G & Al, 2010).

Early recurrence of bacteriuria following treatment is the norm, with as many as 50% of men or women experiencing recurrence within 6 weeks of therapy (Nicolle LE & Al, 1983; 1988). The 5 to 10% of nursing home residents managed with long-term indwelling catheters, have a 100% prevalence of asymptomatic bacteriuria, usually with three to five organism isolated at any time (Warren JW & Al, 1982). The reported microbiology of asymptomatic infections is summarized in Table 7 and is similar to that of symptomatic infections.

References	Prevalence (%)
Hedin K & Al, 2002	23
Hassanzadeh P & Motamedifar M, 2007	53
Lin YT & Al, 2007	57.8
Aguirre-Avalos G & Al 1999	24.7
Ouslander JG & Al, 1996	43
del Río G & Al, 1992	38.5
Kaye D & Al, 1989	23.5
Boscia JA, 1986	23.5
Rodhe N & Al 2006	14.8
Ricci G & Al, 2010	46,05

Table 6. The prevalence of asymptomatic bacteriuria (reported in published studies)

Bacteria (percentage of total isolates)	Hedding K & Al, 2002	Rahav G & Al, 2003	Lin YT & Al, 2006	Hassanzadeh P & Motamedifar M 2007	Ricci & Al, 2010
Escherichia coli	67.27	49.0	29.7	45.3	59.2
Proteus Mirabilis	9.09	2.0	-	13.2	14.11
Klebsiella pneumoniae	10.90	2.0	21.6	13.2	7.06
Providencia spp	-	-	16.2	-	-
Morganella Morganii	-	-	-	-	0.61
Enterobacter cloacae	1.81	2.0	-	3.8	0.31
Citrobacter spp	-	1.8	-	-	0.92
Pseudomonas aeruginosa	-	9.0	13.5	5.7	2.15
Enterococcus faecalis	7.27	8.0	-	-	2.15
Coagulase-neg Staphylococci	-	4.0	-	-	-
Staphylococcus aureus	-	6.0	-	5.7	-

Table 7. Bacteria reported in published studies as etiologic agents in asymptomatic bacteriuria

3.1.4 Skin and soft tissue infections in nursing homes

3.1.4.1 Pressure ulcers

The frequency of pressure ulcers (also termed "decubitus ulcers") in nursing homes patients reflects the quality of nursing home care (Shepard M & Al, 1987; Allman R, 1988). The reported prevalence of pressure ulcers, has varied from 1,6 to up of 20% in different institutions (Michocki RJ & Lamy PP, 1976; Spector WD & Al, 1988; Branders GH & Al, 1990; Young JB & Dobrzanski S, 1992; Nicolle LE & Al, 1994a; Berlowitz DR & Al, 1996; Coleman EA & Al, 2002; Zulkowski K & Al, 2005), with an incidence as high as 10 to 30% patient per year (Berlowitz DR & Wilking SVB, 1989; Branders GH & Al, 1990), and as low as 3,4 to 4,8 episodes per 100000 resident days (Nicolle LE & Al, 1994b). Pressure ulcers are associated with increased mortality (Branders GH & Al, 1990; Livesley NJ & Chow A, 2002; Garcia AD

& Thomas DR, 2006). Infected ulcers are reported to occur from 0,1 to 0,3 episodes per 1000 resident days (Farber BF & Al, 1984; Scheckler W & Peterson P, 1986) or 1,4 per 1000 ulcer days (Nicolle LE & Al, 1994b). Infected pressure ulcers often are deep soft tissue and may have underlying osteomyelitis, cellulitis and bacteremia. Muder RR & Al (1992) reported that 36% of bacteremic skin and soft tissue infections was due to infected decubiti with a case/fatality ratio of 14% for all skin infections, and Livesley NJ & Chow AW (2002) reported that secondary bacteremic infections have a 50% mortality.

Medical factors predisposing to pressure ulcers have been delineated (Berlowitz DR & Wilking SVB, 1989; Garcia AD & Thomas DR, 2006) and include immobility, pressure, friction, shear, moisture, steroids, incontinence, sensory impairment, malnutrition and infections; reduced nursing time can also increase the risk of developing pressure ulcers. Several of these factors may be partially preventable (i.e. malnutrition and fecal incontinence). Prevention of pressure ulcers involves developing a plan for turning, positioning, eliminating focal pressure, reducing shearing forces and keeping skin dry. Attention to nutrition, using disposable briefs and identifying residents at a high risk using prediction tools, can also prevent new pressure ulcers (Smith PW & Al, 2008). The goals are to treat infection, promote wound healing and prevent future ulcers. Many physical and chemical products are now available for the purpose of skin protection, debridement and packing, although controlled study are lacking in the area of pressure ulcer prevention and healing (Lyder CH, 2003) and a variety of products may be also used to relieve or distribute pressure, or to protect the skin (Smith PW & Al, 2008).

Because pressure ulcers, like the skin, are frequently colonized with several different bacteria, antibiotic therapy is not appropriate for a surface swab culture without sign and symptoms of infection (Smith PW & Al, 2008). Surface cultures yield a polymicrobial flora of gram positive and gram negative, aerobic and anaerobic species (Allman R, 1988; Nicolle LE & Al, 1994b). Therefore, surface cultures are not considered reliable to identify infection or, when infection is clinically present, in identify infecting organisms. Non intact skin is more likely to be colonized with pathogens; so some authors obtained positive results for 97% of cultures of superficial swab specimens (Rudelsky B & Al, 1992) even if there were a poor concordance between the different bacterial species identified by biopsy and those identified by aspiration (43% of positive specimens) and swab culture (63% of positive specimens). Another study compared deep-tissue biopsy with aspiration of draining pressure ulcers (Ehrenkranz NJ & Al, 1990). Compared with deep-tissue biopsy, this technique had a sensivity of 93% and a specificity of 99% Ehrenkranz NJ & Al, 1990). Similar species were identified by irrigation-aspiration and deep tissue biopsy. However, aspirates samples of clinically non infected ulcers have also been shown to contain bacteria in 30% of cases (Nicolle LE & Al, 1994b). Culture results must be interpreted with caution, because should not be used as the sole criterion for infections, without clinical or histopathological evidence of infection (Hirshberg J & Al, 2000). Despite the aforementioned information, there is agreement on the most frequently isolated bacteria, including Staphylococcus aureus, beta-Hemolytic Streptococci, Gram negative organisms (including Enterobacteriaceae and Pseudomonas spp, and other Gram positive organisms such Enterococcus spp) and Anaerobic organisms (Chow AW & Al, 1977; Sapico FI & Al, 1986; Muder RR & Al, 1992; Nicolle LE & Al, 1994b; Smith DM & Al, 2010; Lund-Nielsen B & Al, 2011). Colonization with Methicillin-Resistant Staphylococcus Aureus occurs frequently in institutions with

Endemic Methicillin-Resistant Staphylococcus Aureus (Bradley SF & Al, 1991; Strausbaugh LJ & Al, 1991)

3.1.4.2 Cellulitis

Cellulitis (infection of the skin and soft tissue) can occur either at the site of a previous skin break (pressure ulcer) or spontaneously. Skin infections generally are caused by group A Streptococci or Staphylococcus Aureus. However, in cases in which cellulitis is a complication of pressure ulcers or chronic foot ulcers in patients with diabetes or peripheral vascular impairment, infections with other agents, including members of the Enterobacteriaceae, anaerobes or polymicrobial flora are common. Outbreaks of group A streptococcal infections have been described, presenting as cellulitis, pharyngitis, pneumonia or septicemia (Auerbach SB & Al, 1992; Schwartz B & Ussery XT, 1992; Green CM & Al, 2005)

3.1.4.3 Conjunctivitis

Conjunctivitis in the adult presents as ocular pain, redness and discharge. Conjunctivitis has been reported frequently as a common infection in nursing home, but the frequency is variable in different institutions. A prevalence of 0.3 to 3.4% has been reported in different surveys (Garibaldi RA & Al, 1981; Schleckler W & Peterson P, 1986 ; Magaziner J & Al, 1991) while, the incidence of conjunctivitis on different units varied from 0.6 to 3.5 per 1,000 patient-days (Boustcha E & Nicolle LE, 1995). Conjunctivitis occurs more frequently in elderly residents with greater functional impairment (Garibaldi RA & Al, 1981; Boustcha E & Nicolle LE, 1995). It is likely that a high proportion of conjunctivitis cases are noninfectious but are due to irritative, viruses or other factors (Boustcha E & Nicolle LE, 1995). In the nursing homes cases may be sporadic or outbreak-associated (Garibaldi RA & Al, 1981). The batteriology of endemic conjunctivitis is not well studied, but Staphylococcus aureus appears to be the most frequent organism isolated (Boustcha E & Nicolle LE, 1995); infections with upper respiratory flora such as Moraxella catharralis and Haemophilus spp are also reported (Boustcha E & Nicolle LE, 1995). These organisms may be isolated, however, from the conjunctivae of patients without clinical conjunctivitis in the nursing home (Boustcha E & Nicolle LE, 1995). Conjunctivitis has been reported as a clinical presentation for some patients in outbreaks caused by group-A beta-Hemolytic Streptococcus and Methicillin-Resistant Staphylococcus aureus (Center for Disease Control, 1990a; Brennen C & Muder R, 1990). Epidemic conjunctivitis may spread rapidly through the nursing home. Transmission may occur by contaminated eye drops or hand cross contamination. Gloves should be worn for contact with eyes or ocular secretions, with hand hygiene performed immediately after removing gloves (Smith PW & Al, 2008)

3.1.5 Gastrointestinal infections

No surveys have identified either the incidence or the prevalence of infectious diarrhea in non epidemic setting. Most episodes of diarrhea in the nursing home patient are probably noninfectious in origin and are related to the patient's underlying disease, medications (including antibiotics) or diet, especially high protein supplements. Toxigenic Clostridium difficile has been reported to be endemic in some nursing homes (Bentley DW, 1990b; Thomas DB & Al, 1990): the prevalence of Clostridium difficile stool carriage has been reported to be 9 to 26%, with higher rates identified after antibiotic therapy. It is uncertain whether this phenomenon is limited to selected nursing homes or is generalizable. In those nursing homes with a high rates of colonization with endemic Clostridium difficile, most patients are asymptomatic, but carriage may persist for an extended time (Bentley DW, 1990b).

3.1.6 Bacteremia

Bacteremia in the nursing homes, although rarely detected, may be primary or secondary to an infection at another site: the most common source is urinary tract, with Escherichia coli being the culprit in over 50% of cases (Setia U & Al, 1984; Mylotte JM & Al, 2002). The majority of non urinary cases are secondary to skin or soft tissue infections or pneumonia. The incidence of bacteremia is reported to vary widely, from 4 to 39 episodes per 100000 resident days. The reported variation likely reflects differences in patient populations and interventions in different institutions. The case/fatality ratio for bacteremic patients is 21 to 35% (Setia U & Al, 1984; Rudman D & Al, 1988; Muder RR & Al, 1992; Nicolle LE & Al, 1994a) and is consistent with reports of mortality rates in other populations in which similar organisms have been isolated. (Table 8) From 9 to 22% of episodes are polymicrobial, with a soft tissue source most frequently associated with polymicrobial bacteremia.

Bacteria (percentage of total isolates)	Setia U & Al, 1984	Rudman D & Al, 1988	Muder RR & Al, 1992	Nicolle LE & Al, 1994	Siegman-Igra Y & Al, 2002	Mylotte JM & Al, 2002
Staphylococcus aureus	13	9.1	15	10	5	13
Methicillin-resistant S. aureus	-	7	5	-	9	5
Enterococcus spp	3.7	9.1	7.9	3.3	9	9
Coagulase-neg staphylococcus	0.9	-	3.9	-	-	-
ß-hemolitic streptococcus	3.7	-	4.4	6.7	-	-
Streptococcus pneumoniae	0.9	9.1	3.9	13	7	6
Other Gram-positive bacteria	2.8	-	0.5	-	-	-
Escherichia coli	32	15	13	37	24	27
Providencia stuartii	5.6	24	13	-	-	1
Proteus spp	14	18	8.9	10	21	13
Klebsiella pneumoniae	10	-	5.4	6.7	12	3
Pseudomonas aeruginosa	7.4	6.1	3	-	-	3
Morganella morganii	-	-	3.9	-	-	-
Other gram-negative bacteria	1.9	9.1	4.4	3.3	-	-
Anaerobes	3.7	-	-	10	-	-
Mortality (% subjects)	35	21	21	24	35	18

Table 8. Bacteria reported in published studies as etiologic agents in bloodstream infections and mortality rate

In recent years, the acuity of illness in nursing home residents has risen with a most frequent use of central/peripheral venous catheters and an increased of related bacteremic complications. The CDC Guidelines for prevention of intravascular catheter-related infections is a useful resource and generally applicable to nursing homes (O'Grady NO & Al, 2002). Relevant points include aseptic insertion of the intravascular cannula, daily inspection of the intravascular catheter for complications such as phlebitis, and quality control of intravascular fluids and administration sets.

3.2 Outbreaks of bacterial infections in nursing homes

Most of nursing homes infections are sporadic; many are caused by colonizing organism with relatively low virulence. However the nursing home, provides a milieu that is conductive in outbreaks of infectious diseases due to close proximity of susceptible patients in the institutional setting and subsequent cross-transmission of organisms among patients through contact with staff members or environmental contamination. An outbreak or transmission within facility may occur explosively, with many clinical cases appearing within a few days, or may, for example, involve an unusual clustering of Methicillin-Resistant Staphylococcus Aureus clinical isolates on a single nursing unit over several months. On the other hand, a case of Methicillin-Resistant Staphylococcus Aureus infection may follow a prolonged period of asymptomatic colonization after an aspiration event or development of a necrotic wound (Drinka PJ & Al, 2005). Tissue invasion may also be facilitated by the presence of a urinary catheter or chronic wounds. Outbreaks in nursing homes, accounted for a substantial proportion (15%) of reported epidemics (Centers for Disease Control and Prevention, 1989a). Clustering of urinary tracts infections, diarrhea, skin and soft tissue infection, conjunctivitis, and antibiotic resistant bacteriuria have been noted (Strausbaugh, L.J., & Al, 2003). Major outbreak of bacterial infection have also been ascribed to Clostridium difficile (Bentley DW, 1990b; Simor AE & Al, 2002;), Salmonella spp. (Standaert SM & Al, 1994), Escherichia coli (Ryan CA & Al, 1986; Carter AO & Al, 1987), group A Streptococcus (Center for Disease Control, 1990a; Auerbach SB & Al, 1992; Harkness GA & Al, 1992; Schwartz B & Ussery XT, 1992; Arnold KE & Al, 2006), Chlamydia pneumoniae (Troy CJ & Al, 1997; Nakashima K & Al, 2006), Staphylococcus aureus (Bradley SF & Al, 1991; Hsu CCS, 1991) and other pathogens (Table 9).

Nursing homes accounted for 2% of all foodborne disease outbreaks reported to the Centers for Disease Control (1975-1987) and 19% of outbreak associated death (Levine WJ & Al, 1991). Transmissible gastrointestinal pathogens may be introduced to the facility by contaminated food or water or infected individuals. High rate of fecal incontinence, as well as gastric hypochlorhydria, make the nursing home ideal for secondary fecal-oral transmission, underscoring the vulnerability of elderly to infections, as well as the role of cross infection in residents with devices, open wounds or incontinence. In addition, mobile residents with poor hygiene, may interact directly facilitating the spread of infections (Standaert SM & Al, 1994; Musher DM & Al, 2004)

3.2.1 Gastrointestinal infections

Bacterial gastroenteritis (caused by Clostridium difficile, Bacillus cereus, Escherichia coli, Campylobacter spp, Clostridium perfrigens or Salmonella spp) as well as viral and parasitic gastroenteritis are well-known causes of diarrhea outbreaks in nursing homes (Carter OA & Al, 1987; White KE & Al, 1989; Slotwiner-Nie PK & Brandt LI, 2001; Olsen SJ & Al, 2001; Winquist AG & Al, 2001; Simor AF & Al, 2002).

Bacteria	Reference(s)
Staphylococcus aureus	Johnson ET, 1983; Storch GA & Al, 1987; Thomas JC & Al, 1989; Bradley SF & Al, 1991; Hsu CCS, 1991; Levine WJ & Al, 1991; Muder RR, 1991; Strausbaugh LJ & Al, 1991
Group A Streptococcus	Reid RT & Al, 1983; Ruben FC & Al, 1984; Center for Disease Control, 1990a; Auerbach SB & Al, 1992; Harkness GA & Al, 1992; Schwartz B & Ussery XT, 1992; Arnold KE & Al, 2006
Escherichia coli O157:H7	Ryan CA & Al, 1986; Carter AO & Al, 1987
Salmonella spp.	Baine WE & Al, 1973; Levine WJ & Al, 1991; Jackson M, 1992; Standaert SM & Al, 1994
Shigella spp.	Levine WJ & Al, 1991
Bordetella pertussis	Addis DG & Al, 1991
Haemophilus influenzae	Smith PF & Al, 1988
Campylobacter jejuni	Levine WJ & Al, 1991
Aeromonas hydrophila	Bloom H & Bottone E, 1990
Antimicrobial agent-resistant gram-negative bacilli	Shlaes DM & Al, 1986; Rice LB, 1990; John JE & Ribner B 1991; Wingard F & Al, 1993
Clostridium perfrigens	Levine WJ & Al, 1991
Clostridium difficile	Bentley DW, 1984; 1990b; Simor AE & Al, 2002
Bacillus cereus	Levine WJ & Al, 1991
Mycobacterium tuberculosis	Stead W, 1981; Narain JJ & Al, 1985; Bentley D, 1990a; Stead W & Al, 1985
Chlamydia pneumoniae	Troy CJ & Al, 1997; Nakashima K & Al, 2006
Legionella spp	Seenivasan MH & Al, 2005

Table 9. Bacteria reported to have caused outbreaks in nursing homes (published studies)

The elderly are at increased risk of infectious gastroenteritis due to age-related decrease in gastric acid. In fact, while food products are usually the vehicle for introduction of the organism, subsequent person to person spread often occurs, prolonging the duration of the outbreak.

In a population with high prevalence of incontinence, the risk of cross infections is substantial, particularly due to shared bathroom, dining and rehabilitation facilities (Bennet RG, 1993). Foodborne disease outbreaks are very common in this setting, most often caused by Salmonella spp or Staphylococcus aureus (Levine W & Al, 1991; Centre for Diseases Control and Prevention, 2004).

E coli 0157:H7 and Giardia also may cause foodborne outbreaks, underscoring the importance of proper food preparation and storage. Some gastroenteritis outbreaks due to Salmonella spp and enterohemorragic E coli, have had a reported case/fatality ratios up to 12% (Levine W & Al, 1991); by contrast, the case/fatality ratio for most other pathogens is low.

3.2.2 Group-A Streptococcus

Outbreak of Group-A Streptococcal infection (Streptococcus pyogenes) have been frequently reported in nursing homes (Center for Disease Control, 1990a; Reid RT & Al, 1983; Ruben FC & Al, 1984; Auerbach SB & Al, 1992; Schwartz B & Ussery XT, 1992). Infected patients may present with bacteremia, pneumonia, cellulitis, wound infection, pharyngitis or conjunctivitis (Schwartz B & Ussery XT, 1992). Rarely, a toxic shock-like syndrome occurs.

Residents with skin ulcers and wounds are at greater risk of invasive infection. In most outbreaks, geographic localization to a floor or wing of the nursing home occurs (Schwartz B & Ussery XT, 1992).

3.2.3 Others outbreaks

A recent paper by Utsumi and co-workers (2010) identified between 1966 and 2008, six hundred and one articles or reports in English, dealing with outbreaks in nursing homes.

Thirty-seven pathogens (21 types of bacteria) were associated with 206 outbreaks. In addition to the above mentioned bacteria, were involved Chlamydia Pneumoniae , Haemophilus Influentiae, Bordetella Pertussis, Neisseria Meningitidis, Aeromonas Hydrophila, and Bacillus Cereus.

The reported median attack rate (proportion of persons who developed infection among those exposed) and their reference lists were reported in Table 10.

Bacteria	Attack rate	References
Chlamydia Pneumoniae	46%	Rice LB & Al, 1990; Miyashita N & Al, 2005; Nakashima K & Al, 2006
Haemophilus Influentiae	11%	Smith PF & Al, 1988
Bordetella Pertussis	36%	Addis DG & Al, (1991)
Neisseria Meningitidis	3%	Anonymus, 1998
Aeromonas Hydrophila	17%	McAnulty JM & Al, 2000
Bacillus Cereus	24%	Halvorsrud J & Orstavik I , 1980

Table 10. Attack rate of outbreaks as reported in published studies

Mycobacterium tuberculosis is responsible for outbreaks spreading from one facility to another (Ijaz, K & Al, 2002). The high frequency of prior infection with Mycobacterium tuberculosis in the elderly population, coupled with the immunological decline, characteristic of elderly persons, foments higher rates of tuberculosis in the nursing home setting. A survey of 15379 reported cases in 29 state indicated that the incidence of tuberculosis among nursing home residents was 39,2 cases per 100000 population, compared with 21,5 cases per 100000 population among elderly persons living in community (Center for Disease Control, 1990b). Residents who develop reactivated disease and residents who develop active tuberculosis after exposure to those with reactivated disease, constitute the source for facility-wide outbreaks. Because many infected older residents do not present with the classic features of tuberculosis (Rajagopalan S & Yoshikawa TT, 2000), infection in residents may remain unrecognized for prolonged period of time, which sustains transmission. Accordingly, a number of tuberculosis outbreaks involving both residents and staff have been reported (Centers for Disease Control, 1990b; Rajagopalan S & Yoshikawa TT, 2000; Kashef I & Al, 2002). The Centers for Disease Control (1990b) has published specific guidelines for the prevention of tuberculosis in nursing homes.

Since 1990, ten reports have described outbreaks of Streptococcus pneumoniae in nursing homes (Gleinch S & Al, 2000). These have frequently occurred in facilities with low pneumococcal vaccination rates. Multidrug-resistant strains of Streptococcus pneumonia accounted for 4 of these outbreaks. The largest, involved a 100-bed nursing home in Oklahoma (Nuorti JP, 1998). Eleven of 84 residents (13%) developed pneumonia, and 3 residents died. The outbreak strain, serotype "23F", exhibited resistance to penicillin, other ß-lactam antibiotics, trimethoprim-sulfamethoxazole, erythromycin, clindamycin and tetracycline.

Additional reports besides that of Loeb and colleagues (2000) document the occurrence of outbreaks caused by Chlamydia pneumoniae. The attack rate for 3 outbreaks caused by Chlamydia pneumoniae in Ontario nursing homes ranged from 44% to 68% among residents and it was 34% among the staff of one nursing home (Troy CJ & Al, 1997). Of the 302 residents affected, 16 developed pneumonia and 6 died.

Single report identify 5 other respiratory tract pathogens that have caused outbreak in nursing home residents: Chlamydia psittaci (Smith PW, 1994), Legionella pneumophila (Stout JE & Al, 2000), Haemophilus influenza type B (Smith PF, 1988) and Bordetella pertussis (Addis DG & Al, 1991).

4. Antibiotic resistance

Because infections occur frequently in nursing homes, residents are exposed to antimicrobial agents (Nicolle LE & Al, 1984, 1996; Finnegan TP & Al, 1985; Magaziner J & Al, 1991; Jackson M & Al, 1992). With mostly broad-spectrum antibiotics available and in wide use, resistance problems has been repeatedly documented since the early 1970s.

Indeed, numerous studies based on routine surveillance data, indicate a strong relationship between use and resistance (van de Sande-Bruinsma N & Al, 2008) but, nowadays, the epidemiology of antimicrobial resistance in nursing homes remains poorly understood (Lautenbach E & Al, 2009).

4.1 Sources of antibiotic resistance

Antimicrobial agent-resistant bacteria may be introduced into nursing homes by two different routes. They may emerge endogenously in patient flora during courses of antimicrobial therapy, or they may enter with new residents who are already colonized or infected (Bradley SF & Al, 1991; Mulhausen PL & Al, 1996; Muder RR & Al, 1999). Emergence may reflect selection of resistant strains or acquisition of genetic determinants that confer resistance by either spontaneous mutation or gene transfer. Spontaneous mutations that confer resistance are thought to be rare, but two studies have suggested that gene transfer plays a an important role in long-term care facilities. In an outbreak caused by ceftazidime-resistant bacteria in a chronic-care facility in Massachusetts, Rice and colleagues (1990) reported that the outbreak arose from plasmid transmission among different species and genera of Enterobacteriaceae, and not from dissemination of a single resistant isolate. The outbreak, which involved 29 patients, was caused by strains of Klebsiella pneumonia, Enterobacter cloacae, Escherichia coli, Serratia spp., Enterobacter agglomerans and Citrobacter diversus, that produced similar extended-spectrum ß-lactamases whose genes were located on closely related plasmids. The outbreaks had followed the introduction of ceftazidime into the facility, and its widespread empiric use. Similar observation were reported in a study of gentamicin-resistant gram negative bacilli in a Veterans' Administration nursing home care unit (Shlaes DM & Al, 1990). One Escherichia coli plasmid, which conferred resistance to ampicillin, carbenicillin, tetracycline and sulfonamides, proved identical to plasmids from two Citrobacter freundii strains and a Providencia stuartii strain isolated from three different patients. The introduction of resistant strain by colonized or infected patients who are admitted from other facilities has also been documented: one study reported the entry of an Methicillin-Resistant Staphylococcus aureus strain into the nursing home by a patient who was colonized at the referring hospital (Strausbaugh LJ & Al, 1991). Another study, revealed that 8 of 10 patients admitted to an intermediate-care ward were already colonized with strains of members of the Enterobacteriaceae carrying a plasmid encoding a novel ß-lactamase (Shlaes DM & Al, 1988). Regarding of the route of entry for resistant pathogens into the nursing home, antimicrobial use drives selection pressure for new acquisitions. Bjork and colleagues (1984) reported that in 10 patients with chronic indwelling urinary catheters residing in a Veterans' Administration nursing home care unit in North Dakota over 30 months, 70% of 63 antibiotic courses resulted in bacteriuria with organism resistant to the antibiotic that had been administred. As 40% of the positive urine cultures were polymicrobial, it is likely that antimicrobial therapy merely selected out the more resistant strains. The authors identified cross-infection in only one case and a greater percentage of Escherichia coli strains isolated from nursing home residents were resistant to ampicillin, tetracycline and trimethoprim-sulfamethoxazole, than Escherichia coli strains isolated from patients in the adjoining hospital.

4.2 Risk factors for acquisition of antibiotic resistance

Few studies have examined risk factors for infection with antimicrobial pathogens in nursing home patients. Infections with antibiotic resistant bacteria appears to occur most often in nursing home patients with antecedent colonization (Bradley SF & Al, 1991; Muder RR & Al, 1991; Mulhausen PL & Al, 1996). However, risk factors for colonization and infection are not necessarily the same. Overall infection with resistant bacteria was more likely to occur in nursing home residents who had been hospitalized recently or who a substantial decline in functional status (Terpenning MS & Al, 1994). Muder and colleagues (1991) reported risk factors for Methicillin-Resistant Staphylococcus Aureus (MRSA) infection in residents of their intermediated-care ward and nursing home care unit. In a stepwise logistic regression analysis, both persistent Methicillin-Resistant Staphylococcus Aureus colonization and dialysis were independent risk factor for Methicillin-Resistant

Staphylococcus Aureus infection. Terpenning and colleagues (1994) in an Ann Arbor, Michigan, identified risk factors for infection caused by both Methicillin-Resistant Staphylococcus Aureus and resistant Gram negative bacilli. By stepwise logistic regression analysis, diabetes mellitus and peripheral vascular disease were significant independent risk factors for Methicillin-Resistant Staphylococcus Aureus infection. Moreover, the presence of an indwelling urinary catheter or intermittent urinary catheterization, pressure ulcers and prior antibiotic use were significant independent risk factors for infection caused by resistant Gram-negative bacilli (Terpenning MS & Al, 1994; Muder & Al, 1997) . In a cross-sectional survey among 1,215 residents of long-term care facilities in Jerusalem, the Vancomycin-Resistant Enterococci (VRE) carriage rate was 9.6%. Previous hospitalization and antibiotic treatment were associated with elevated Vancomycin-Resistant Enterococci colonization rate. In contrast, moderate and severe levels of dependency and prolonged stay in a nursing home were associated with a decrease in the Vancomycin-Resistant Enterococci colonization rate. (Benenson S & Al, 2009).

In a prospective cohort study a total of 3339 patients with invasive pneumococcal infection were identified between 1995 and 2002. Multivariate modeling revealed that risk factors for infection with penicillin-resistant as opposed to penicillin-susceptible pneumococci were year of infection, absence of chronic organ system disease and previous use of penicillin, trimethoprim-sulfamethoxazole and azithromycin. Infection with trimethoprim-sulfamethoxazole-resistant pneumococci was associated with absence of chronic organ system disease and with previous use of penicillin, trimethoprim-sulfamethoxazole, and azithromycin. Infection with macrolide-resistant isolates was associated with previous use of penicillin, trimethoprim-sulfamethoxazole, clarithromycin, and azithromycin. Infection with fluoroquinolone-resistant pneumococci was associated with previous use of fluoroquinolones, current residence in a nursing home, and nosocomial acquisition of pneumococcal infection (Vanderkooi OG, 2005).

4.3 Risk factors for colonization

Given the high prevalence of colonization with antibiotic-resistant strains in nursing homes, why do some patients never become colonized and others become persistent carriers? When colonized nursing home residents have been compared with non carriers, underlying illness, presence of intravenous, urinary or enteral feeding devices, antibiotic use, presence of wounds, decline in functional status and increased intensity of nursing care have been associated to various degrees with High-level Gentamicin-Resistant Enterococci, Vancomycin-Resistant Enterococci, Drug-Resistant Streptococcus Pneumoniae and Methicillin-Resistant Staphylococcus Aureus (Zervos MJ & Al, 1987; Bradley SF & Al, 1991; Chenoweth CE & Al, 1994; Terpenning MS & Al, 1994; Brennen C & Al, 1998). Similar risk factors for the carriage of resistant Gram Negative Bacilli have been found. Nursing home residents colonized with resistant Gram Negative Bacilli were significantly more likely to have lived in a large skilled nursing facility, have had prior antibiotic treatment, or have had urinary incontinence or a catheter, than non colonized persons in nursing homes or the community (Gaynes RP & Al, 1985). Colonization with Gram Negative Bacilli resistant to Gentamicin, trimethoprim or cefriaxone, has been associated to varying degrees with increased length of stay, increased debility, need for a urinary device, prior pneumonia, presence of wound or chronic disease (Huovinen P, 1984; Shlaes DM, 1986; MacArthur RD

& Al, 1988; Bradley SF & Al, 1991; Wingard E & Al, 1993; Terpenning MS & Al, 1994). Given the overlap in risk factors, it is not surprising to find that many nursing home residents are colonized with more than one antibiotic-resistant pathogen (Chenoweth CE & Al, 1994; Terpenning MS & Al, 1994; Brennen C & Al, 1998)

4.4 Occurrence: organisms and antibiotic resistance

Even though interest in the epidemiology of antibiotic resistance in healthcare setting outside hospital is on the increase, the extend of antibiotic resistance in nursing home is still relatively unknown. Most information is derived from surveillance studies of infections in nursing home residents or outbreak investigations. No studies have defined the overall magnitude of this problem in a systematic manner, but available data suggest that antimicrobial agent resistant pathogens are frequently encountered in this setting. In fact nursing homes residents have an high frequency of colonization with antimicrobial-resistant organisms, including Methicillin-Resistant Staphylococcus Aureus, Vancomycin-Resistant Enterococci, Enterococci with high-level Gentamicin-Resistance, Extended-Spectrum ß-Lactamase-Fluoroquinolone-Resistant Gram-Negative Pathogens, Gram-Negative Uropathogens, , Penicillin-Resistant Pneumococci.

4.4.1 Methicillin-Resistant Staphylococcus Aureus (MRSA)

Methicillin-Resistant Staphylococcus Aureus was first described in 1961, and since then it has become a worldwide problem (Jevons MP, 1961; Tansel & Al, 2003; Diekema DJ & Al, 2004; Corrente M & Al, 2005). The presence of Methicillin-Resistant Staphylococcus Aureus in nursing homes was first reported in 1970 by O'Tool (O'Toole & Al, 1970). Methicillin-Resistant Staphylococcus Aureus is a frequent colonizer of debilitated patients; on this point, Bradley observed that the rate of colonization with Methicillin-Resistant Staphylococcus Aureus was <25% (Bradley SF & Al, 1991). The same Author showed that in two of the most common sites of colonization, nares and wound, colonization rates range from 8 to 53% and from 30 to 82% respectively (Bradley SF, 1999). Lee YL and colleagues (1997) reported a one-year prospective surveillance study of Staphylococcus Aureus colonization and infection. Nasal and stool or rectal screening cultures were done on admission, and all patients underwent screening on at least a quarterly basis for one year. Overall, 35% of patients were colonized at least once with Staphylococcus Aureus (72% Methicillin-Susceptible; 25% Methicillin-Resistant; 3% mixed phenotype). Mendelson evaluated the rate of colonization by Staphylococcus Aureus, especially Methicillin-Resistant Staphylococcus Aureus, in 270 elderly residents of a large long-term care facility. The Authors showed that 23,3% of residents were carriers of Staphylococcus Aureus and 27% of those had Methicillin-Resistant Staphylococcus Aureus (Mendelson G & Al, 2003). It is estimated that residents of nursing homes who are colonized with Methicillin-Resistant Staphylococcus Aureus have a 4 to 6 fold increase in infection rate. In a study by Muder RR and colleagues (1991), 25% of Methicillin-Resistant Staphylococcus Aureus carriers had an episode of staphylococcal infection, versus only 4% of Methicillin-Susceptible Staphylococcus Aureus carriers.

In a retrospective cohort study, Capitano showed that the median infection management cost of a Methicillin-Resistant Staphylococcus Aureus infection was six times greater than that of a Methicillin-Susceptible Staphylococcus Aureus infection, whereas the median associated nursing care cost was two times greater. The median overall infection cost associated with Methicillin-Resistant Staphylococcus Aureus was 1,95 times greater than that associated with Methicillin-Susceptible Staphylococcus Aureus. Nursing care cost constituted the major portion of the overall infection cost for both groups (Methicillin-Susceptible Staphylococcus Aureus = 51%; Methicillin-Resistant Staphylococcus Aureus = 48%) (Capitano B & Al, 2003).

Risk factors for Methicillin-Resistant Staphylococcus Aureus colonization include: residence in a medical ward or medical intensive care unit or prolonged hospitalization (13 weeks), advanced age and a history of invasive procedures (Asensio A & Al, 1996). In a study by O'Sullivan, the risk factors significantly associated with Methicillin-Resistant Staphylococcus Aureus colonization were male sex, age over 80 years, residence in the nursing home for more than six months, hospitalization during the previous six months, peripheral vascular disease, pressure ulcers, steroid therapy, poor general skin condition, antibiotic therapy during the previous three months and a mental test score of less than 14. Multivariate analysis identified male sex and pressure ulcers as independent variables (O'Sullivan NP & Keane CT, 2000). In a case control study conducted in a community nursing home, Thomas reported that nasogastric intubation and antibiotic therapy in the previous 6 months were the most important factors associated with Methicillin-Resistant Staphylococcus Aureus colonization (Thomas JC & Al, 1989). Other risk factors are indwelling urinary catheters and urinary incontinence (Terpenning MS & Al, 1994).

4.4.2 Vancomycin-Resistant Enterococci (VRE)

First described in 1987 in Europe Vancomycin Resistant Enterococci have recently emerged as important nosomial pathogens and in the last years have become among the most feared pathogens in US hospitals. Studies dealing with the emergence of Vancomycin-Resistant Enterococci in the United States, revealed that most patients with Vancomycin-Resistant Enterococci were in Intensive Care Units (Clark NC & Al, 1993). Colonization with Vancomycin-resistant Enterococcus has been reported from community settings in the United States, including, to a limited extend, long-term care facilities (Coque TM & Al, 1996; Bonten MJ & Al, 1998). Bonilla showed that prevalence of Vancomycin-Resistant Enterococcus colonization among patients in the long-term care facilities at the Ann Arbor Department of Veterans Affairs Medical Center, exceeded the prevalence in the intensive care unit and in the general medical wards (Bonilla HF & Al, 1997). Brennan decribed the epidemiology of Vancomycin-Resistant Enterococcus colonization in a 400 bed long-term care facility for veterans. The author observed that 24 of 36 patients were colonized with Vancomycin-Resistant Enterococcus that persisted for 67 days and were associated with antibiotic administration (Brennan C & Al, 1998). In a prospective cohort study, 45% (45 of 100 patients) were colonized with Vancomycin-Resistant Enterococcus. The risk factors identified by univariate analysis were: hospitalization in the prior 60 days, an admission diagnosis of infection, inability to ambulate, presence of a feeding tube or urinary catheter or decubitus ulcer and documented more probable antibiotic use in the previous 60 days (particularly the use of Vancomycin and third generation cephalosporins). Stepwise logistic regression analysis identified the presence of decubitus ulcer or hospital admission, and documented a probable antibiotic use in the 60 days before admission, as significant risk factors for colonization with Vancomycin-Resistant Enterococcus at the time of admission (Elizaga ML & Al, 2002).

4.4.3 Enterococci with high-level gentamicin resistance

Two studies, both from the Ann Arbor Veterans Administration nursing home care unit have identified risk factors for colonization with Gentamicin-Resistant Strains of Enterococci. In the first study a one-day prevalence survey reported by Zervos and colleagues, the need for advanced nursing care and antibiotic therapy in the prior 3 months were independent risk factors for colonization (Zervos MJ & Al, 1987). In the second study, presence of wounds, renal failure, intermittent catheterization, low Katz functional status and low serum albumin were independent risk factors for colonization with strains possessing high-level resistance to gentamicin (Terpenning MS & Al, 1994).

4.4.4 Extended-spectrum ß-lactamase gram-negative pathogens (ESBLs)

The first report of Extended-Spectrum ß-Lactamase Gram-Negative bacilli, came from Europe and were quickly followed by reports in the United States. This type of antimicrobial resistance is now recognized worldwide. The prevalence of Extended-Spectrum ß-Lactamase Gram-Negative Pathogens in long-term care facilities is becoming alarming. The first reported outbreak of bacteria resistant to ceftazidime in the United States occurred in 1990 among patients in a chronic care facility in Massachusetts (Rice LB & Al, 1990). In a study of ceftazidime-resistant Escherichia coli and Klebsiella pneumonia in Chicago, 31 of 35 patients from 8 nursing facilities harboured an Extended-Spectrum ß-Lactamase producing enteric pathogen. (Weiner J & Al, 1999). Weiner reported that prior exposure to ciprofloxacin or trimethoprim-sulfamethoxazole was an independent predictor of colonization with Escherichia coli resistant to ceftazidime among nursing home residents. Molecular analysis of isolates, showed that a particular resistance-conferring plasmid appeared frequently, thus supporting the growing concern that long-term facilities may act a reservoir for antimicrobial drug-resistant organisms. Several studies have evaluated the risk factors for colonization or infections with Extended-Spectrum ß-Lactamase-producing organisms in the hospitalized patients. Reported risk factors include the presence of intravascular catheters, emergency intra-abdominal surgery, gastrotomy or jejunostomy tube, gastrointestinal colonization, length of hospital or intensive care unit stay, prior antibiotics (including third generation cephalosporins), severity of illness, presence of an urinary catheter, and ventilator assistance (Schiappa DA & Al, 1996). In a case-control study, Sandoval and colleagues (2004) showed that exposure to any cephalosporin and percentage of residents using gastrotomy tubes within the nursing home, were associated with having a clinical isolate resistant to third-generation cephalosporin (Sandoval C & Al, 2004). Nursing home residents would appear to have several additional risk factors for infection with Extended-Spectrum ß-Lactamase- Gram-Negative producing organisms. It has been well documented that hand-washing rates are low among nursing home personnel (Denman SJ & Burton JR, 1992). Urinary catheterization and decubitus ulcers are frequent, and have been associated with colonization of non- Extended-Spectrum ß-Lactamase producing, antibiotic-resistant gram negative bacilli (Muder RR & Al, 1991; SmithPW & Al, 2000).

4.4.5 Fluoroquinolone-resistant gram-negative pathogens

Resistance in fluoroquinolones has been increasing over time in long-term care facilities. In a correlational longitudinal survey study, Viray showed that Escherichia Coli fluoroquinone-resistance rates was high but variable, and were generally increasing over time (Viray M &

Al, 2005). In a case control study, Cohen showed that Fluoroquinone-Resistant Escherichia coli urinary tract infection was more common with prior fluoroquinolone use (Cohen AE & Al, 2006). Maslow conducted a cross-sectional study to determine the prevalence of, and risk factors for colonization with Fluoroquinone-Resistant Escherichia coli in residents of a long-term care facility. Fluoroquinone-Resistant Escherichia coli were identified from rectal swabs for 25 of 49 (51%) partecipants at study entry. On multivariate analyses, prior fluoroquinolone use was the only independent risk factor for Fluoroquinone-Resistant Escherichia coli carriage and was consistent for fluoroquinolone exposures in the previous 3, 6, 9 or 12 months. Pulsed-field gel electrophoresis of Fluoroquinone-Resistant Escherichia coli identified clonal spread of one strain among 16 residents (Maslow JN & Al, 2005).

4.4.6 Gram-negative uropathogens

Shlaes and colleagues identified risk factors for urinary colonization with Gentamicin-Resistant Gram-negative Bacilli in patients of a Veteran Administration nursing home care unit near Cleveland, Ohio, using stepwise logistic regression (Shlaes DM & Al, 1986). Perineal or rectal colonization with Gentamicin-Resistant strains and presence of a urinary catheter were significant independent risk factors. Another study at the same institution by Wingard and colleagues, examined carriage of Trimethoprim-Resistant Gram-negative Bacilli (Wingard E & Al, 1993). Functional status and length of stay were significant independent risk factors for colonization: functional status was the most important risk factor for acquiring Trimethoprim-Resistant strains by cross-colonization. Gaynes, studying colonization with multiply resistant Gram-negative bacilli in patients admitted to the hospital from community nursing homes, reported that bladder dysfunction, residence in large nursing homes, age and prior antibiotic use were independent risk factors (Gaynes RP & Al, 1985). Terpenning identified intermittent catheterization, inflammatory bowel disease, chronic renal disease, presence of wounds and prior pneumonia, to be independent risk factors for colonization with Gentamicin and/or Ceftriaxone-Resistant Gram-negative Bacilli in a stepwise regression analysis (Terpenning MS & Al, 1994).

4.4.7 Penicillin-Resistant Pneumococci

Penicillin resistance is common in Streptococcus Pneumoniae and is a problem all over the world, both in the community and in hospital setting. In 2002, the European Antimicrobial Resistance Surveillance project (http://www.earss.rivm.nl) reported five countries with a prevalence of Penicillin-Resistant Pneumococci of greater than or equal to 30%. Overall, in 2002, the European Antimicrobial Resistance Surveillance Project reported 11% of Streptococcus Pneumoniae strains as non susceptible to penicillin and 17% non susceptible to erythromycin. Two events have occurred since 2000 that may have reducc the selective pressure driving antimicrobial resistance: the more appropriate use of antimicrobial and the pneumococcal conjugate vaccine (Klugman KP, 2004).The earlier study reports by Millar and Denton were among the first to describe Penicillin-Resistant Pneumococcal infection in elderly institutionalized and debilitated patients (Denton M & Al, 1993; Millar MR & Al, 1994). Nuorti reported a significant outbreak of Penicillin-Resistant Pneumococci in a long-term care facility in rural Oklaoma. The Author observed that 13% of the residents developed pneumonia, and that the mortality rate was 23%. Resistant isolates were recovered from 64% of residents with pneumonia and from 23% of non infected residents (Nuorti JP & Al, 1998).

4.4.8 Others organisms

In addition to those listed above, there are other kinds of antimicrobial-resistant pathogens. Smith and colleagues described an outbreak caused by an Ampicillin-Resistant strain of Haemophilus influenzae, involving six patients in a nursing home and adjoining hospital during a 1-month period (Smith PF & Al, 1988). Two patients were bacteremic and one died. All patients had personal contact with at least one other case patient, suggesting person-to-person spread. Sturm and colleagues reported a similar outbreak involving 15 subjects in a pulmonary rehabilitation centre in the Netherlands (Sturm AW & Al, 1990). The outbreak strain of Haemophilus influenza was resistant to amoxicillin, thrimethoprim-sulfamethoxazole, chloramphenicol and tetracycline. Choi described a nursing home outbreak caused by Salmonella Heidelberg serotype, frequently expressing multiple resistance (Choi AT & Al, 1990). Forty-four (22%) of the 199 residents were affected. Patients treated with antibiotics excreted the outbreak strain for a median duration of 14 weeks, prolonging the presence of a potential source for additional cases.

Although Acinetobacter infections in long-term care facilities and nursing homes are not well described, during the last decade, increasingly resistant strains of Acinetobacter, necessitating greater use of broad-spectrum antibiotics, such imipenem and ampicillin-sulbactam (Jain R & Danziger LH, 2004; Bassetti M & Al, 2008).

Sengstock and colleague in a six-year period reported in an increase of Multi-Drug-Resistant Acinetobacter baumannii, a link between increasing antibiotic-resistance, morbidity and mortality, and a transfer between hospital and nursing home and viceversa (Sengstock DM & Al, 2010). The article demonstrated that Acinetobacter baumannii is widespread including hospitals, long-term acute-care and nursing homes, and that the transfer of multidrug-resistant strains among health care facilities is bidirectional. These data confirm previous report (Gould CV & Al, 2006; Saeed S & Al, 2006; Stephens C & Al, 2007; Furuno JP & Al, 2008)

5. Conclusions

In the nursing home setting, antimicrobial use is an important issue, relevant to antimicrobial resistance. Previous study have found relatively high rates of antimicrobial use and substantial inappropriate use of antimicrobial agents in nursing homes and long-term care facilities (Zimmer JG & Al, 1986; Crossley K & Al 1987; Jones SR & Al, 1987; Katz PR & Al, 1990; Warren JW & Al, 1991; Yakabowich MR & Al, 1994; Pickering TD & Al, 1994; Montgomery P & Al, 1995). In addition to increasing the risk of colonization or infection with antimicrobial-resistant organisms, inappropriate antimicrobial use adds cost to resident care and may place the patient at increased risk for drug adverse reactions (Mylotte JM, 1999). Recommendations for improving antimicrobial use have included development of a formulary and continuing review of antimicrobial use and prevalence of antimicrobial resistance in cultures obtained from patients with suspected infections. In the last decades, an increasing number of nursing homes have developed infections control programs with surveillance and control activities (Smith PW, 1999). A major contribution to this development was the publication of guidelines by the Association for Professional in Infection Control and Epidemiology (APIC) – Society for Healthcare Epidemiologists of America (SHEA) in 1997 (Smith PW & Rusnak PG, 1997), revisited in 2008 (Smith PW & Al, 2008).

5.1 Prevention and control of infections in nursing homes

Most nursing homes have infection control programs, even if the components of these programs vary among different institutions and countries. (Garibaldi RA & Al, 1981; Crossley K & Al, 1985; Kabbuz RF & Tenney JH, 1988; Campbell B, 1991). The overall goal of the infection control program is to prevent infections and, when that is not possible, to limit interpatient transmission of potential pathogens (Nicolle LE & Garibaldi RA, 1995). Surveillance for infections in the nursing home is integral to the program (Smith PW, 1987). Valid infection surveillance requires the use of standard definitions, appropriate for the nursing home (McGeer AB & Al, 1991), effective case finding measures, systematic analysis and reporting of data, and an awareness to identify potential outbreaks as easy as possible. The optimal method for surveillance in nursing home is not identified, because it differs depending on the characteristics of each nursing home, staffing and patients populations.

Infection prevention and control is important for continuum of care and their main functions are (a) to obtain and manage clinical data, including surveillance information for endemic and epidemic infections; (b) to develop and recommend policies and procedures; (c) to intervene directly to prevent infections and (d) to educate and train health care workers, patients and caregivers. (Table 11)

An effective infection control program includes a method of surveillance for infections and antimicrobial-resistant pathogens, an outbreak control plan for epidemics, isolation and standard precautions, hand hygiene, staff education, an employee health program, a resident health program, policy formation and periodic review with audits, and a policy to communicate reportable diseases to public health authorities.

Infection surveillance in nursing homes involves collection of data on nursing home-acquired infections (Do AM & Al, 1999). Surveillance can be limited to a particular objective or may be a facility-wide goal. Surveillance often is based on individual patient risk factors, focused on a unit or based on a particular pathogen or infection type.

Surveillance may be either passive or active; in passive surveillance ("routine surveillance"), an infection control professional uses data collected for routine patient care. Although less costly in term of resources, passive surveillance is inherently biased. It may underestimate the magnitude of outcomes measured and delay detection of outbreaks. The feasibility of passive surveillance has been demonstrated and has led to continuing education opportunities.

Active surveillance uses multiple data sources to detect infections and antimicrobial resistance early, but data in nursing homes are lacking. Hospital definitions may not be applicable in nursing home setting; modified nursing home specific criteria were developed by a Canadian Consensus Conference, which took into account the unique limitations of the nursing home setting (McGeer A & Al, 1991). These criteria have been used widely but not uniformly (Danzig LE & Al, 1995). In addition a facility must have clear goals and aims for setting up a surveillance program. These goals, like other elements of an infection control program have to be reviewed periodically to reflect changes in the facility's population, pathogens of interest and changing antimicrobial resistance patterns. In addition, plans to analyse the data and use them to design and implement proven preventive measures, must be made in advance. The analysis and reporting of infection rates in nursing homes must be conducted monthly, quarterly and annually to detect trends. Because the length of stay in nursing home is long, and each resident is at risk for a prolonged duration, infection rates (infections/1000 resident days) can be calculated by using resident days or average resident census for the surveillance period as the denominator. These data can be used to estabilish endemic baselines rates and recognize variations from the baseline that could represent an outbreak. Feed back to the nursing home staff is critical to the success of the surveillance program, and this information should lead to specific infection control initiatives and follow up surveillance.

The Centers for Disease Control and Prevention's Healthcare Infection Control and Prevention Advisory Committee (HICPAC) proposes use of "Standard Precautions" which have been designed for the care of all patients in hospitals (Garner JS, 1996). "Standard Precautions" apply to blood, all body fluids, secretions and excretions regardless of whether they contain visible blood, skin that is not intact, or mucous membrane material. Designed to reduce the risk of transmission of pathogens from apparent and ambiguous source of infection, these precautions include hand hygiene compliance, glove use, masks, eye protection, gown and avoidance of injuries from sharp materials. Transmission-based precautions are intended for use with patients who may be infected with highly transmissible or epidemiologically significant pathogens. These include airborne precautions, droplet precautions and contact precautions.

Although these guidelines were designed for acute care setting, several of them, especially the universal precautions, apply to nursing home setting as well. However, facilities should evaluate these guidelines and individualize the plan to obtain cultures based on the population they serve.

Healthcare workers may play an important role in the dissemination of antibiotic-resistant bacteria in nursing homes (Thomas JC & Al, 1989): contamination of the hand of healthcare workers has been recognized as playing a role in the transmission of pathogenetic bacteria to patients since the observations of Holmes, Semmelweis and other, more than 100 years ago (Otherson MJ & Otherson HB, 1987). Hand antisepsis remains the most effective and last expansive measure to prevent transmission of nosocomial infections. However, compliance with hand washing recommendations among healthcare workers averages only 30-50% and improves only modestly following educational interventions (Mody L & Al, 2003). Healthcare workers frequently reported poor compliance with hand hygiene measures because of skin irritation from frequent washing, too little time because of a heavy workload, and simply forgetting. Introduction of alcohol-based hand rubs have been shown to enhance compliance with hand hygiene in the nursing home setting, and should be used to complement educational initiatives (Mody L & Al, 2003).

While the cost of introducing alcohol-based hand rubs could be a concern of nursing homes, recent data in acute care have shown that the total costs of a hand hygiene promotion campaign, including alcohol-based hand rubs, corresponded to less than 1% of costs that could be attributed to nosocomial infections (Pittet D & Al, 2004). Introducing the alcohol-based hand rubs must take into account some problems: alcohol-based hand rubs should not be used if hands are visibly soiled, in which case hand hygiene with antimicrobial soup and water is recommended. Alcohol-based hand rubs can cause dry skin; however recent data on rubs containing emollients have shown to cause less skin irritation and dryness (Centers for Disease Control , 2002).

Management strategies	
Infection control program	
Surveillance	• Review microbiology data • Maintain line listing of cases • Prevalence surveys of residents, staff or new admissions • Identify readmission cases

Outbreak investigation
    Policies, isolates, environment
    Staff education
Antimicrobial utilization program
Employee health program	

Patient care strategies	
Optimal management of comorbidities Optimal nutrition Avoidance of invasive devices	
Vaccination	• Influenza • Pneumococcus • Tetanus
Screening	• Hepatitis B and C virus • Tuberculosis (selected cases)
Precautions	• Hand-washing, antimicrobial soaps • Environment decontamination • Private room for colonized/infected residents • Barrier precautions for colonized/infected residents • Strict isolation for colonized/infected residents • Isolation of new admission • Special placement colonized/infected residents • Cohort colonized/infected residents • Cohort colonized personnel • Establish isolation ward
Reduction of reservoir	• Exclusion of colonized/infected residents from facility • Rapid discharge of colonized/infected residents • Decolonization therapy of residents, personnel o new admissions
Outbreak management	

Mechanism for early identification
    Policies for laboratory utilization
    Case finding and analysis
    Isolation and cohorting
    Specific therapy	

Table 11. Recommended approaches to the prevention and minimization of infections and outbreaks in nursing home

Another key point of the infection control program is staff education. Ongoing staff education is critical in health care setting, because of the plethora of literature published every year, advancements in technology and regulatory demands. The infection control program plays a vital role in educating nursing home personnel on various infection control measures, particularly in view of rapid staff turnover. Informal education and quality improvement meeting should be complemented with in-service education on various topics, including hand hygiene compliance, antimicrobial usage and antimicrobial resistance, appropriate and early diagnosis of infections, infection control and prevention measures, isolation precautions and policies.

5.1.2 Patient care practices

Patient-specific strategies to prevent infection are targeted to increase general and specific immunity and, hence, limit susceptibility to infection. These include maintenance of adequate nutrition and optimal management of associated chronic diseases. For example, nursing care practices should attempt to minimize or prevent the occurrence of aspiration in patients with neurologic impairment, avoid trauma to neuropathic feet, and prevent the occurrence of pressure ulcers in patients with limited mobility. Ensuring optimal use of immunizing agents is important, including pneumococcal vaccination (Center for Disease Control, 1989b). Use of invasive devices should be limited to those situations in which they are essential for patient care. When tube feeding is necessary to maintain nutritional status, percutaneous gastrostomy or jejunostomy feeding tubes may be preferred over nasogastric tubes because of a reported decreased occurrence of aspiration pneumonia (Fay DE & Al, 1991), even if other studies have not supported this observation (Clocon JO & Al, 1988; Peak A & Al, 1990). It has been suggested that use of external condom catheters for incontinence in men may be associated with a lower incidence of invasive urinary tract infections compared with long-term indwelling catheters, but this, too, is controversial, because of reported increased incidence of phimosis and skin irritation that predisposes to urinary infections (Flerer J & Ekstrom M, 1981).

5.1.3 Outbreaks management

Outbreaks of infection should be anticipated in the nursing home setting and policies to respond to a suspected or proven outbreak must be developed prior to occurrence. Such policies should include general aspects of outbreak management including identification, communication and authority, as well as specific issues related to the most frequent organisms likely to occur. Adequate management requires ongoing surveillance for infection to ensure early identification, specific criteria to identify a potential outbreak, case finding strategies and laboratory backup to identify the etiologic agent and plan appropriate interventions. Authority within the facility to initiate appropriate measures to control an outbreak should be clearly defined. Early notification and ongoing communication within the institution and with appropriate public health authorities must be outlined clearly prior to the crisis of an epidemic.

The response to the outbreak must include immediate control measures to identify and isolate cases, as appropriate, and limit patient and staff exposure. Control measures will include use of patient isolation, limitations in patient movement and interaction with the facility and, frequently, specific therapy. Compliance with isolation practices leads to special problems in nursing homes. As patients' room are their permanent residence, transfer within the institution for isolation purposes is disruptive for patients and family. Cognitive impaired residents will not be able to understand the reasons for and practices of isolation and it may be difficult to restrict movement for some of these patients. Policies developed, should acknowledge these potential problems and identify the methods by which they will be addressed. An integral part of outbreak management is a review and analysis of the course of the outbreak, impact and potential problem areas that may be changed to improve management in the future.

6. References

Addis, D.G., Davis, J.P., Meade, R.D., Burstyn, D.G., Meissner, M., Zastrow, J.A., Berg, J.L., Drinka, P., & Phillips, R. (1991) A pertussis outbreak in a WInsconsin nursing home. *J Infect Dis* 164: 704-710

Aguirre-Avalos, G., Zavala-Silva, M.L., Díaz-Nava, A., Amaya-Tapia, G., Aguilar-Benavides, S. (1999) Asymptomatic bacteriuria and inflammatory response to urinary tract infection of elderly ambulatory women in nursing homes. *Arch Med Res* 30 (1): 29-32

Ahlbrecht, H., Shearen, C., Degelau, J., & Guay, D.R. (1999) Team approach to infection prevention and control in nursing home setting. *Am J Infect Control* 27: 64-70

Ahmed, A. ,Allman, R.M., & DeLong, J.F. (2003) Predictors of nursing home admission for older adults hospitalized with heart failure. *Arch Gerontol Geriatr* 36 (2): 117-126

Allman, R. (1988) Pressure ulcers among the elderly. *N Engl J Med* 320: 850-853

Alvarez, S., Shell, C., Woolley, T., Berk, S., & Smith, J. (1988) Nosocomial infections in long-term care facilities. *J Gerontol* 43: M9-M17

Andresen, M. & Puggaard, L. (2009) Autonomy among physically frail older people in nursing home settting: a study protocol for an intervention study. *BMC Geriatrics* 8:32

Anonymus (1998) Outbreaks of group B Meningococcal disease – Florida, 1995 and 1997. *Morbil Mortal Weekly Rep* 47: 833-837

Arnold, K.E., Schweitzer, J.L., Wallace, B, Salter, M., Neeman, R., & Hlady, W.G (2006) Tightly clustered outbreak of group A streptococcal disease at a long term care facility. *Infect Control Hosp Epidemiol* 27: 1377-1384

Asensio, A., Guerriero, A., Quereda, C., Lizan, M., & Martinez-Ferrer, M. (1996) Colonization and infection with Methicillin-Resistant Staphylococcus Aureus: associated factors and eradication. *Infect Control Hosp Epidemiol* 17: 20-28

Asha NJ Tompkins, D., & Wilcox, M.H. (2006) Comparative analysis of prevalence, risk factors, and molecular epidemiology of antibiotic-associated diarrhea due to Clostridium difficile, Clostridium perfringens, and Staphylococcus aureus. *J Clin Microbiol* 2006 Aug; 44(8): 2785-2791.

Aspinall, R. & Andrew, D. (2000) Thymic involution in aging. *J Clin Immunol* 20 (4): 250–256

Aspinall, R. Del Giudice, G., Effros, R.B., Grubeck-Loebenstein, B., & Sambhara, S. (2007) Challenges for vaccination in the elderly. *Immun Ageing* 4; 9-18

Auerbach, S.B., Schwartz, B., Williams, D., Fiorilli, M.G., Adimora, A.A., & Breiman, R.F.Al (1992) Outbreak of invasive group A streptococcal infections in a nursing home: leson on prevention and control. *Arch Intern Med* 152: 1017-1022

Baine, W.E., Gagarosa, J., Bennet, J & Barker, W.Jr. (1973) Institutional salmonellosis. *J Infect Dis* 128: 357-360

Bajekal, M. (2002) Survey for England 2000: Characteristics of care homes and their residents. London: the Stationery Office, 2002

Banaszak-Koll, Fendrick, A. Mark., Foster., N.L., Herzog, A.R., Kabeto, M.U., Kent, D.M., Straus, W. L, & Langa, K.M. (2004) Predicting nursing home admission: estimates from a 7-year-follow up of a nationally representative sample o folder Americans. Alzh Dis Assoc Disord 18 (2): 83-89

Bartholomeyczik, S., Reuther, S., Luft, L., van Nie, N., Meijers, J., Schols, J., & Halfens, R. (2010) Prevalence of malnutrition, interventions and quality indicators in German nursing homes - first results of a nationwide pilot study. *Gesundheitswesen* 2010 Dec; 72(12): 868-74.

Bassetti, M., Righi, E., Esposito, S., Petrosillo, N., & Nicolini, L. (2008) Drug treatment for multidrug treatment-resistant Acinetobacter baumannii. *Future Microbiol* 3: 649-660

Bates ,C.J. Prentice, A., Cole, T.J., van der Pols, J.C., Doyle, W., Finch, S., Smithers, G., & Clarke, P.C. (1999a) Micronutrients: highlights and research challenges from the 1994-1995 National Diet and Nutrition Survey of people aged 65 years and over. *Br J Nutr* 82: 7-15

Bates, C.J., Prentice, A., & Finch, S. (1999b) Gender differences in food and nutrient intakes and status indices from the National Diet and Nutrition Survey of people aged 65 years and over. *J Clin Nutr* 53: 694-699

Beck-Sague, C., Banerjee, S., & Jarvis, W.R. (1993) Infectious diseases and mortality among US nursing home residents. *Am J Public Health*. 1993 Dec; 83(12): 1739-1742.

Beck-Sague, C., Villarino, E., Giuliano, D., Welbel, S., Latts, L., Manangan L.M., Sinkowitz, R.L. & Jarvis, W.R. (1994) Infectious diseases and death among nursing home residents: results of surveillance in 13 nursing homes. Infect *Control Hosp Epidemiol* 15: 494-496

Beers, M.H., Ouslander, J.G., Fingold, S.F., Morgenstern, H., Reuben, D.B., Rogers, W., Zeffren, M.J., & Beck, J.C. (1992) Inappropriate medication prescribing in skilled-nursing facilities. *Ann Intern Med* 117: 684-689

Benenson, S., Cohen, M.J., Block, C., Stern, S., Weiss, Y., Moses, A.E. & JIRMI Group (2009) Vancomycin-resistant enterococci in long-term care facilities. *Infect Control Hosp Epidemiol*. 30(8): 786-789

Bennet, R.G. (1993) Diarrhea among residents of long-term care facilities. *Infect Control Hosp Epidemiol* 14: 397-404

Bentley, D,W., (1984) Bacterial pneumonia in the elderly: clinical features, diagnosis, etiology and treatment. *Gerontology*30: 297-307

Bentley, D.W., (1990a) Tuberculosis in long-term care facilities. *Infect Control Hosp Epidemiol* 11: 42-46

Bentley, D.W., (1990b) Clostridium difficile-associated disease in long-term care facilities. *Infect Control Hosp Epidemiol* 11:434-438

Bentley, D.W., Bradley, S., High, K., Schoenbaum, S., Taler, G., & Yoshinawa, T.T. (2000) Practice guideline for evaluation of fever and infection in long-term care facilities. *Clin Infect Dis* 31: 640-653

Ben-Yehuda, A., & Weksler, M.E. (1992) Host resistance and the immune system. *Clin Geriatr Med* 8:701-711

Berland, B. & Gleckman, R.A. (1992): Fever of unknown origin in the elderly: A sequential approach to diagnosis. *Postgrad Med* 92:197–210.

Berlowitz, D.R. & Wilking, S.V.B. (1989) Risk factors for pressure sores. . *J Am Geriatr Soc* 37: 1043-1050

Berlowitz, D.R., Brandeis, G.H., Brand, H.K., Halpern, J., Ash, A.S., & Moskowitz, M.A. (1996) Evaluating pressure ulcer occurrence in long term care. Pitfalls in interpreting administrative data. *J Clin Epidemiol* 49: 289-292

Bertoni, A.G., Saydah, S., & Brancati, F,L. (2001) Diabetes and the risk of infection-related mortality in the United States. *Diabetes Care*. 24:1044-1049

Bettelli, G. (2011) Preoperative evaluation in geriatric surgery: comorbidity, functional status and pharmacological history. Minerva *Anestesiol 77: 1-2*

Bjork, D.T., Pelletler, L.L., & Tight, R.R. (1984) Urinary infections with antibiotic resistant organisms in catheterized nursing home patients. *Infect Control* 5: 173-176

Blandford, G., Watkins, L.B., & Mulvihill, M.N. (1998) Assessing abnormal feeding behavior in dementia: a taxonomy and initial finding. In: *Weight Loss and Eating Behavior in Alzheimer's Patients. Research and Practice in AD*. Eds Vellas B, Riviere S, Fitte J. New York: Serdi Publishing Company

Bloom, H., & Bottone, E. (1990) Aeromonas hydrphila diarrhea in a long-term care setting. *J Am Geriatr Soc* 38: 804-806

Bonilla, H.F., Zervos, M.A., Lyons, M.J., Bradley, S.F., Hedderwick, S.A:, Ramsey, M.A., Paul, L.K., & Kauffman, C.A. (1997) Colonization with Vancomycin-resistant Enterococcus faecium: comparison of a long-term care unit with an acute-care hospital. *Infect Control Hosp Epidemiol* 18: 333-339

Bonten, M.J., Slaughter, S., Hayden, M.K., Nathan, C., Van Voorhis, J., & Weinstein, R.A. (1998) External sources of Vancomycin-resistant Enterococci for intensive care units. *Crit Care Med* 26: 2001-2004

Boog, C.J.P. (2009) Principles of vaccination and possible development strategies for rational design. *Immunol Lett* 122: 104-107

Boscia, J.A., Kobasa, W.D., Knight, R.A., Abrutyn, E., Levison, M.E., Kaye, D. (1986) Epidemiology of bacteriuria in an elderly ambulatory population. *Am J Med* 80 (2): 208-214

Boström, A.M., Van Soest, D., Kolewaski, B., Milke, D.L., & Estabrooks, C.A. (2011) Nutrition Status Among Residents Living in a Veterans' Long-Term Care Facility in Western Canada: A Pilot Study. *J Am Med Dir Assoc* 12 (3): 217-225

Boustcha, E. & Nicolle, L.E. (1995) Conjunctivitis in a long-term care facility. *Infect Control Hosp Epidemiol* 16(4): 210-6.

Bowman, C., Whistler, J., & Ellerby, M. (2004) A national census of care home residents. *Age Ageing* 33: 561-566

Bradley, S.F. (1999) Methicillin-resistant Staphylococcus Aureus long-term concerns. *Am J Med* 106: 2-10

Bradley, S.F., Terpenning, M.S., Ramsey, M.A., Zarins, L.T., Jorgensen, K.A., Sottile, W.S., Scheberg. D.R., & Kauffman, C.A. (1991) Methicillin-resistant Staphylococcus Aureus: colonization and infection in a long-term care facility. *Ann Intern Med* 115: 417-422

Branders, G.H., Norris, J.N., Nash, D.V., & Lipsitz, L.A. (1990) The epidemiology and natural history of pressure ulcers in elderly nursing home residents. *J Am Med Assoc* 264: 2905-2909

Brennan, C., Wagner, M.M., & Muder, R.R. (1998) Vancomycin-resistant Enterococcus faecium in a long-term care facility. *J Am Geriatr Soc* 46: 157-160

Brennen, C. & Muder, R. (1990) Conjunctivitis associated with methicillin-resistant staphylococcus aureus in a long-term care facility. *Am J Med* 88 (suppl 5): 14N-17N

Brennen, C., Muder, R.R., & Muraca, P. (1988) Occult endemic tuberculosis in a chronic care facility. *Infect Control Hosp Epidemiol* 9: 548-552

Brennen, C.,Wagener, M.M., & Muder, R.R. (1998) Vancomycin-resistant Enterococcus faecium in a long-term care facility. *J Am Geriatr Soc* 46: 157-160

Brusaferro, S. & Moro, M.L. (2005) Le residenze assistenziali per anziani: una nuova sfida per il controllo delle infezioni correlate alle pratiche assistenziali. *Giorn It Inf Osp* Gennaio- Marzo 2005; 12: 8-21

Bruunsgaard, H., Pedersen, A.N., Schroll, M., & Skinhøj, P., Pedersen, BK. (2001). "Decreased natural killer cell activity is associated with atherosclerosis in elderly humans". *Exp Gerontol* 37 (1): 127–136

Calverley, P.M., Anderson, J.A., Celli, B., Ferguson, G.T., Jenkins, C., Jones, P.W., Yates, J.C., & Vestbo, J., TORCH investigators. (2007) Salmeterol and fluticasone propionate and survival in chronic obstructive pulmonary disease. *N Engl J Med* 356: 775-789

Cambier, J. (2005). Immunosenescence: a problem of lymphopoiesis, homeostasis, microenvironment, and signaling. *Immunological Reviews* 205: 5–6.

Campbell, B. (1991) Surveillance and control of infections in long-term care: the Canadian experience. *Am J Med* 91 (Suppl 3B): 3B – 286S-288S

Cantrell, M. & Norman, D.C. (2010) Practice of Geriatrics Chapter 38 Infections in "Free Medical Textbook" October 5, 2010. Avaible at: *http://medtextfree.wordpress.com/2010/10/05/chapter-38-infections/*

Capitano, B., Leshem, O.A., Nightingale, C.H., & Nicolau, D.P. (2003) Cost effect of managing Methicillin-Resistant Staphylococcus Aureus in a long-term care facility. *J Am Geriatr Soc* 51: 10-16

Carmeli, Y., Eliopoulous, G.M., Mozaffari, E., & Samore, M. (2002) Health and economic outcomes of vancomycin-resistant enterococci. *Arch Intern Med* 162(19): 2223-2228

Carratalà, J., Mykietiuk, A., Fernandez-Sabé, N., Suàrez, C., Dorca, J., Verdaguer, R., Manresa, F., & Gudiol, F. (2007) Health care-associated pneumonia requiring hospital admission. Epidemiology, antibiotic therapy and clinical outcomes. *Arch Intern Med* 167: 1393-1399

Carter, A.O., Borczyk, A.A., Carlson, J.A.K., Harvey, B., Hockin, J.C., Karmali, M.A., Kriehan, C., Korn, D.A., & Lior, H. (1987) A severe outbreak of Escherichia coli O157:H7 associated hemorrhagic colitis in a nursing home. *N Engl J Med* 317; 1496-1500

Carter, O.A., Borcyk, A.A., Carlson, J.A., Harvey, B., Hockin, J.C., & Karmali, M.A. (1987) Infectious diarrhea in the elderly. *N Engl J Med* 317: 1495-1500

Castle, S.C., Norman, D., Yeh, M., Miller, D., & Yoshikawa, T. (1991): Fever response in elderly nursing home residents: Are the older truly colder? *J Am Geriatr Soc* 39: 853–857.

Centers for Disease Control and Prevention (1989a) Surveillance for epidemics. *Morbid Mortal Weekly Rep* 38: 694-696

Centers for Disease Control and Prevention (1989b) Recomendations of the Immunization Practices Advisory Committee. Pneumococcal polysaccharide vaccine. *Morbid Mortal Weekly Rep* 38: 64-67

Centers for Disease Control and Prevention (1990a) Nursing home outbreaks of invasive group-A streptococcal infections – Illinois, Kansas, Noth Carolina and Texas. *Morbid Mortal Weekly Rep* 39: 577-579

Centers for Disease Control and Prevention (1990b) Prevention and control of tuberculosis in facilities providing long-term care to the elderly: recommendations of the Advisory Committee for Elimination of Tuberculosis. *Morb Mortal Wkly Rep* 39 (RR-10): 7-20

Centers for Diseases Control and Prevention (2004) Diagnosis and management of foodborne illnesses. A primer for physicians and other health care professionals. *Morbid Mortal Weekly Recomm Rep* 53: 1-33

Centers for Diseases Control and Prevention. (2002) Guidelines for hand hygiene in healthcare settings: recommendation of the health infection control practices advisory committee and the HICPAC/SHEA/APIC/IDSA hand hygiene task force. *Morbid Mortal Weekly Recomm Rep* 21: S3-S40

Centers for Diseases Control and Prevention. (2003) Public Health and Aging – United States and worldwide. *MMWR Morb Mortal Wkly Rep* 2003 february 14; 52(6):101-106

Centers for Medicare and Medicaid (CMS) Manual System, State Operations Manual. *Appendix*. 2005. pp. 183–4

Chan, K.M., Wong, S.F., & Yoong, T. (1998) Nursing home applications: reason and possible interventions. *Singapore Med J* 39(10): 451-455

Chang, C.C. & Roberts, B.L. (2011) Malnutrition and feeding difficulty in Taiwanese older with dementia. *J Clin Nurs* 2011 apr 26; doi: 10.1111/j.1365-2702.2010.03686.x.

Chenoweth, C.E., Bradley, S.F., Terpenning, M.S., Zarins, L.T., Ramsey, M.A., & Schaberg, D.R. (1994) Colonization and transmission of high level gentamicin-resistant enterococci in a long-term care facility. *Infect Control Hosp Epidemiol* 15: 703-709

Choi, A.T., Yoshikawa, T., Bridge, J., Schlaffer, A., Osterwell, D., Reid, D., & Norman, D.C. (1990) Salmonella outbreak in a nursing home. *J Am Geriatr Soc* 38: 531-534

Chong, W.F., Ding, Y. Y., & Heng, B.H. (2011) A comparison of comorbidities obtained from hospital administrative data and medical chart in older patients with pneumonia. *BMC Health Serv Res* 11: 105

Chow, A.W., Galpin, J.E., & Guze, L.B. (1977) Clindamycin for treatment of sepsis caused by decubitus ulcers. *J Infect Dis* 735: 565-568

Clark, N.C., Cooksey, R.C., Hill, B.C., Swenson, J.M., & Tenover, F.C. (1993) Characterization of glycopeptides-resistant enterococci from US hospitals. *Antimicrob Agents Chemiother* 37: 2311-2317

Clocon, J.O., Silverstone, F.A., Graver, L.M., & Foley, C.J. (1988) Tube feedings in elderly patients: indications, benefits and complications. *Arch Intern Med* 148: 429-433

Cohen, E., Hierholzer, W., Schilling, C., & Snydman, D. (1979) Nosocomial infections in skilled nursing facilities: a preliminary survey. *Public Health Rep* 94: 162-165

Cohen, E., Lautenbach, E., Morales, K.H., & Linkin, K.H. (2006) Fluoroquinolone-resistant Escherichia coli in the long-term care setting. *Am J Med* 119: 958-963

Coleman, E.A., Martau, J.M., Lin, M.K., & Kramer, A.M. (2002) Pressure ulcers prevalence in long-term nursing home residents since the implementation of OBRA '87. Omnibus Budget Reconciliation Act (comment). . *J Am Geriatr Soc* 50: 728-732

Coque, T.M., Tomayko, J.F., Ricke, S.C., Okhyusen, P.C., & Murray, B.E. (1996) Vancomycin-Resistant Enterococci from nosocomial, community and animal sources in the United States. *Antimicrob Agents Chemiother 40: 2605-2609*

Corrente, M., Monno, R., Totaro, M., Martella, V., Buonavoglia, D., Rizzo, C., Ricci, D., Rizzo, G., & Buonavoglia C (2005) Characterization of methicillin-resistant Staphylococcus Aureus (MRSA) isolated at the Policlinico Hospital fo Bary (Italy). *New Microbiol* 28 (1): 57-65

Cosgrove, S.E., Kaye, K.S., Eliopoulous, G.M., & Carmeli, Y. (2002) Health and economic outcomes of the emergence of third-generation cephalosporin resistance in Enterobacter Species. *Arch Intern Med* 162(2): 185-190

Cosgrove, S.E., Kaye, K.S., Harbarth, S., Karchmer, A.W., & Carmeli, Y. (2005) The impact of methicillin resistance in Staphylococcus aureus bacterieremia on patients outcome: mortality, length of stay and hospital charges. *Infect Control Hosp Epidemiol* 26 (2) : 166-174

Crossley, K., Henry, K., Irvine, P., & Willenbring, K. (1987) Antibiotic use in nursing homes: prevalence, cost and utilization review. *Bull NY Acad Med* 63: 510-518

Crossley, K., Irvine, P., Kaszar, D.J. & Loewenson, R.B. (1985) Infection control practices in Minnesota nursing homes. *J Am Med Assoc* 254: 2918-2921

Curns, A.T., Holman, R.C., Sejvar, J.J., Owing, M.F., & Schonberger, L.B. (2005) Infectious disease hospitalizations among older adults in the United States from 1990 to 2002. *Arch Intern Med* 165 (21); 2005 nov 28: 2514-2520

D'Agata, E. & Mitchell, S.L. (2008) Pattern of antimicrobial use among nursing home residents with advanced dementia. *Arch Intern Med* 2008 Febbruary 25; 168 (4): 357-362

Daly, P.B., Smith, P.W., Rusnak, P.G., & Woods, G.L. (1991) A microbiologic survey of long-term care facilities. *Nebr Med J* 76: 161-165

Danzig, L.E., Short, L.J. & Collins, K. (1995) Bloodstream infections associated with a needless intravenous infusion system in patients receiving home infusion therapy. *J Am Med Assoc* 273: 1862-1864

Darnowsky, S., Gordon, M., & Simor, A. (1991) Two years infection surveillance in a geriatric long-term care facility. *Am J Infect Control 19: 185*-190

Das, R., Perrelli, E., Towle, V., van Ness, P.H., & Juthani-Meta, M. (2009) Antimicrobial susceptibility of bacteria isolated from urine sample obtained from nursing home residents. *Infect Control Hosp Epidemiol* 30 (11): 116-119

del Río, G., Mestre, J., & Dalet, F. (1992) Prevalence and treatment of bacteriuria in the geriatric population. *Enferm Infecc Microbiol Clin* 10(10): 602-606

Denman, S.J., & Burton, J.R. (1992) Fluid intake and urinary tract infection in the elderly. *J Am Med Assoc* 267: 2245-2249

Denton , M., Hawkey, P.M., Hoy, C.M., & Porter, C (1993) Co-existent cross-infection with Streptococcus pneumonia and Group B Streptococci on an adult oncology unit. *J Hosp Infect* 23: 271-278

Diekema, D.J., Bootsmiller, B.J., Vaughn, T.E., Woolson, R.F., Yankey, J.W., Ernst, E.J., Flach, S.D., Ward, M.M., Franciscus, C.L., Pfaller, M.A., & Doebbeling, B.G.N. (2004) Antimicrobial resistance trends and outbreak frequency in United States Hospitals. *Clin Infect Dis* 38: 78-85

Dixon, W.G., Kezouh, A., Bernatsky, S., & Suissa, S. (2011) The influence of systemic glucocorticoid therapy upon the risk of non-serious infection in older patients with rheumatoid arthritis: a nested case-control study. *Ann Rheum Dis.* 2011 Jun; 70(6): 956-960.

Do, A.N., Ray, B.J., & Banerjee, S.N. (1999) Bloodstream infection associated with needless device use and importance of infection control practices in the home health setting. *J Infect Dis* 179: 442-448

Donini, L.M., DeFelice, R., Tagliaccica, A., Palazzotto, A., De Bemardini, L., & Cannella, C. (2000) MNA predictive value in long-term care. *Age & Nutrition* 11:2–5

Doshi, J.A., Shaffer, T., Briesacher, B.A. (2005) National estimates of medication use in nursing homes: findings from the 1997 Medicare Current Beneficiary Survey and the 1996 Medical Expenditure Survey. *J Am Geriatr Soc* 53: 438-443

Drinka, P.J., Stemper, M.E., Gauerke, C.D., Miller, J.E., Goodman, B.M., & Reed, K.D. (2005) Clustering of multiple endemic strins of methicillin-resistant Staphylococcus aureus in a nursing home: an 8-year study. *Infect Control Hosp Epidemiol* 26: 215-218

Drummond, M.B., Dasenbrook, C.E., Pitz, N.W., Murphy, D.J., & Fan, E. (2008) Inhaled corticosterois in patients with stable chronic obstructive pulmonary disease: a systematic review and meta-analysis. *J Am Med Assoc* 300: 2407-2416

Duffy, L.M., Cleary, J., Ahern, S., Kuskowski, M.A., West, M., & Wheeler, L. (1995) Clean intermittent catheterization: safe, cost-effective bladder management for male residents of VA nursing homes. *J Am Geriatr Soc* 43: 865-870

Durand, M., & Joseph, M. (2005) Infections of the upper respiratory tract. Available at: *http://www.mheducation.com/HOL2_chapters/HOL_chapters/chapter30.htm* Accessed July 12, 2005

Earhart, K.C. & Baugh, W.P., (2005) Rhinocerebral mucormycosis. Available at: *http://www.emedicine.com/med/topic2026.htm* Accessed July 12, 2005

Eberle, C.M., Winsemius, D., Garibaldi, R.A. (1993) Risk factors and consequences of bacteriuria in non-catheterized nursing home residents. *J Gerontol.* 48(6): M266–M271.

Ehrenkranz, N.J., Alfonso, B., & Nerenberg, D. (1990) Irrigation-aspiration for culturing draining decubitus ulcers: correlation of bacteriological findings with a clinical inflammatory scoring index. *J Clin Microbiol* 28: 2389-2393

Eikelenboom-Boskamp, A., Cox-Claessens, J.H., Boom-Poels, P.G., Drabbe, M.I., Koopmans, R.T, & Voss, A. (2011) Three-year prevalence of healthcare-associated infections in Dutch nursing homes. *J Hosp Infect* 78 (1): 59-62

Elizaga, M.L., Weinstein, R.A., & Hayden, M.K. (2002) Patients in long-term care facilities: a reservoir for Vancomycin Resistant Enterococci. *Clin Infect Dis* 34: 441-446

Elphick, H.L., Elphick, D.A., & Sanders, D.S. (2006) Small bowel bacterial overgrowth. An unrecognized cause of malnutrition in older adults. *Geriatrics* 2006 sept; 61 (9): 21-26

El-Sohl, A.A., Aquilina, A.T., Dhillon, R.S., Ramadan, F., Nowak, P., & Davies, N. (2002) Impact of invasive strategy on management of antimicrobial treatment failure in institutionalized older people with severe pneumonia. *Am J Resp Crit Care Med* 166: 1038-1043

El-Sohl, A.A., Pietrantoni, C., Bhat, A., Bhora, M., & Berbary, E. (2004) Indicators of potentially drug-resistant bacteria in severe nursing home-acquired pneumonia. *Clin Infect Dis* 39: 474-480

Ely, J.W., Osheroff, J.A., Chambliss, M.L., & Ebell, M.H. (2006). Approach to leg edema of unclear etiology. *J Am Board Fam Med* 19(2):148-160.

Eom, C.S., Jeon, C.Y., Lim, J.W., Cho, E.G., Park, S.M., & Lee, K.S. (2011) Use of acid-suppressive drugs and risk of pneumonia: a systematic review and meta-analysis. *Can Med Assoc J* 2011 Feb 22; 183(3): 310-319

Eriksen, H.M., Koch, A.M., Elstrøm, P., Nilsen, R.M., Harthug, S., & Aavitsland, P. (2007) Healthcare-associated infection among residents of long term care facilities: a cohort and nested case-control study. *Journal of Hospital Infection* 65 (4): 334-340

Ernst, P., Gonzalez, A.V., Brassard, P., & Suissa, S. (2007) Inhaled corticosterois use in chronic obstructive pulmonary disease and the risk of hospitalization for pneumonia. *Am J Respir Crit Care Med* 176: 162-166

Farage, M.A. & Maibach, H.I. (2011) Morphology and physiological changes of genital skin and mucosa. *Curr Probl Dermatol*. Febb, 10, 2011; 40:9-19

Farber, B.F., Poplausky, M., Gruber, M., & Brody, J.P. (1984) A prospective study of nosocomial infections in a chronic care facility. *J Am Geriatr Soc* 32: 499-502

Fay, D.E., Poplausky, M., Gruber, M., & Lance, P. (1991) Long term enteral feeding: a retrospective comparison of delivery via percutaneous endoscopic gastrostomy and nasoenteric tubes. *Am J Gastroenterol* 86: 1604-1609

Finnegan, T.P., Austin, T.W., & Cape, R.D. (1985) A 12-month fever surveillance study in a veterans' long-stay institution. *J Am Geriatr Soc* 33: 590-594

Flacker, J.M. & Kiely, D.K. (2003) Mortality-related factors and 1-year survival in nursing home residents. *J Am Geriatr Soc* 51: 213-221

Flamm, R.K., Weaver, M.K., Thornsberry, C., Jones, M.E., Karlowsky, J.A. & Sahm, D.F. (2004) Factors associated with relative rate of antibiotic resistance in Pseudomonas aeruginosa isolated tested in clinical laboratories in the United States from 1999 to 2002. *Antimicrob Agents Chemiother* 48 (7): 2431-2436

Flerer, J. & Ekstrom, M. (1981) An outbreak of Providencia stuartii urinary tract infections: patients with condom catheters are a reservoir of the bacteria. *J Am Med Assoc* 245: 1553-1555

Flournoy, D.J. (1994) Antimicrobial susceptibilities of bacteria from nursing home residents in Oklahoma. *Gerontology* 40: 53-56

Franceschi, C., Bonafè, M., & Valensin, S. (2000b) Human immunosenescence: the prevailing of innate immunity, the failing of clonotypic immunity, and the filling of immunological space. *Vaccine* 18 (16): 1717-1720

Franceschi, C., Bonafè, M., Valensin, S., Olivieri, F., De Luca, M., Ottaviani, E., & De Benedictis, G. (2000a) Inflamm-aging: An Evolutionary Perspective on Immunosenescence". *Ann N Y Acad Sci* 908: 244-254

Franceschi, C., Valensin, S., Fagnoni, F., Barbi, C., & Bonafè, M. (1999) Biomarkers of immunosenescence within an evolutionary perspective: the challenge of heterogeneity and the role of antigenic load. *Experimental Gerontolgy* 34: 911-921

Franson, T., Duthie, E., Cooper Jr.J., van Oudenhove, G., & Hoff, R. (1986) Prevalence survey of infections and their predisposing factors at a hospital-based nursing home care unit. *J Am Geriatr Soc* 34: 95-100

Freedland, C.P., Roller, R.D., Wolfe, B.M., & Flynn, N.M. (1989) Microbial contamination of continuous drip feeding. *J Parenter Enter Nutr* 13: 18-22

Fridkin, S.K., Hageman, J.C., Morrison, M., Sanza, L.T., Como-Sabetti, K., Jernigan, J.A., Harriman, K., Harrison, L.H., Lynfield, R., & Farley, M.M., Active Bacterial Core Surveillance Program of the Emerging Infections Program Network. (2005). Methicillin-resistant Staphylococcus aureus disease in three communities. *N Engl J Med* 352:1436-1444

Fry, A.M., Shay, D.K., Holman, R.C., Curns, A.T., & Anderson, L.J. (2005) Trends in hospitalizations for pneumonia among persons aged 65 years or older in the United States, 1988-2002. *J Am Med Assoc* 294 (21); 2005 Dec 7: 2712-2719

Fulop, T., Gagné, D., Goulet, A.C., Desgeorges, S., Lacombe, G., Arcand, M., & Dupuis, G. (1999) Age-related impairment of p56lck and ZAP-70 activities in human T lymphocytes activated through the TcR/CD3 complex. *Exp Gerontol* 34 (2): 197–216.

Furniss, L., Craig, S.K., Burns, A. (1998) Medication use in nursing homes for the elderly. *Int J Geriatr Psychiatry* 13: 433-439

Furuno, J.P., Hebden, J.N., & Standiford, H.C. (2008) Prevalence of methicillin-resistant Staphylococcus aureus and Acinetobacter baumannii in long-term acute care facility. *Am J Infect Control* 36: 468-471

Galvin, J. (2002) An audit of pressure ulcer incidence in a palliative care setting. Int J Palliat Nurs 8(5):214-221

Gambert, S.R., Duthie, E.H. Jr., Priefer, B., & Rabinovitch, R.A. (1982) Bacterial infections in hospital-based skilled nursing facility. *J Chron Dis* 35: 781-786

Gammack, J.K. (2003) Use and management of chronic urinary catheters in long term care: much controversy, little consensus. *J Am Med Dir Assoc* 4(2 Suppl) S52-S59

Garb, J., Brown, R., Garb, J., & Tuthill, R. (1978) Differences in etiology of pneumonias in nursing home and community patients. *J Am Med Assoc* 240: 2169-2172

Garcia, A.D. & Thomas, D.R. (2006) Assessmet and management of chronic pressure ulcers in the elderly. *Med Clin North Am* 90: 925-944

Garibaldi, R.A. (1999) Residential care and the elderly: the burden of infection. J *Hosp Infect* 1999 Dec; 43 Suppl: S9-18.

Garibaldi, R.A., Brodine, S., & Matsumiya, S. (1981) Infections among patients in nursing homes. Policies, prevalence and problems. *N Eng J Med* 305: 731-735

Garner, J.S. (1996) The Hospital Infection Control Practices Advisory Committee, guideline for isolation precautions in hospitals. *Infect Control Hosp Epidemiol* 17: 53-80

Gau, J.T., Acharya, U., Khan, S., Heh, V., Mody, L., & Kao, T.C. (2011) Pharmacotherapy and the risk for community-acquired pneumonia. *BMC Geriatrics* 10: 45

Gaugler, J.E., Duval, S., Anderson, K.A., & Kane, R.L. (2007) Predicting nursing home admission in U.S.: A meta-analysis. *BMC Geriatrics* 7: 13

Gavazzi, G., Krause, K.H. (2002) Ageing and infection. *Lancet Infect Dis* 2(11): 659-666

Gaynes, R.P., Weinstein, R.A., Chamberlain, W., & Kabins, S.A. (1985) Antibiotic resistant flora in nursing home patients admitted to the hospital. *Arch Intern Med* 145: 1804-1807

Ghadially, R., Brown, B.E., Sequeira-Martin, S.M., Feingold, K.R., & Elias, P.M. (1995). The aged epidermal permeability barrier. Structural, functional, and lipid biochemical abnormalities in humans and a senescent murine model. J *Clin Invest.* 95:2281–2290

Gillchrest, B.A. (1999) Aging of the skin. In: *Principles of geriatric medicine and gerontology.* Hazard WR, Blass JP, Ettinger WH, Halter JB, Ouslander JG (eds.) 4th edition, Mc Graw Hill: 1999;573-590

Ginaldi, L., Loreto, M.F., Corsi, M.P., Modesti, M., & De Martinis, M. ,(2001). Immunosenescence and infectious diseases. *Microbes and Infection* 3 (10): 851–857

Girodon, F., Lombard, M., Galan, P., Brunet-Lecomte, P., Monget, A.L., Arnaud, J., Preziosi, P., & Hercberg, S. (1997) Effect of micronutrient supplementation on infection in institutionalized elderly subjects: a controlled trial. *Ann Nutr Metab* 41: 98-107

Gleckman, B. & Hibert, D. (1982) Afebrile bacteriemia: a phenomenon in geriatric patients. *J Am Med Assoc* 248: 1478-1481

Gleich, S., Morad, Y., & Echague, R (2000) Streptococcus pneumonia serotype 4 outbreaks in a home for the aged: report and review of recent outbreaks. *Infect Control Hosp Epidemiol* 21: 711-717

Gordon, W.Z., Kane, R.L., & Rothemberg, R. (1985) Acute hospitalization in a home for the aged. *J Am Geriatr Soc* 35: 519-523

Gosney, M.A., Hammond, M.F., Shenkin, A., & Allsup, S. (2008) Effect of micronutrient supplementation on mood in nursing home residents. *Gerontology* 54: 292-299

Gould, C-V-, Rothemberg, R., & Steinberg, J.P. (2006) Antibiotic resistance in long-term acute care hospitals: the perfect storm. *Infect Control Hosp Epidemiol* 27: 920-925

Green, C.M., van Beneden, C:A., Javadi, M., Skoff, T.H., Beall, B., & Facklam, R. (2005) Cluster of death from Group A streptococcus in a long-term care facility – Georgia 2001. *Am J Infect Contro*l 33: 108-113

Greenow, J.E., Christenson, E.J., & Montos, P. (1989) Contamination of enteral nutrition system during prolonged use. J Parenter Enter Nutr 13: 23-25

Gross, J.S., Neufeld, R.R., Libow, L.S., Gerber, I., & Rodstein, M. (1988) Autopsy study of the elderly institutionalized patient. *Arch Intern Med* 148: 173-176

Grude, N., Tveten, Y & Kristiansen, B.E. (2001) Urinary tract infections in Norway: bacterial etiology and susceptibility. A retrospective study of clinical isolates. *Clin Microbiol Infect* 7: 543-547

Gulmez, S.E., Holm, A., Frederiksen, H., Jensen, T.G., Pedersen, C., & Hallas, J. (2007) Use of proton pump inhibitors and the risk of community-acquired pneumonia: a population-based case-control study. *Arch Intern Med* 167: 950-955

Ha, U.S. & Cho, Y.H. (2006) Catheter-associated urinary tract infections: new aspects of novel urinary catheters. *Int J Antimicrob Agents.* 2006 Dec; 28(6): 485-90.

Hakim, F.T. & Gress, R.E. (2007) Immunosenescence: deficits in adaptive immunity in elderly. *Tissue antigens* 70 (3): 179–189

Hall, K.E. & Wiley, J.W. (1999) Age-associated changes in gastrointestinal function. In: *Principles of geriatric medicine and gerontology.* Hazard, W.R., Blass, J.P., Ettinger, W.H., Halter, J.B., Ouslander, J.G. (eds.) 4th edition, Mc Graw Hill: 1999; 835-842

Halvorsrud, J., & Orstavik, I. (1980) An epidemic of rotavirus-associated gastroenteritidis in a nursing home for te elderly. *Scand J Infect Dis* 12: 161-164

Han, S., Yang, K., Ozen, Z., Peng, W., Marinova, E., Kelsoe, G., & Zheng, B. (2003). "Enhanced differentiation of splenic plasma cells but diminished long-lived high-affinity bone marrow plasma cells in aged mice". *J Immunol* 170 (3): 1267–1273

Harkness, G.A., Bentley, D.W., Mottley, M., & Lee, J. (1992) Streptococcus pyogenes outbreak in a long term care facility. *Am J Infect Control* 20: 142-148

Harper, C. & Newton, P. (1989) Clinical aspects of pneumonia in the elderly veterans. *J Am Geriatr Soc* 37:867-872

Hassanzadeh, P., & Motamedifar, M. (2007) The prevalence of asymptomatic bacteriuria in long term care facility residents in Shiraz, Southwest Iran: a cross-sectional study. *Pak J Biol Sci* 10 (21): 3890-3894

He, Z., Sun, Z., Liu, S., Zhang, Q., & Tan, Z. (2009) Effect of early malnutrition on mental system, metabolic syndrome and immunity and the gastrointestinal tract. *J Vet med Sci* 71 (9): 1143-1150

Hedin, K., Petersson, C., Widebäck, K., Kahlmeter, G., & Mölstad, S. (2002) Asymptomatic bacteriuria in a population of elderly in municipal institutional care. *Scand J Prim Health Care* 20 (3): 166-168

Henoch, I. & Gustaffson, M. (2003) Pressure ulcers in palliative care: development of a hospice pressure ulcer risk assessment scale. *Int J Palliat Nurs* 9(11):474-484

High, K. (2007) Immunization in older adults. *Clin Geriatr Med* 2007; August; 23 (3): 669-685. Viii-ix

High, K., Bradley, S., Gravenstein, S., Mehr, D.R., Quagliariello, V.J., Richards, C., & & Yoshinawa, T.T. (2009) Clinical practice guideline for the evaluation of fever and infection in older adult residents of long-term care facilities: 2008 Update by the Infectious Disease Society of America. *Clin Infect Dis* 48: 149-171

High, K., Bradley, S., Loeb, M., Palmer, R., Quagliariello, V., & Yoshinawa, T.T. (2005) A new paradigm for clinical investigation of infectious syndromes in older adults: assessment of functional status as a risk factor and outcome measure. *Clin Infect Dis* 40: 114-122

Hildebrandt, G.H., Dominguez, B.L., Schork, M.A., Loesche, W.J. (1997) Functional units, chewing, swallowing and food avoidance among elderly. *J Prosthet Dent* 77: 588-595

Hing, E. & Bloom, B. (1990) Long-term care for the functionally dependent elderly. *Vital Health Stat* n°104, 1990

Hirshberg, J., Rees, R.S., Marchant, B., & Dean, S. (2000) Osteomyelitis related to pressure ulcers: the cost of neglect. *Adv Skin Wound Care* 13: 25-29

Hoffman, N., Jenkins, R., & Putney, K. (1990) Nosocomial infection rates during a one-year period in a nursing home care unit of a Veterans Administration hospital. *Am J Infect Control* 18: 55-63

Hsu, C.C:S. (1991) Serial survey of Methicillin-resistant Staphylococcus aureus nasal carriage among residents in a nursing home. *Infect Control Hosp Epidemiol* 12: 416-421

Huovinen, P. (1984) Trimethoprim-resistant Escherichia coli in a geriatric hospital. *J Infect* 8: 145-148

Ijaz, K., Dillaha, J.A, & Yang, Z (2002) Unrecognized tuberculosis in a nursing home causing death with spread of tuberculosis to the community. *J Am Geriatr Soc* (2002) 50; 1213-1218

IKED (Initiative for quality improvement and Epidemiology of Diabetes) Report, 2007. National Public Health Institute, Brussel, Belgium 2007

Incalzi, R.A., Maini, C.L., Fuso, L., Giordano, A., Carbonin, P.U., Galli, G. (1989) Effect of aging on mucociliary clearance. *Compr Gerontol* [A] 3: 65-68

Irvine, P., van Buren, N., & Crossley, K. (1984) Causes for hospitalization of nursing homes residents. *J Am Geriatr Soc* 32: 103-105

Ito, K Hirao, A., Arai, F., Matsuoka, S., Takubo, K., Hamaguchi, I., Nomiyama, K., Hosokawa, K., Sakurada, K., Nakagata, N., Ikeda, Y., Mak, T.W., & Suda, T. (2004) Regulation of oxidative stress by ATM is required for self-renewal of haematopoietic stem cells". *Nature* 431 (7011): 997–1002

Jackson, M., Fierer, J., Barrett-Connor, E., Fraser, D., Klauber, M.R., Hatch, R., Burkhart, B., & Jones, M. (1992) Intensive surveillance for infections in a three-year study of nursing home patients. *Am J Epidemiol* 135: 685-696

Jackson, M.L., ., Neuzil, K.M., & Thompson, W.W. (2004) The burden of community acquired pneumonia in seniors: results of a population-based study. *Clin Infect Dis* 39 (11); 2004 Dec: 1642-1650

Jackson, M.L., Nelson, J.C., Weiss, N.S., Neuzil, K.M., Barlow, W., & Jackson, L.A. (2008) Influenza vaccination and risk of community-acquired pneumonia in immunocompetent elderly people: population-based, nested case-control study. *Lancet* 372: 398-405

Jacobson, C. & Strausbaugh, L.J. (1990) Incidence and impact of infection in a nursing home care unit. *Am J Infect Control 18: 151-159*

Jain, R., & Danziger, L.H. (2004) Multidrug-resistant Acinetobacter infections: an emerging challenge to clinician. *Ann Pharmacother* 38: 1449-1459

Jankowski, I.M. (2010) Tips for protecting critically ill patients from pressure ulcers. *Crit Care Nurse* 30 (2): S7-S9

Jette, A.M., Branch, L.G., Sleeper, L.A., Feldman, H., Sullivan, L.M. (1992) High risk profile for nursing home admission. *The Gerontologist* 32(5): 634-640

Jevons, M.P. (1961) "Celbein-resistant" staphylococci. *Br Med J* 1: 124-125

John, J.E., & Ribner, B.S. (1991) Antibiotic resistance in long-term care facilities. *Infect Control Hosp Epidemiol* 12: 245-250

Johnson, E.T. (1983) The condom catheter: urinary tract infection and other complications. *South Med J* 76: 579-582

Jones, A.L., Dwyer, L.L., Bercovitz, A.R., & Strahan, G.W. (2009) The National Nursing Home Survey: 2004 overview. *Vital Health Stat* 2009; 167: 1–155

Jones, S.R., Parker, D.F., Kiebow, E.S., Kimbrough, R.C., & Freur R.S. (1987) Appropriateness of antimicrobial therapy in long-term care facilities. *Am J Med* 83: 499-502

Juthani-Mehta, M. & Quagliariello, V.J., (2010) Infectious diseases in the Nursing Home setting: challenges and opportunities for clinical investigation. *Clin Infect Dis* 15; 51(8) 2010 October: 931-938

Kabbuz, R.F., & Tenney, J.H., (1988) Infection control in Maryland nursing homes. *Infect Control Hosp Epidemiol* 9: 159-162

Kaganski, N., Berner, Y., Koren-Morag, N., Perelman, L., Knobler, H., & Levy, S. (2005) Poor nutritional habits are predictors of poor outcome in very old hospitalized patients. *Am J Clin Nutr* 82: 784-791

Kardos, P., Wencker, M., Glaab, T., & Vogelmeier, C. (2007) Impact of salmeterol/fluticasone propionate versus salmeterol on exacerbations in severe chronic obstructive pulmonary disease. *Am J Respir Crit Care Med* 175: 144-149

Kashef, I., Dillaha, J.A., Yang, Z., Cave, M.D., & Bates, J.H. (2002) Unrecognized tuberculosis in a nursing home causing death with spread of tuberculosis to the community. *J Am Geriatr Soc* 50: 1213-1218

Katz, P.R., Beam, T.R., Brand, F., & Boyer, K (1990) Antibiotic use in the nursing home. Physician practice patterns. *Arch Intern Med* 150: 1465-1468

Keating, M.J. 3rd., Klimek, J.J., Levine, D.S., & Kiernan, F.J. (1984): Effect of aging on the clinical significance of fever in ambulatory adult patients. *J Am Geriatr Soc* 32: 282-287

Kelly, F.J., Dunster, C., & Mudway, I. (2003) Air pollution and the elderly oxidant/antioxidant issues with consideration. *Eur Resp J* Suppl. 40: 70S-75S

Kerr, H. & Byrd, J. (1991) Nursing home patients transferred by ambulance to a VA emergency department. *J Am Geriatr Soc* 39: 132-136

Kersten, H., Ruths, S., & Wyller TB (2009) Pharmacotherapy in nursing homes. *Tidsskr Nor Laegeforen* 2009 Sep 10; 129(17): 1732-1735

Kinsella, K., & Velkoff, V.A. (2001) International population report (series P95/01-1) Washington DC. US Government Printing Office, 2001

Klontz, K.C., Adler, W.H., & Potter, M. (1997) Age-dependent resistance factors in the pathogenesis of foodborne infectious disease. *Aging* (Milano) 9: 320-326

Kluger, M.J., Kozak, W., Conn, C.A., Leon, L.R., & Soszynski, D. (1996): The adaptive value of fever. *Infect Dis Clin North Am* 10: 1-20

Klugman, K.P. (2004) Vaccination: a novel approach to reduce antibiotic resistance. *Clin Infect Dis* 39: 649-651

Knockaert, D.C., Vanneste, L.J., & Bobbaers, H.J. (1993): Fever of unknown origin in elderly patients. *J Am Geriatr Soc* 32: 282-287.

Knol, W., van Marum, R.J., Jansen, P.A., Souverein, P.C., Schobben, A.F., & Egberts, A.C. (2008) Antipsychotic drug use and risk of pneumonia in elderly people. *J Am Geriatr Soc* 56: 661-666

Kothe, H., Bauer, T., Marre, R., Suttorp, N., Welte, T., Dalhoff, K., & The Competence Network for Community-Acquired Pneumonia study group (2008) Outcome of community-acquired pneumonia: influence of age, residence status and antimicrobial treatment. *Eur Respir J* 32: 139-146

Krauss, N.A. & Altman, B.M. (2004) Research findings *5: Characteristics of nursing home residents, 1996. December 2004. Agency for Healthcare Research and Quality, Rockville, MD. Available at: *http://www.meps.ahrq.gov/mepsweb7data_file7pubications7rf57rf5.shtml*

Kunin, C.M., Douthitt, S., Dancing, J., Anderson, J., & Moeschberger, M. (1992) The association between the use of urinary catheters and morbidity and mortality among elderly patients in nursing homes. *Am J Epidemiol* 135: 291-301

Laheji, R.J., Sturkenboom, M.C., Hassing, R.J., Dieleman, J., Stricker, B.H., & Jansen, J.B. (2004) Risk of community-acquired pneumonia and use of gastric acid-suppressive drugs. *J Am Med Assoc* 292: 1955-1960

Lamy, M., Mojon, P., Kalykakis, G., Legrand, R., & Butz-Jorgensen, E. (1999) Oral status and nutrition in the institutionalized elderly. *J Dent* 27: 443-448

Laria, A., Zoli, A., Gremese, E., & Ferraccioli, G.F. (2011) Proton pump inhibitors in rheumatic diseases: clinical practice, drug interactions, bone fractures and risk of infections. *Reumatismo* 2011 Mar;63(1):5-10.

Lautenbach, E., Marsicano, R., Tolomeo, P., Heard, M., Serrano, S., & Stieritz, D.D. (2009) Epidemiology of Gram negative antimicrobial resistance in a multi-state network of long-term care facilities. Infect Control Hosp Epidemiol 30 (8): 790-793

Lee, Y.L., Cesario, T., Gupta, G., Flionis, L., Tran, C., Decker, M., & Thrupp, L.D. (1997) Surveillance of colonization and infection with Staphylococcus Aureus susceptible or resistant to Methicillin in a community skilled-nursing facility. Am J Infect Control 25: 312-321

Lee, Y.L., Thrupp, L.D., & Nothvogel, S. (1996) Infection surveillance and antibiotic utilization in a community-based skilled nursing facility. Aging Clin Exp Res 8: 113-122

Lelovics, Z. (2009) Nutritional status and nutritional rehabilitation of elderly people living in long-term care institutions. Orv Hetil 2009 Nov 1; 150(44): 2028-2036.

Leung, F.W. & Schnelle, J.F. (2008) Urinary and fecal incontinence in nursing home residents. Gastroenterol Clin North Am 37(3) 697

Levine, W.J., Smart, J., Archer, D., Bean, N., & Tauxe, R. (1991) Foodborne disease outbreaks in nursing homes, 1975 trough 1987. J. Am. Med. Assoc. 266: 2105-2109

Lim, W.S. & Macfarlane, J.T. (2001) A prospective comparison of nursing home acquired pneumonia with community acquired pneumonia. Eur Resp J 18: 362-368

Lin, Y.T., Chen, L.K., Lin, M.H., & Hwang, S.J. (2006) Asymptomatic bacteriuria among the institutionalized elderly. J Chin Med Assoc 69 (5): 213-217

Linton, P., Lustgarten, J., & Thoman, M. (2006) T cell function in the aged: Lessons learned from animal models. Clinical and Applied Immunology Reviews 6: 73–97

Livesley, N.J. & Chow, A.W. (2002) Infected pressure ulcers in elderly individuals. Clin Infect Dis 35: 1390-1396

Loeb, M., , McGeer, A., McArthur, M., Peeling, R.W., Petric, M., & Simor, A.E. (2000) Surveillance for outbreaks of respiratory tract infections in nursing homes. Can Med Assoc J 162: 1113-1117

Loeb, M., Bentley, D.W., Bradley, S., Crossley, K., Garibaldi, R., Gantz, N., McGeer, A., Muder, R.R., Mylotte, J., Nicolle, L.E., Nurse, B., Paton, S., Simor, A.E., Smith, P., & Strausbaugh, L. (2001b) Development of minimum criteria for the initiation of antibiotics in residents of long-term-care facilities: results of a consensus conference. Infect Control Hosp Epidemiol 22(2): 120–124

Loeb, M., Simor, A.E., & Walter, S. (2001a) Antibiotic use in Ontario facilities that provide chronic care. J Gen Intern Med 16: 376-383

Lord, J.M., Butcher, S., Killampali, V., Lascelles, D., & Salmon, M. (2001) Neutrophil ageing and immunesenescence. Mech Ageing Dev 122 (14): 1521–1535

Luman, W., Kwek, K.R., Loi, K.L., Chiam, M.A., Cheung, W.K., & Ng, H.S. (2001) Percutaneous endoscopic gastrostomy--indications and outcome of our experience at the Singapore General Hospital. Singapore Med J. 2001 Oct; 42(10): 460-465.

Lund-Nielsen, B., Adamsen, L., Gottrup, F., Rorth, M., Tolver, A., & Kolmos, H.J. (2011) Qualitative bacteriology in malignant wounds. A prospective, randomized, clinical study to compare the effect of honey and silver dressings. Ostomy Wound Manag 57(7): 28-36

Lyder, C.H. (2003) Pressure ulcer prevention and management. J Am Med Assoc 289: 223-226

MacArthur, M.D., Lehman, M.H., Currie-McCumber, C.A., & Shlaes, D.M. (1988) The epidemiology of gentamicin-resistant Pseudomonas aeruginosa on an intermediate care unit. *Am J Epidemiol* 128: 821-827

Magaziner, J., Tenney, J.H., DeForge, B., Hebel, R., Muncie, H.L., & Warren, J.W. (1991) Prevalence and characteristics of nursing home-acquired infection in the aged. *J Am Geriatr Soc* 39: 1071-1078

Magnussen, M. & Robb, S. (1980) Nosocomial infections in a long-term care facility. *Am J Infect Control* 8: 12-17

Magri, F., Borza, A., del Vecchio, S., Chytiris, S., Cuzzoni, G., Busconi, L., Rebesco, A., & Ferrari, E. (2003) Nutritional assessment of demented patients: a descriptive study. *Aging Clin Exp Res* 15: 148-153

Mandal, S.K., & Ray, A.K., (1987) Vitamin C status of elderly patients on admission into an assessment geriatric ward. *J Int Med Res* 15: 96-98

Marin, A., Monsó, E., Garcia-Nuñez, M., Sauleda, J., Noguera, A., Pons, J., Agustí, A., & Morera, J. (2010) Variability and effects of bronchial colonization in patients with moderate COPD. *Eur Respir J* 35: 295-302

Marrie, T.J., Durant, H., & Kwan, C. (1986) Nursing home-acquired pneumonia: a case-control study. *J Am Geriatr Soc* 34: 697-702

Maslow, J.N., Lee, B., & Lautenbach, E. (2005) Fluoroquinone-resistant Escherichia coli carriage in long term care facility. *Emerg Infect Dis* 11: 889-894

Mathai, D., Jones, R.N., Pfaller, M-A- & the SENTRY Partecipant Group North America (2001) Epidemiology and frequency of resistance among pathogens causing urinary tract infections in 1510 hospitalized patients: a report from the SENTRY Antimicrobial Surveillance Program (North America). Diagnostic Microbiol Infect Dis 40 (3): 129-136

Mc Evoy, A.J., Dutton, A.J., & James, O.F.W. (1983) Bacterial contamination of the small intestine is an important cause of occult malasorption in the elderly. *Br Med J* 287: 789-793

Mc Geer, A., Campbell, A.B., Eckert, D.G., Emori, T.G., Hierholzer, W.J., Jackson, M.M., Nicolle, L.E., Peppler, C., Rivera, A., Simor, A.E., Smith, P.W., & Wang, E. (1991) Definitions of infections for surveillance in long-term care facilities. *Am J Infect Control* 19: 1-7

Mc Nabney, M.K., Wolff, J.L., Semanick, L.M., Kasper, J.D., & Boult, C. (2007) Care needs of higher functioning nursing home residents. *J Am Med Dir Assoc* 8(6): 409-412

McAnulty, J.M., Keene, W.E., & Leland, D. (2000) Contaminated drinking water in one town manifesting as an outbreak of cryptosporidiosis in another. *Epidemiol Infect* 125: 79-86

Mendelson, G., Yearmack, Y., Granot, E., Ben-Israel, J., Colodner, R., & Raz, R. (2003) Staphylococcus Aureus carrier state among elderly residents of a lont-term care facility. *J Am Med Assoc* 4: 125-127

Meyer, K.C. (2001) The role of immunity in susceptibility to respiratory infection in the aging lung. *Respir Physiol* 1: 23-31

Meyer, K.C., Ershler, W., & Rosenthal, N.S. (1996) Immune dysregulation in the aging human lung. *Am J Respir Crit Care Med* 153: 1072-1079

Meyers, B., Sherman, E., Mendelson, M., Velasquez, G., Srulevitch-Chin, E., & Hubbard, M. (1989) Bloodstream infection in the elderly. *Am J Med* 86; 379-384

Michocki, R.J. & Lamy, P.P. (1976) The problem of pressure sores in a nursing home population: statistical data. *J Am Geriatr Soc* 24: 323-328

Millar,M.R., Brown, N.M., Tobin, G.W., Murphy, P.J., Winsdor, A.C.M., & Speller, D.C.E. (1994) Outbreak of infection with penicillin-resistant Streptococcus pneumonia in a hospital for the elderly. *J Hosp Infect* 27: 99-104

Miller, L.G., Perdreau-Remington, F., Rieg, G., Mehdi, S., Perlroth, J., Bayer, A.S., Tang, A.W., Phung, T.O.,& Spellberg, B. (2005) Necrotizing fasciitis caused by community-associated methicillin-resistant Staphylococcus aureus in Los Angeles. *N Engl J Med* 352:1445-1453

Miller, S.C., Prohaska, T.R., Furner, S.E., Freels, S., Brody, J.A., & Levy, P.S. (1998) Time to nursing home admission for persons with Alzheimer's disease: the effect of health care systems characteristics. *J Gerontol B Psychol Sci Soc Sci* 53B: S341-S353

Min, H., Montecino-Rodriguez, E., Dorshkind, K. (2004) Reduction in the developmental potential of intrathymic T cell progenitors with age". *J Immunol* 173 (1): 245–250

Mittman, C., Edelman, N.H., & Norris, A.H. (1965) Relationship between chest wall and pulmonary compliance with age. *J Appl Physiol* 20; 1211-1216

Miyashita, N., Ouch, K., & Shoji H. (2005) Outbreak of Chlamydophila pneumonia infection in long-term care facilities and an affiliated hospital. *J Med Microbiol* 54: 1243-1247

Mocchegiani, E. & Malavolta, M. (2004). NK and NKT cell functions in immunosenescence. *Aging Cell* 3 (4): 177–1

Mocchegiani, E., Costarelli, L., Giacconi, R., Piacenza, F., Basso, A., & Malavolta, M. (2011) Zinc, metallothioneins and immunosenescence: effect of zinc supply as nutrigenomic approach. *Biogerontology* 2011 Apr 19; DOI: 10.1007/s10522-011-9337-4

Mody, L., Kaufman, S.R., Donabedian, S., Zervos, M., & Bradley, S.F. (2008) Epidemiology of staphylococcus aureus colonization in nursing home residents. *Clin Infect Dis* 2008 may 1st; 46 (9): 1368-1373

Mody, L., Maheshwari, S., Galecki, A., Kauffman, C.A., & Bradley, S.F. (2007) Indwelling device use and antibiotic resistance in nursing homes: identifying a high-risk group. *J Am Geriatr Soc* 2007 Dec; 55(12): 1921-1926

Mody, L., McNeil, S.A., & Sun, R. (2003) Introduction of a waterless alcohol-based hand rub in a long-term care facility. *Infect Control Hosp Epidemiol* 24: 165-171

Montgomery, P., Semenchuk, M., & Nicolle, L.E. (1995) Antimicrobial use in nursing homes in Manitoba. *J Geriatr Drug Ther* 9: 55-74

Morrison, R.R., Ahronheim, J.C., & Morrison, G.R. (1998) Pain and discomfort associated with common hospital procedures and experiences. *J Pain Symptom Manage* 15 (2): 61-101

Muder, R.R., Brennen, C., Drennings, S.D., Stout, J.E., Wagener, M.M. (1997) Multiply antibiotic-resistant Gram negative bacilli in a long-term care facility: a case-control study of patient risk factors and prior antibiotic use. *Infect Control Hosp Epidemiol* 18: 809-813

Muder, R.R., Brennen, C., Wagener, M.M., & Goetz, A.M. (1992) Bacteriemia in long-term care facility: a five year prospective study of 163 consecutive episodes. *Clin Infect Dis* 14: 647-654

Muder, R.R., Brennen, C., Wagener, M.M., Vickers, R.M., Rihs, J.D., Hancock, G.A., Yee, Y.C., Miller, J.M. & Yu, V.L. (1991) Methicillin-resistant Staphylococcal colonization and infection in a long-term care facility. *Ann Intern Med* 114: 107-112

Mulhausen, P.L., Harrell, I.J., Weinberger, M., Kochersberger, G.G., & Feusser, J.R. (1996) Contrasting methicillin-resistant Staphylococcus aureus colonization in Veterans' Affairs and community nursing homes. *AM J Med* 100: 24-31

Murciano, C., Villamón, E., Yáñez, A., O'Connor, J.E., Gozalbo, D., & Gil, ML. (2006). Impaired immune response to Candida albicans in aged mice. *J Med Microbiol* 55 (Pt 12): 1649–1656

Musher, D.M., & Musher B.L. (2004) Contagious acute gastrointestinal infections. *N Engl J Med* 351: 2417-2427

Muszkat, M., Greenbaum, E., Ben-Yehuda, A., Oster, M., Yeu'l, E., Heimann, S., Levy, R., Friedman, G., & Zakay-Rones, Z. (2003) Local and systemic immune response in nursing-home elderly following intranasal or intramuscular immunization with inactivated influenza vaccine. *Vaccine* 21 (11-12): 1180–1186

Mylotte, J.M., Tayara, A., & Goodnough, S. (2002) Epidemiology of bloodstream infection in nursing home residents: evaluation in a large cohort from multiple homes. *Clin Infect Dis* 35: 1484-1490

Mylotte, J.M. (1996) Measuring antibiotic use in a long-term care facility. *Am J Infect Control* 24: 174-179

Mylotte, J.M. (1999) Antimicrobial prescribing in long-term care facilities. *Infect Control Hosp Epidemiol* 27: 10-19

Nakamura, H., Fukushima, H., Miwa, Y., Shiraki, M., Gomi, I., Saito, M., Mawatari, K., Kobayashi, H., Kato, M., & Moriwaki, H. (2006) A longitudinal study on the nutritional state of elderly women at a nursing home in Japan. *Intern Med* DOI:10.2169/internalmedicine.45.1743

Nakashima, K., Tanaka, T., Kramer, M.H., Takahashi, H., Ohyama, T., & Kishimoto, T. (2006) Outbreak of Chlamydia pneumonia infection in a Japanese nursing home, 1999-2000. *Infect Control Hosp Epidemiol* 27: 1171-1177

Narain, J.J., Lofgren, J., Warren, E & Stead, W. (1985) Epidemic tuberculosis in a nursing home: a retrospective cohort study. *J Am Geriatr Soc* 33: 258-263 & Al, 1985;

Naylor, K., Li, G., Vallejo, A.N., Lee, W.W., Koetz, K., Bryl, E., Witkowski, J., Fulbright, J., Weyand, C.M., & Goronzy, J.J. (2005) The influence of age on T cell generation and TCR diversity. *J Immunol* 174 (11): 7446–7452

Nickel, J.C. (2003) Benign prostatic hyperplasia: does prostate mass matter? *Rev Urol* 5 (suppl 4); S12-S17

Nicolle, L.E. (2000) Urinary tract infections in long-term-care facility residents. *Clin Infect Dis* 31: 757-761

Nicolle, L.E. (2001) Preventing infection in non hospital settings: Long-term care. *Emerging Infect Dis* 2001; 7 (2), march-april 2001: 205-207

Nicolle, L.E. (2002) Urinary tract infections in geriatric and institutionalized patients. *Curr Opin Urol* 12: 51-55

Nicolle, L.E., Evans, G., Laverdieve, M., Phillips, P., Quan, C., & Rotstein, C. (2005b) Complicated urinary tract infection in adults Can J Infect Dis Med Microbiol 16: 349-360

Nicolle, L.E., & Garibaldi, R.A. (1995) Infection control in long-term care facilities. *Infect Control Hosp Epidemiol* 16: 348-353

Nicolle, L.E., Bjornson, J., Harding, G., & Mac Donell, J. (1983) Bacteriuria in elderly institutionalized men. *New Engl J Med* 309: 1420-1425

Nicolle, L.E., Bradley, S., Colgan, R., Rice, J.C., Schaeffer, A., & Hooton, T.M. (2005) Infectious diseases Society of America Guidelines for the diagnosis and treatment of asymptomatic bacteriuria in adults. *Clin Infect Dis* 40: 643-654

Nicolle, L.E., Henderson, E., Bjornson, J., McIntyre, M., Harding, G., & Mac Donell, J. (1987a) The association of bacteriuria with resident characteristics and survival in elderly institutionalized med. *Arch Intern Med* 106: 682-686

Nicolle, L.E., Mayhew, W.J., & Bryan, L. (1987b) Prospective, randomized comparison of therapy and no therapy for asymptomatic bacteriuria in institutionalized elderly women. *Am J Med* 83: 27

Nicolle, L.E., Mayhew, W.J., & Bryan, L. (1988) Outcome following antimicrobial therapy for asymptomatic bacteriuria. *Age Ageing* 17: 187-192

Nicolle, L.E., McIntyre, M., Hoban, D., & Murray, D. (1994a) Bacteriemia in a long-term care facility. *Can J Infect Dis* 5: 130

Nicolle, L.E., McIntyre, M., Zacharias, I.L., & Mac Donell, J. (1984) Twelve month surveillance of infections in institutionalized elderly men. *J Am Geriatr Soc* 32: 513-519

Nicolle, L.E., Orr, P., Duckworth, H., Brunks, J., Kennedy, J., Urias, B., Murray, D., & Al Harding, G. (1994b) Prospective study of decubitus ulcers in two long term care facilities. *Can J Infect Control* 9: 35-38

Nicolle, L.E., Strausbaugh, L.J., & Garibaldi, R.A. (1996) Infections and antibiotic resistance in nursing homes. *Clin Microbiol Rev* 9: 1-7

Norman, D. & Yoshikawa, T.T. (1996) Fever in the elderly. *Infect Dis Clin North Am* 10: 93-100

Norman, D. & Toledo, S. (1992) Infections in elderly persons: an altered clinical presentation. *Clin Geriatr Med* 8: 713-719

Norman, R.A. (2003) Geriatric dermatology. *Dermatol Ther* 16:260-268

Notice to readers: National Nursing Home Week – May 8-14, 2005. *MMWR Morb Mortal Wkly Rep* 2005 May 6; 54(17): 438

Nuorti, J.P., Butler, J.C. & Crutcher, J.M. (1998) An outbreak of multidrug-resistant pneumococcal pneumonia and bacteria among unvaccinated nursing home residents. *N Engl J Med* 338: 1861-1868

O'Grady, N.O., Alexander, M., Dellinger, E.P., Gerberding, J.L., Heard, S.O., & Maki, D.G. (2002) Guidelines for prevention of intravascular catheter-related infections. Centers for Disease Control and Prevention. *MMWR Recomm Rep* 51: 1-29

O'Sullivan, N.P., Keane, C.T. (2000) Risk factors for colonization with Methicillin-Resistant Staphylococcus Aureus among nursing home residents. *J Hosp Infect* 45: 206-210

O'Toole, R.D., Drew, W.L., Dahlgren, B.J. & Beaty, H.N. (1970) An outbreak of methicillin resistant Staphylococcus aureus infection. Observation in hospital and in nursing home. *J Am Med Associa* 213: 257-263

Olsen, S.J., DeBess, E.E., McGivern, T.E., Marano, N., Eby, T., & Mauvais, S. (2001) Noscomial outbreak of fluoroquinolone-resistant Salmonella infection. *N Engl J Med* 344: 1572-1579

Omran, M.L. & Morley, J.E. (2000) Assessment of protein energy malnutrition in older persons. Part I: history, examination, body composition, and screening tools. *Nutrition* 16: 50-63

Ordòñez, J., De Antonio Veira, J.A., Pou Soler, C., Navarro Calero, J, Rubio Navarro, J., Marcos Olivares, S., López Ventura, M. (2010) Efecto de un suplemento nutricional oral hiperproteico en pacientes desnutridos ubicados en residencias geriátricas. *Nutr Hosp* July-Aug. 2010; 25 (4): 549-554

Otherson, M.J., & Otherson, H.B. (1987) A history of handwashing seven hundred years at a snail's pace. *The Pharos* 50: 23-27

Ouslander, J. & Schnelle, J.F. (1995) Incontinence in the nursing home. *Ann Intern Med* 122: 438-449

Ouslander, J. (1989) Medical care in the nursing home. *J Am Med Assoc* 262: 2582-2590

Ouslander, J., Greengold, B., & Chen, S. (1987) Complication of chronic indwelling urinary catheters among male nursing home patients: a perspective study. *J Urol* 138: 1191-1195

Ouslander, J.G., Schapira, M., Schnelle, J.F., Fingold, S. (1996) Pyuria among chronically incontinent but otherwise asymptomatic nursing home residents. *J Am Geriatr Soc* 44(4): 420-423

Ouyang, Q., Wagner, W.M., Voehringer, D., Wikby, A., Klatt, T., Walter, S., Müller, C.A., Pircher, H., & Pawelec, G. (2003) Age-associated accumulation of CMV-specific CD8+ T cells expressing the inhibitory killer cell lectin-like receptor G1 (KLRG1). *Exp Gerontol* 38 (8): 911–920.

Pagliari, P., Cosso, P., Ricci, G., & Ianes, A.B. (2011) Quale antibiotico per la terapia delle cistiti nell'anziano in RSA? *G Gerontol* 57: 498

Pauly., L., Stehle, P., & Volkert, D. (2007) Nutritional situation of elderly nursing home residents. *Z Gerontol Geriatr.* 40 (1): 3–12.

Pawelec, G. (1999). Immunosenescence: impact in the young as well as the old? *Mech Ageing Dev 108: 1-7*

Peak, A., Cohen, C.E., & Mulvihill, M.N. (1990) Long-term enteral feeding of aged demented nursing home patients. *J Am Geriatr Soc* 38: 1195-1198

Perez-Stable, E.J., Flaherty, D., Schecter, G., Slutkin, G., & Hopewell, D.C. (1988) Conversion and reversion of tuberculin reaction in nursing home residents. *Am Rev Respir Dis* 137: 801-804

Peterson, P.K., Stein, D., Guay, D.R.P., Logan, G., Obald, S., Gruninger, R., Davies, S., & Breitenbucher, R. (1988) Prospective study of lower respiratory tract infections in an extended-care nursing home program: potential role of oral ciprofloxacin. *Arch Intern Med* 85: 164-171

Phair, J., Kauffman, C.A., Bjorson, A., Adams, L., & Linuetmann, C. Jr. (1978) Failure to respond to influenza vaccine in the aged: correlation with B-cell number and function. *J Lab Clin Med* 92: 822-828

Philip, W., Bennett, G., Bradley, S., Drinka, P., Lautenbach, E., Marx, J., Mody, L., Nicolle, L.E. & Stevenson, K. (2008) SHEA/APIC Guideline: Infection prevention and control in the long-term care facility, July 2008. *Infect Control Hosp Epidemiol* Sept. 2008; 29 (9): 785-814

Phillips, S.K. & Branaman-Phillips, M.A. (1993) The use of intramuscular cefoperazone versus intramuscular ceftriaxone in patients with nursing home acquired pneumonia. *Am J Med* 41: 1071-1074

PHS D. (Ed.) US Department of Health and Human Services (DHHS) PHS. National Center for Health Statistics. Health United States 1985. Hyattsville, MD: 1985 p. 86-1232

Pickering, T.D., Gurwitz, J.H., Zaleznik, D., Noonan, J. P., & Avorn, J. (1994) The appropriateness of oral fluoroquinolone prescribing in long-term care setting. *J Am Geriatr Soc* 42: 28-32

Pittet, D., Sax, H., & Hugonnet, S. (2004) Cost implications of successful hand hygiene promotion. *Infect Control Hosp Epidemiol* 25: 264-266

Pourat, N. (1995) Ethnic/racial differences in the use of nursing home services among the elderly. *Annual Research Meeting of the Academy for Health Service Research and Health Policy.* Abstract Book, Chicago, IL, June 4-6 1995

Pressure Ulcer Advisory Panel/European Pressure Ulcer Advisory Panel Pressure Ulcer Prevention and Treatment Clinical Practice Guideline. Washington, DC: National Pressure Ulcer Advisory Panel; 2009

Rajagopalan, S., & Yoshikawa, TT. (2000) Tuberculosis in long-term care facilities. *Infect Control Hosp Epidemiol* 21: 611-615

Raz, R., Schiller, D., & Nicolle, L.E. (2000) Chronic indwelling catheter replacement before antimicrobial therapy for symptomatic urinary tract infection. *J Urol* 164: 1254-1258

Regal, R.E., Pham, C.Q., & Bostwick, T.R. (2006) Urinary tract infections in extended care facilities: preventive management strategies. Consult Pharm. 2006 May; 21(5): 400-409.

Reid, R.T., Briggs, R.S., Seal, D.V., & Pearson, A.D. (1983) Virulent Streptococcus pyogenes outbreak and spread in a geriatric unit. *J Infect* 6: 219-225

Ribeiro, B.J. & Smith, S.R. (1985) Evaluation of urinary catheterization and urinary incontinence in a general nursing home population. *J Am Geriatr Soc* 33: 479-482

Ricci, G., Cosso, P., Leonetti, A., Pagliari, P., & Ianes, A.B. (2009) I disturbi psicocomportamentali nella demenza: studio di un campione di soggetti anziani residenti in Residenza Sanitaria Assistenziale. *G Gerontol* 57: 70-77

Ricci, G., Cosso, P., Pagliari, P., & Ianes, A.B. (2010) Le infezioni delle basse vie urinarie nell'anziano in residenza sanitaria assistenziale: studio osservazionale di 54 mesi. *G Gerontol* 58: 270-278

Rice, L.B., Willey, S.H., Papanicolaou, G.A., Medeiros, A.A., Eliopoulos, G.M., Moellering, R.C., & Jacoby, G.A. (1990) Outbreak of ceftazidime resistance caused by estende-spectrum-ß-lactamases at a Massachusetts chronic-care facility. *Antimicrob Agents Chemiother* 34: 2193-2199

Richards, C.L. (2004) Urinary tract infections in the frail elderly: issues for diagnosis, treatment and prevention. *Int Urol Nephrol* 36(3): 457-63

Rodhe, N., Mőlstad , S., Englund, L., & Svärdsudd, K. (2006) Asymptomatic bacteriuria in apopulation of elderly resident living in a community setting: prevalence characteristics and associated factors. *Fam Pract* doi:10-1093/fampra/cml007

Rogers, M.A., Mody, L., Chenoweth, C., Kaufman, S.R. & Saint, S. (2008) Incidence of antibiotic resistant infection in long-term residents of skilled nursing facilities. *Am J Infect Control* 2008 sept; 36 (7): 472-475

Ruben, F.C:, Norden, B., Heisler, B., & Korica, Y (1984) An outbreak of Streptococcus pyogenes infections in a nursing home. *Ann Intern Med* 101: 494-496

Rudelsky, B., Lipschits, M., Isaacsohn, M., & Sonnenblick, M. (1992) Infected pressure sores: comparison of methods for bacterial identification. *South Med J* 85: 901-903

Rudman, D., Hontanosas, A., Cohen, C., & Mattson, D. (1988) Clinical correlates of bacteriemia in a Veterans Administration extended care facility. *J Am Geriatr Soc* 36: 726-732

Ryan, C.A., Tauxe, R.V., Hosek, G.W., Wells, J.G., Stoesz, P.A., & McFadden, H.W.Jr. (1986) Escherichia coli O157:H7 diarrhea in a nursing home: clinical, epidemiological and pathological findings. *J Infect Dis* 154: 631-638

Saeed, S., Fakih, M.G., Riederer, K., Shah, A.R., & Khatib, R. (2006) Interinstitutional and intrainstitutional transmission of a strain of Acinetobacter Baumannii detected by molecular analysis: comparison of pulsed-field gel electrophoresis and repetitive sequence-based polymerase chain reaction. *Infect Control Hosp Epidemiol* 27: 981-983

Saint, S., Kaufman, S.R., Rogers, M.A., Baker, P.D., Ossenkop, K., & Lipsky, B.A. (2006) Condom versus indwelling urinary catheters: a randomized trial. *J Am Geriatr Soc* 54: 1055-1061

Saletti, A., Lindgren, E.Y., Johansson, L., & Cederholm, T. (2000) Nutritional status according to mini nutritional assessment in an institutionalized elderly population in Sweden. *Gerontology* 46(3):139–145

Sandoval, C., Walter, S.D., MCGeer, A., Simor, A.E., Bradley, S.F., Moss. L.M., & Loeb, M.B. (2004) Nursing home residents and Enterobacteraceae Resistant to third-generation Cephalosporins. *Emerg Infect Dis* 10: 1050-1055

Sapico, F.I., Ginunas, V.J., & Thornhill-Joynes, M.T. (1986) Quantitative microbiology of pressure sores in different stages of healing. *Diagn Microbiol Infect Dis* 5: 31-38

Schaeffer, A.J., & Schaeffer, E.M. (2007) Infections of the urinary tract. In: Wein, A.J., et Al. Campbell-Walsh *Urology*. *9th ed.* Philadelphia, Pa.: Saunders; 2007. *http://www.mdconsult.com/das/book/body/202281144-2/0/1445/0.html.*

Scheckler, W. & Peterson, P. (1986) Infections and infections control among residents of eight rural Wisconsin nursing homes. *Arch Intern Med* 146: 1981-1984

Schiappa, D.A:, Hayden, M.J., Matushek, M.G., Hashemi, F.N., Sullivan, J., Smith, K.Y., Miyashiro, D., Quinn, J.P., Weinstein, R.A., & Trenholme, G.M. (1996) Ceftazidime-resistant Klebsiella pneumoniae and Escherichia coli bloodstream infection: a case-control and molecular epidemiology investigation. *J Infect Dis* 174: 529-536

Schicker, J.M., Franson, T.R., Duthie, Jr., E.H., & LeClair, S.M. (1988) Comparison of methods for calculation and depiction of incidence infection rates in long-term care facilities. *J Clin Epidemiol* 41: 757-761

Schnelle, J.F., Adamson, G.M., Cruise, P.A., al-Samarrai, N., Sarbaugh, F.C., Uman, G., & Ouslander, J.G. (1997) Skin disorders and moisture in incontinent nursing home resident: intervention implications. *J Am Geriatr Soc* 45 (10) 1182.1188

Schumm, K. & Lam, T.B. (2008) Types of urethral catheters for management of short-term voiding problems in hospitalized adults: a short version Cochrane review. *Neurourol Urodyn* 27(8): 738-746

Schwartz, B. & Ussery, X. (1992) Group A streptococcal outbreaks in nursing homes. *Infect Control Hosp Epidemiol* 13: 742-747

Seenivasan, M.H., Yu, V.L., & Muder, R.R. (2005) Legionnaires' disease in long-term care facilities: overview and proposed solutions. *J Am Geriatr Soc* 53: 875-880

Selbaek, G., Kirkevold, Ø., & Engedal, K. (2007) The prevalence of psychiatric symptoms and behavioural disturbances and the use of psychotropic drugs in Norwegian nursing homes. *Int J Geriatr Psychiatry* 22: 843-849

Sengstock, D.M., Thyagarajan, R., Apalara, J., Mira, A., Chopra, T., & Kaye, K.S. (2010) Multi-drug resistant Acinetobacter baumannii: an emerging pathogen among older adults in community hospital and nursing homes. *Clin Infect Dis* 50 (12) 1611-1616

Setia, U., Serventi, I., & Lorenz, P. (1984) Bacteremia in a long-term care facility: spectrum and mortality. *Arch Intern Med* 144: 1633-1635

Setia, U., Serventi, I., & Lorenz, P. (1985) Nosocomial infections among patients in long-term care facility: spectrum, prevalence, and risk factors. *Am J Infect Control* 13: 67-62

Shah, B.R. & Hux, J.E. (2003) Quantifying the risk of infectious diseases for people with diabetes. *Diabetes Care.* 26:510-513

Shahin, E.S., Meijers, J.M., Schols, J.M., Tannen, A., Halfens, R.J., & Dassen, T. (2010) The relationship between malnutrition parameters and pressure ulcers in hospital and nursing homes. *Nutrition* 2010 sept; 26 (9): 886-889

Shepard, M., Parker, D., & DeClerque, N. (1987) The underreporting of pressure sores in patients transferred between hospital and nursing home. *J Am Geriatr Soc* 35: 159-160

Shindo, Y., Sato, S., Maruyama, E., Ohashi, T., Ogawa, M., Hashimoto, N., Imaizumi, K., Sato, T., & Hasegawa, Y. (2009) Health-care-associated pneumonia among hospitalized patients in a Japanese community hospital. *Chest* 135: 633-640

Shlaes, D.M., Currie-McCumber, C.A., & Lehman, M.H. (1988) Introdution of a plasmid encoding the OHIO-1 ß-lactamase to an intermediate care ward by patient transfer. *Infect Control Hosp Epidemiol* 9: 317-319

Shlaes, D.M., Lehman, M.H., Currie-McCumber, C.A., Kim, C.H., & Floyd, R. (1986) Prevalence of colonization with antibiotic resistant gram-negative bacilli in a nursing home care unit: the importance of cross-colonization as documented by plasmid analysis. *Infect Control* 7: 538-545

Shlaes, D.M., Lehman, M.H., Currie-McCumber, C.A., Kim, C.H., & Floyd, R. (1986) Prevalence of colonization with antibiotic resistant gram-negative bacilli in a nursing home care unit: the importance of cross-colonization as documented by plasmid analysis. *Infect Control* 7: 538-545

Sieggreen, M.Y. & Kline, R.A. (2004) Arterial insufficiency and ulceration: diagnosis and treatment options. *Nurs Pract.* 29 (9): 46-52.

Siegman-Igra, Y., Fourer, B., & Orni-Wasserlauf, R (2002) Reappraisal of community-acquired bacteremia: a proposal of a new classification for the spectrum of acquisition of bacteremia. *Clin Infect Dis* 34: 1431-1439

Simor, A.F., Bradley, S.F., Strausbaugh, L.J., Crossley, K., & Nicolle, L.E., SHEA Long-Term Care Commitee (2002) Clostridium difficile in long-term care facilities for the elderly. *Infect Control Hosp Epidemiol* 23: 696-703

Singh, S., Amin, A.V., & Loke, Y.K. (2009) Long-term use of inhaled corticosteroids and the risk of pneumonia in chronic obstructive pulmonary disease: a meta-analysis. *Arch Intern Med* 169: 219-229

Slotwiner-Nie, P.K. & Brandt, L.I. (2001) Infectious diarrhea in the elderly. *Gastroenterol Clin North Am* 30: 625-635

Smith, D.M., Snow, D.E., Rees, E., Zischkau, A.M., Hanson, J.D., Walcott, R.D., Sun, Y., White, J., Kumar, S., & Dowd, S.E. (2010) Evaluation of the bacteria diversity of pressure ulcers using bTEFAP pyro-sequencing. *BMC Med Genomics* 3: 41

Smith, P.F., Stricof, R.L., Shayegani, M., & Morse, D.L. (1988) Cluster of Haemophilus influenza type B infection in adults. *J Am Med Assoc* 260: 1446-1448

Smith, P.W. (1985) Infections in long-term care facilities. *Infect Control* 6: 435-436

Smith, P.W. (1987) Consensus conference on nosocomial infections in long-term care facilities. *Am J Infect Control* 15: 97-100

Smith, P.W. (1999) Development of nursing home infection control. *Infect Control Hosp Epidemiol* 20: 303-305

Smith, P.W. (Ed) (1994) *Infections control in long term care facilities*, 2nd ed. Delmar Publisher Inc., Albany, NY, pp 131-146

Smith, P.W., & Rusnak, P.G. (1997) Infection prevention and control in the long-term care facility. SHEA long-term-care Committee and APIC Guidelines Committee. *Infect Control Hosp Epidemiol* 18; 831-849

Smith, P.W., Bennett, G., Bradley, S., Drinka, P., Lautenbach, E., Marx, J., Mody, L., Nicolle, L.E., & Stevenson, K. (2008) SHEA/APIC Guidelines: Infection prevention and control in the long-term care facility, July 2008. *Infect Control Hosp Epidemiol* 29 (9): 785-814

Smith, P.W., Daly, P.B., & Roccaforte, J.S. (1991) Current status of nosocomial infection control in extended care facilities. *Am Med J* 91: S281-S285

Smith, P.W., Seip, C.W., Schaefer, S.C:, & Bell-Dixon, C (2000) Microbiologic survey of long-term care facilities. *Am J Infect Control* 28: 8-13

Smitten, A.L., Choi, H.K., Hochberg, M.C., Suissa, S., Simon, T.A., Testa, M.A., & Chan, K.A. (2008) The risk of hospitalized infection in patients with rheumatoid arthritis. *J Rheumatol* 35:387–93

Spector, WD., Kapp, W.D., Tucker, R.J., & Sternberg, J. (1988) Factors associated with presence of decubitus ulcers at admission to nursing homes. *Gerontologist* 28: 830-834

Stamm, W.E. & Hooton, T.M. (1993) Management of urinary tract infections in adults. *N Engl J Med* 329:1328-1334

Standaert, S.M., Hutcheson, R.H., Schaffener, W. (1994) Nosocomial transmission of Salmonella gastroenteritis to laundry workers in a nursing home. *Infect Control Hosp Epidemiol* 15: 22-26

Standfast, S.J., Michelsen, P.B., Baltch, A.I., Smith, R.P., Latham, F.K., Spellacy, A.B., Venezia, R.A., & Andritz, M.H. (1984) A prevalence survey of infections in a combined acute and long-term care hospital. *Infect Control* 5: 177-184

Stead, W. (1981) Tuberculosis among elderly persons: an outbreak in nursing home. *Ann Intern Med* 94: 606-610

Stead,W., Lofgren, J., Warren, E., & Thomas, C. (1985) Tuberculosis as an endemic and nosocomial infection among the elderly in nursing homes. *N Engl J Med* 312: 1483-1487

Steinmiller, A., Robb, S., & Muder, R. (1991) Prevalence of nosocomial infections in long-term care Veterans medical centers. *Am J Infect Control* 19: 143-146

Stephens, C., Franceis, S.J., Abell, V., DiPersio, J.R., & Wells, P. (2007) Emergence of Acinetobacter baumannii in critically ill patients within an acute care teaching hospital and a long-term acute care hospital. *Am J Infect Control* 35: 212-215

Stevenson, K.B., Moore, J., Colwell, H., & Sleeper, B. (2005) Standardized infection surveillance in long-term care: interfacility comparison from a regional cohort facilities. *Infect Control Hosp Epidemiol* 26: 231-238

Storch, G.A., Radcliff, J.L., Meyer, P.L. & Hirinchs, J,H. (1987) Methicillin-resistant Staphylococcus aureus in a nursing home. *Infect Control* 8: 24-29

Stout, J.E., Brennen, C., & Muder, R.R. (2000) Legionnaires' disease in a newly constructed long-term care facility. *J Am Geriatr Soc* 48: 1589-1592

Stratton, R.J., King, C.L., Stroud, M.A., Jackson, A.A., & Elia, M. (2006) "Malnutrition Universal Screening Tool' predicts mortality and length of hospital stay in acutely ill elderly. *Br J Nutr* 95(2): 325-330

Strausbaugh, L.J. & Joseph, C.J. (1999) Epidemiology and prevention of infections in residents of long term care facilities. In: Mayhall, C.G., editor. *Hospital epidemiology and infection control*. 2nd ed. Philadelphia: Lippincott Williams & Wilkins; 1999. p. 1461

Strausbaugh, L.J., & Joseph, C.J. (2000) The burden of infection in long-term care. *Infect Control Hosp Epidemiol* 21: 674-679

Strausbaugh, L.J., Jacobson, C., Sewell, D.L., Potter, S., & Ward, T.T. (1991) Methicillin-resistant Staphylococcus Aureus in extended care facilities: experiences in a Veteran's Affairs Nursing Home and review of the literature. *Infect Control Hosp Epidemiol* 12: 151-159

Strausbaugh, L.J., Sukumar, S.R., Joseph, C.L. (2003) Infectious disease outbreaks in nursing homes: an unappreciated hazard for frail elderly persons. *Clin Infect Dis* 36: 36: 870-876

Strout, R.D. & Suttles, J. (2005) Immunosenescence and macrophage functional plasticity: dysregulation of macrophage function by age-associated microenvironmental changes". *Immunol Rev* 205: 60–71

Sturm, A.W., Monstert, R., Roning, P.J.E., van Klingeren, B., & van Alphen, L. (1990) Outbreak of multiresistant nonencapsulated Haemophilus influenza infection in a pulmonary rehabilitation centre. *Lancet* 335: 214-216

Suderkotter, C. & Kalden, H. (1997) Aging and the skin immune system. *Arch Dermatol* 133 (10): 1256–1262

Sutcliffe, C., Burns, A., Challis, D., Mozley, C.G., Cordingley, L., Bagley, H.,& Huxley, P. (2007) Depressed mood, cognitive impairment, and survival in older people admitted to care homes in England. *Am J Geriatr Psychiatry* 15: 708-715

Tan, J.S. (2000) Infectious complications in patients with diabetes mellitus. *Int Diabetes Monitor* 12: 1-7

Tansel, O., Kugoglu, F., Mutlu, B., Anthony, R.M., Uyar, A., Vahaboglu, H., & French, G.L. (2003) A methicillin-resistant staphylococcus aureus outbreak in a new University hospital due to a strain transferred with an infected patient from another city, six month previously. *New Microbiol* 26 (2): 175-180

Terpenning, M.S., Bradley, S.F., Wan, J.Y., Chenoweth, C.E., Jorgenson, K.A. & Kauffman, C.A. (1994) Colonization and infection with antibiotic-resistant bacteria in a long-term care facility. *J Am Geriatr Soc* 42: 1062-1069

Thomas, D.B., Bennett, R.G., Laughon, B.E., Greenough, W.B., & Barlett, J.G. (1990) Post-antibiotic colonization with Clostridium difficile in nursing home patients. *J Am Geriatr Soc* 38: 415-420

Thomas, J.C., Bridge, J., Waterman, S., Vogt, J., Kilman, L., & Hancock, G. (1989) Transmission and control of methicillin-resistant Staphylococcus aureus in a skilled nursing facility. *Infect Control Hosp Epidemiol* 10: 106-110

Thomas, J.C., Bridge, J., Waterman, S., Vogt, J., Kilman, L., & Hancock, G. (1989) Transmission and control of methicillinn-resistant Staphylococcus aureus in a skilled nursing facility. *Infect Control Hosp Epidemiol* 10: 106-110

Topinkovà, E., Neuwirth, J., Stanková, M., Mellanová, A., & Haas, T. (1997) Urinary and fecal incontinence in geriatric facilities in the Czech Republic. *Cas Lek Cesk* 136 (18): 573-577

Troy, C.J., Peeling, R.W., Ellis, A.G., Hockin, J.C., Bennet, D.A., & Murphy, M.R. (1997) Chlamydia pneumoniae as a new source of infectious outbreaks in nursing homes. *J Am Med Assoc* 277: 1214-1218

Tsan, L., Langberg, R., Davis, C., Phillips, Y., Pierce, J., Hojlo, C., Gibert, C., Gaynes, R., Montgomery, O., Bradley, S., Danko, L., & Roselle, G. (2008) Prevalence of nursing home-associated infections in the Department of Veterans Affairs nursing home care units. Am J Infect Control. 2008 Apr; 36(3): 173-9.

Tsan, L., Langberg, R., Davis, C., Phillips, Y., Pierce, J., Hojlo, C., Gibert, C., Gaynes, R., Montgomery, O., Bradley, S., Danko, L., & Roselle, G. (2010) Nursing home-associated infections in Department of Veterans Affairs community living centers. *Am J Infect Control.* 2010 Aug; 38(6): 461-466

Utsumi, M., Makimoto, K., Quroshi, N., & Ashida N. (2010) Types of infectious outbreaks and their impact in elderly care facilities: a review of the literature. *Age Ageing* 39: 299-305

Uyemura, K., Castle, S.C., & Makinodan, T. (2002) The frail elderly: role of dendritic cells in the susceptibility of infection. *Mech Ageing Dev* 123 (8): 955–962

Valdez, R., Narayan, K.M., Geiss, L.S., & Engelgau, M.M. (1999). Impact of diabetes mellitus on mortality associated with pneumonia and influenza among non-Hispanic black and white US adults. *Am J Public Health* 89:1715-1721.

Valiyeva, E.,. Russell, L.B., Miller ,J.E., & Safford, M.M. (2006) Lifestyle-related risk factors and risk of future nursing home admission. *Arch Intern Med* 166(9): 985-990

van de Sande-Bruinsma, N., Grundmann, N., Verloo, D., Tiemersma, E., Monen, J., & Goossens H. (2008) Antimicrobial use and resistance in Europe. *Emerg Infect Dis* 14: 1722-1730

Van Duin, D., Mohanty, S., & Thomas, V. (2007b). Age-associated deficits in human TLR-1/2 function. *J Immunol* 178 (2), 2007 Jan 15: 970-975

Van Duin, D., Allore, H.G. & Mohanty, S. (2007a). Prevaccine determination of the expression of costimulatory B7 molecules in activated monocytes predicts influentia vaccine responses in young and older adults. *J Infect Dis* 195 (11) june 2007; 1590-1597

Van Rensbergen, G. & Nawrot, T. (2010) Medical conditions of nursing homes admission. *BMC Geriatrics* 10:46

Vanderkooi, O.G., Low, D.E., Green, K., Powis, J.E., McGeer, A. & Toronto Invasive Bacterial Disease Network. (2005) Predicting antimicrobial resistance in invasive pneumococcal infections. *Clin Infect Dis* 40(9):1288-1297.

Vergese, A. & Berk, S. (Eds) (1990) *Infections in nursing homes and long-term care facilities.* Karger, Basel, 1990

Viahov, D., Tenney, J., Cervino, K., & Shamer, D. (1987) Routine surveillance for infections in nursing homes: experience at two facilities. *Am J Infect Control* 15: 47-53

Viray, M., Linkin, D., Maslow, J.N., Stieritz, D.D., Carson, L.S., Bilker, W.B., & Lautenbach, E. (2005) Longitudinal trends in antimicrobial susceptibilities across long-term care facilities: emergence of fluoroquinolone resistance. *Infect Control Hosp Epidemiol* 26: 56-62

Voehringer, D., Koschella, M., Pircher, H. (2002) Lack of proliferative capacity of human effector and memory T cells expressing killer cell lectin-like receptor G1 (KLRG1) *Blood* 100 (10): 3698–3702

Votey, S.R. & Peters, A.L. (2005) Diabetes mellitus, type 2 - a review. Available at: *http://www.emedicine.com/emerg/topic134.htm* Accessed July 12, 2005

Warren, J.W., Tenney, J., Hoopes, J.M., Muncie, H.L., & Antony, W.C. (1982) A prospective microbiologic study of bacteriuria in patients with chronic indwelling catheters. *J Infect Dis* 146: 719-723

Warren, J.W., Damron, D., Tenney, J., Hoopes, J.M., Deforge, R., & Muncie, H.Jr. (1987) Fever, bacteriemia and death as complications of bacteriuria in women with long-term urethral catheters. *J Infect Dis* 155: 1151-1158

Warren, J.W., Muncie, H.Jr. & Hall-Craggs, M. (1988) Acute pyelonephritis associated with bacteriuria during long-term catheterization: a prospective clinico-pathological study. *J Infect Dis* 158: 1341-1346

Warren, J.W., Palumbo, F.B., Fitterman, L., & Speedle, S.M. (1991) Incidence and characteristics of antibiotic use in aged nursing home patients. *J Am Geriatr Soc* 39: 963-972

Warren, J.W., Steinberg, L., Uebel, R., & Tenney, J. (1989) The prevalence of urethral catheterization in Maryland nursing homes. *Arch Intern Med* 149: 1535-1537

Wasserman, M., Levinstein, M., Keller, E., Lee, S., & Yoshikawa, T. (1989): Utility of fever, white blood cell, and differential count in predicting bacterial infections in the elderly. *J Am Geriatr Soc* 37: 534–543

Wayne, S.J., Rhyne, R. L., & Stratton, M. (1992) Longitudinal prescribing patterns in a nursing home population. *J Am Geriatr Soc* 40: 53-56

Weiner, J., Quinn, J.P., Bradford, P.A., Goering, R.V., Nathan, C., Bush, K., & Weinstein, R.A. (1999) Multiple antibiotic resistant Klebsiella and E. Coli in nursing homes. *J Am Med Assoc* 281: 517-523

Weinstein, M.P., Towns, M.L, Quartey, S.M., Mirrett, S., Reimer, L.G., Parmigiani, G., Reller, L.B. (1983): The clinical significance of positive blood cultures: A comprehensive analysis of 500 episodes of bacteremia and fungemia II. Clinical observations with special reference to factors influencing prognosis. *Rev Infect Dis* 5:54–70

Welty, C., Burstin, S., Muspratt, S., & Tager, I.B. (1985) Epidemiology of tuberculosis infections in chronic care population. *Am Rev Respir Dis* 132: 133-136

Weng, N.P. (2006) Aging of the immune system: how much can the adaptive immune system adapt?. *Immunity* 24 (5): 495–499

Werner, H. & Kuntsche, J. (2000) Infection in the elderly--what is different? *Z Gerontol Geriatr*. 2000 Oct; 33(5): 350-356.

White, K.E., Hedberg, C.W., Edmonson, L.M., Jones, D.B., Osterholm, M.T. & MacDonald, K.L. (1989) An outbreak of Giardiasis in a nursing home with evidence for multiple modes of transmission. *J Infect Dis* 160: 298-304

Wingard, F., Shlaes, J., Mortimer, E., & Shlaes, D (1993) Colonization and cross-colonization of nursing home patients with thrimetoprim-resistant gram-negative bacilli. *Clin Infect Dis* 16: 75-81

Winquist, A.G., Roome, A., Mshar R, Fiorentino, T, Mshar, P., & Hadler, J. (2001) Outbreak of campylobacteriosis at a senior center. *J Am Geriatr Soc* 49: 304-307

Wong, E.S. & Hooten, T.M. (1981) Guideline for prevention of catheter-associated urinary tract infections. *Infect Control* 2: 125-130

Yakabowich, M.R., Keeley, G.,& Montgomery, P.R. (1994) Impact of a formulary on personal care homes in Manitoba. *Can Med Assoc J* 150: 1601-1607

Yamaya, M., Yanai M, Ohrui, T., Arai, H., & Sasaki, H. (1991) Interventions to prevent pneumonia among older adults. *J Am Geriatr Soc* 49: 85-90

Yoshikawa, T.T., Nicolle, L.E., & Norman, D.C. (1996) Management of complicated urinary tract infections in older patients. *J Am Geriatr Soc* 44: 1235-1241

Young, J.B. & Dobrzanski, S. (1992) Pressure sores epidemiology and current management concepts. *Drugs Aging* 2: 42-57

Zervos, M.J., Terpenning, M.S., Schaberg, D.R., Therasse, P.M., Mendendorp, S.V., & Kauffman, C.A. (1987) High-level aminoglycoside-resistant enterococci: colonization of nursing home and acute care hospital patients. *Arch Intern Med* 147: 1591-1594

Zhanel, G.G., Nicolle, L.E., & Harding, G.K.M. (1995) Prevalence of asymptomatic bacteriuria and associated host factors in women with diabetes mellitus. *Clin Infect Dis* 21: 316-322

Ziegler, T.R., Cole, C.R. (2007) Small bowel bacterial overgrowth in adults: a potential contributor to intestinal failure. *Curr Gastroenterol Rep* 2007 Dec; 9(6): 463-467

Zimmer, J.G., Bentley, D.W., Valenti, W.M. & Watson, N.M. (1986) Systemic antibiotic use in nursing homes. A quality assessement. *J Am Geriatr Soc* 34: 703-710

Zulkowski, K., Langemo, D., & Posthauer, M. (2005) NUAP. Coming to Consensus on Deep Tissue Injury. *Adv Skin Wound Care* 18: 28-29

4

Stability of Antibiotic Resistance Patterns in Agricultural Pastures: Lessons from Kentucky, USA

Sloane Ritchey, Siva Gandhapudi and Mark Coyne
University of Kentucky,
USA

1. Introduction

Animal and human wastes contain fecal bacteria, including pathogens that can contaminate groundwater, streams, lakes, and reservoirs through runoff and infiltration. Bacterial nonpoint sources of pollution continually impair water quality (Hartel et al., 2002). These pollution sources may come from failed septic systems, large animal operations, land application of wastes, sewage treatment facilities, and wildlife. Fecal pollution of rivers and streams is of great concern due to the direct potential threat to human health, and the increased costs associated with water treatment.

Groundwater contamination from these wastes can be a serious environmental concern in well-drained soils and soils with shallow water tables. Karst topography in Kentucky, for example, constitutes 55% of the land area (KGS, 2002), much of which is in pasture where land application of animal waste is commonly practiced. Of the 4,521 total km (2,810 total mi) of rivers and streams assessed in Kentucky in 2000, 73% were impaired for primary contact (>200 fecal coliforms/100 mL; USEPA, 2000). Similar reports regarding impaired watersheds can be found throughout the United States. Dombek et al. (2000) reported that 47% of assessed river miles in Minnesota were impaired for primary contact due to high levels of fecal coliform bacteria. Graves et al. (2002) reported that approximately 13% of monitored streams and 1% of estuaries in Virginia were impaired, with >60% of the impairments due to fecal contamination. The recurrence of such reports is evidence that tools are needed to identify such pollution sources and facilitate restoration efforts such as implementing total maximum daily loads (TMDLs) or best management practices (BMPs).

The reliance of pollution remediation efforts on TMDLs has been one of the driving forces behind developing techniques to distinguish between human and non-human fecal pollution sources (Johnson et al., 2004). A standard method of assessing water quality impairment based on the potential for pathogenic microbes of intestinal origin is to enumerate commensal bacteria such as coliforms. While total and fecal coliform counts produce an estimate of pollution levels, specific sources of the microbial pollution cannot be determined. Microbial source tracking (MST) techniques offer unique approaches to differentiate nonpoint source pollution. By tracking a pollution source to its origin, resources and management tools may be better allocated to improve water quality. Some issues that affect the usefulness of these MST techniques include the appropriate database portability, size, and temporal characteristics to yield adequate power of prediction given the diversity of antibiotic resistance patterns in a watershed.

The answers to these issues are as yet undetermined. Several reports agree that MST techniques are most applicable to limited geographical areas such as specific watersheds rather than larger geographic regions (Guan et al., 2002; Johnson et al., 2004; Lu et al., 2005; McClellan et al., 2003). There is also no consensus on whether using *Escherichia coli* (EC) or fecal streptococci (FS) is preferred for use as indicator bacteria. Because of the labor-intensive and time-consuming nature of database building, the characteristics of a useful database are critical in the future applicability of MST methodologies.

There is little research that has concluded with any certainty on temporal variability effects on the ability of a host source database to classify nonpoint sources of pollution. There are research papers that have reported on lack of temporal stability due to among-species variation (Caugant et al., 1981; Gordon, 2001). One assumption made for the use of microbial source tracking is temporal stability or the ability to collect samples from the same source over time with little to no change in the outcome. Gordon (2001) reported on the minimal population differentiation in *E. coli* with only 5% of observed diversity derived from among-species variation, and this was considered inadequate. However, with a representative and adequately sized database, is 5% temporal variation significant?

Gordon (2001) continued to report on the most significant problem using *E. coli* in an MST database in which substantial changes in community occur from host to external environment. Caugant et al. (1981) reported that transient and resident strains of *E. coli* are present in the same host and they pose many questions as to the ramifications this may have to the usefulness of MST techniques. Jenkins et al. (2003) reported on the clonal diversity of *E. coli* among the same Black Angus steers sampled four times through one year. They evaluated ribotypes from two herds and discovered that a high clonal diversity index necessitated a large number of isolates (>900) for a database to be independent of temporal variations; however, they were uncertain whether their 20:1 resident to transient ratio could be overcome. Although Wiggins et al. (2003) studied fecal streptococci, they established that separate geographical databases, i.e., several watersheds, could be merged together to create a large, more representative database. Further, they concluded that the profiles were temporally stable for at least one year using antibiotic resistance analysis.

Phenotypic MST techniques such as antibiotic resistance analysis (ARA) have had moderate levels of success in small and relatively simple aquatic systems to differentiate human and nonhuman sources of pollution, or two-way level of classification (Carson et al., 2001; Guan et al., 2002; Graves et al., 2002; Hagedorn et al., 1999; Hartel et al., 2002; Harwood et al., 2000; Ritchey and Coyne, unpublished data; Ritchey and Coyne, 2009; Wiggins et al., 1999). Correct classification rates of ≥50% including five or more sources are considered useful by resource managers and rates of 60-70% are very useful (Harwood et al., 2000). Guan et al. (2002) conducted a study evaluating profiles using 14 antibiotics with a database consisting of 319 EC isolates collected from nine host sources. The database correctly classified 46% of the domestic, 95% of the wildlife, and 55% of the human sources. When the researchers pooled the nonhuman sources and compared the isolates to human sources, the RCC was 86% for human and 92% for nonhuman isolates. Harwood et al. (2000) constructed a database of 6144 fecal coliforms FC and 4619 FS isolates from profiles using 9 antibiotics. For the larger database, when the isolates from the animal sources were analyzed separately, the RCC was 54% for the FC human isolates and 61% for the FS isolates. Pooling the animal sources together increased the human RCCs to 69% for the FC isolates and to 76% for the FS isolates. Reducing the number of sources and pooling the animal sources together, greatly increased RCC values (Carson et al., 2001; Guan et al., 2002; Harwood et al., 2000).

Generally, the primary concern of water resource managers and public health officials is discriminating human and nonhuman sources of contamination followed by secondary information to determine the source of the animal contamination (Harwood et al., 2000). Ritchey and Coyne (unpublished data) reported rates of correct classification of 66% for human and 67% for nonhuman sources at the two-way level of classification. However, caution must be exercised when testing the portability or spatial variability of the database by applying it on a large geographic-scale and in more complex systems. Many researchers (Guan et al., 2002; Johnson et al., 2004; Lu et al., 2005; McLellan et al., 2003) have concluded that because of the importance for an MST database to represent an area, yet exhibit limited temporal variability despite the genetic diversity of bacteria, MST techniques may be more useful when applied to limited geographical areas such as specific watersheds. Work presented by Harwood et al. (2000) with a database of 6144 isolates produced acceptable RCCs. Those RCCs were lower than the RCCs obtained by Wiggins (1996) when using limited geographic areas, but similar to Wiggins et al. (1999) when the geographical area of their study was increased.

Regardless if one is evaluating an aquatic or terrestrial system, the same unresolved issues remain that affect the ability of MST techniques to ascertain the source of contamination from fecal sources to an adequate level of predictability. These issues predominantly lie in the intrinsic resistance and stability, which can vary considerably based on antibiotic profiles chosen, source and type of fecal bacteria, portability, temporal characteristics, and soil and/or water conditions. Based on past and current research, complex environmental systems still require considerable research to adequately evaluate the application of MST.

2. Terrestrial systems and a Kentucky study

Numerous studies show that pollutant concentrations from manure-amended agriculture lands often exceed water quality standards (Howell et al., 1995; Reddy et al., 1981). Bacteria survival also influences bacterial contamination from manure-amended agriculture lands through runoff and infiltration. Some important factors influencing bacteria survival in soil are soil type, moisture, temperature, sunlight, pH, antibiotics, competitive organisms, available nutrients, organic matter, and clay content (Ellis and McCalla, 1978). Few studies have evaluated sod management practices on fecal bacteria survival, but Entry et al. (2000) showed that vegetation type in riparian filter strips had no effect on fecal coliform survival in soils.

Various studies have investigated the correlation behind surface derived fecal sources and elevated fecal levels in groundwater, via infiltration, and surface water, via overland flow or erosion. Several studies have reported that moisture levels play a primary role in determining bacterial growth and duration, while temperature was a secondary factor (Berry and Miller, 2005; Collins, 2004; Sinton et al., 2007; Stoddard et al., 1998; Unc and Goss,

2003). Soil physicochemical characteristics including soil type, structure, depth to water tables, and bedrock, i.e. karstic, should be considered when investigating non point sources of contamination. Stoddard et al. (1998) studied leachate of manure treated and untreated shallow karst tilled and no-tilled soils from central Kentucky (the Bluegrass region). Neither timing of manure application nor tillage method significantly affected leachate concentration of fecal coliforms. Movement of fresh fecal bacteria, within 60 days of application, moved below the root zone upon sufficient rainfall events.

Based on past and current research, complex environmental systems still require considerable research to adequately evaluate the application of MST techniques. Mowing is a common sod management practice that could affect fecal bacteria survival and antibiotic resistance patterns in poultry manure-amended pasture lands because it subjects fecal bacteria to environmental stress. In the Kentucky study Ritchey and Coyne (unpublished data), fecal bacteria survival was examined in frequently mowed, poultry manure-amended sod on Maury silt loam soil for 70 days. Simultaneously evaluated was the efficacy of antibiotic resistance analysis across time for this known animal waste source.

3. Study conditions

The soil consisted of Maury silt loam (fine, mixed, mesic, Typic Paleudalf) in undisturbed sod-covered plots with mixed grass vegetation dominated by fescue. There were 14 experimental units measuring 2.4 m wide by 6 m long, spaced 2.5 m apart. The treatments were undisturbed (n=3), disturbed every week (n=4), and disturbed biweekly (n=4). Disturbance was simulated by using a push mower. Each treatment had one unmanured plot as a control. All treatments received poultry manure at a rate of 20 kg per plot (14 Mg ha^{-1}) in a completely randomized design. Sampling was conducted on day 0, 7, 14, 21, 28, 49, and 70. Because source was known, monitoring the environmental conditions to determine how these sources reacted with the respective condition changes on pasture areas was possible. In this way, behavior of these fecal coliforms with measurable environmental conditions could better be predicted.

Two soil cores, 5 cm deep, were extracted from random locations in each plot, before mowing, at each interval during the experiment. The soil cores were bagged separately and stored at 4 ^{0}C until analysis within 24 h of collection. Each core was separated into vegetative cover and soil for analysis. Fecal coliforms and fecal streptococci from vegetation and soil were enumerated separately. Composite samples of vegetative cover along with the surface residue were prepared from the two cores in each plot and 3 g of composite sample was added to 90 ml of 2 mM phosphate buffer (pH 7.2). The surface 5 cm of soil from each core in each plot was thoroughly mixed and 10 g of field moist soil was added to 90 ml of phosphate buffer. The buffer and samples were agitated on a reciprocating shaker at approximately 160 rpm for 30 min to extract the bacteria. Oven dry weights of vegetative and soil samples were determined and all fecal bacteria concentrations were expressed on a dry weight basis. Samples were analyzed for fecal coliforms and fecal streptococci within 24 h using a spiral plater (Autoplate ® 4000 spiral plater, Spiral Biotech, Inc., Bethesda, MD). Fecal coliforms were incubated on mFC agar (Difco™ mFC Agar, Detroit, MI) at 44.5 °C for 22 h, and fecal streptococci were incubated on KFS agar (Difco ™ KFS Agar, Detroit, MI) at 35 °C for 48 h.

After EC and FS colonies were counted, at least five isolates from each plot were selected at random. To verify the presence of EC and FS, the isolates were grown on EC-MUG broth and mEnterococcus agar, respectively. The positively identified isolates were spiral plated in duplicate onto Mueller Hinton agar. Immediately after plating the *E. coli* isolates, antibiotic diffusion discs (BBL™ Sensi-Disc, Sparks, MD) were placed onto the agar surface using an 8-place dispenser (BBL® Sensi-Disc 8-place dispenser, Cockeysville, MD). Seven antibiotics were evaluated at the following concentrations: ampicillin (10 µg), cephalothin (30 µg), erythromycin (15 µg), rifampin (5 µg), streptomycin (10 µg), tetracycline (30 µg), and trimethoprim (5 µg). The cultures were incubated at 35 °C for 24 h and zones of inhibition for each antibiotic disc were measured at the end of the incubation period. The same procedure was followed for the fecal streptococci isolates except the positively identified isolates were grown in Tryptic Soy Broth (Difco ™ Tryptic Soy Broth, Detroit, MI) at 35 °C for 48 h and then spiral plated onto Mueller Hinton agar that was incubated at 35 °C for 48 h.

Statistical analysis for fecal coliform and fecal streptococci concentrations in sod and soil was performed separately using the PROC MIXED procedure in SAS ® (SAS version 8.2, SAS Institute Inc., Cary, NC) for the analysis of variance and means separation among the treatments were determined by difference in least square means. A linear regression model using a first order decay model (log CFU g^{-1} = K Days + Constant; K= mortality rate) was used to estimate the fecal coliform and fecal streptococci mortality rates in sod and soil. Statistical analysis for *E. coli* and fecal streptococci antibiotic resistance patterns was performed using the PROC GLM procedure in SAS. Repeated measures were used for analysis of variance to detect differences in treatments, collection dates, and interaction of treatments by collection dates. The LSD procedure was used to detect significant pairwise differences. Principle components analysis was performed using the PROC PRINCOMP procedure in SAS. Discriminant analysis was used to evaluate correct rates of classification and was performed using the PROC DISCRIM procedure in SAS.

4. Results and discussion

4.1 Population and survival

The background fecal coliform and fecal streptococci concentrations in the plots were not significantly different from one another prior to manure application. The fecal coliform concentrations in background ranged from non detectable (<1) to 100 CFU g^{-1} in sod and non detectable to 50 CFU g^{-1} in soil. The fecal streptococci concentrations in the background ranged from 1,000 to 16,000 CFU g^{-1} in sod and 100 to 800 CFU g^{-1} in soil. The poultry manure contained approximately 7.9 x 10^8 CFU g^{-1} fecal coliforms, and 2.5 x 10^9 CFU g^{-1} fecal streptococci.

Manure application significantly increased the fecal coliform and fecal streptococci concentrations in sod and soil compared to the respective unmanured controls and remained so for the duration of the experiment. The fecal coliform and fecal streptococci concentrations exceeded 10^6 CFU g^{-1} sod and 10^5 CFU g^{-1} soil seven days after manure application (Tables 1 and 2). Fecal coliform and fecal streptococci concentrations in unmanured control plots also increased after manure application, but this was most likely due to cross contamination resulting from mowing and sample collection. Mowing frequency neither increased nor decreased the fecal coliform and fecal streptococci concentration in either sod or soil in the

Treatment	Day 7	Day 14	Day 21	Day 28	Day 49
Sod					
Never Mowed	6.9a* †	7.9a*	6.4a*	6.0a*	5.1a*
Never Mowed control	4.1	4.0	4.1	4.0	BD
Mowed Biweekly	6.8a*	7.2ab*	6.3a*	6.4a*	4.6a*
Mowed Biweekly control	4.4	3.9	4.2	3.6	1.9
Mowed Weekly	6.6a*	6.9b*	5.7a*	6.1a*	4.5a*
Mowed Weekly control	5.1	4.9	4.4	4.1	3.2
Soil					
Never Mowed	5.5a*	4.1a*	4.4a*	4.0b*	2.6a*
Never Mowed control	2.9	2.4	ND	1.2	BD
Mowed Biweekly	5.1a*	5.1a*	5.1a*	3.8b*	2.6a*
Mowed Biweekly control	3.1	2.4	1.9	BD	BD
Mowed Weekly	5.1a*	4.5a*	4.3a*	4.3a*	3.0a
Mowed Weekly control	3.6	3.3	3.1	3.3	3.6

† Values at each interval and sample type sharing the same letter are not significantly different (p ≥ 0.05). None of the controls were significantly different from one another. * Significantly different (p ≤ 0.05) from unmanured controls. ND- Not determined. BD – Below detection levels.

Table 1. Average fecal coliform concentration (log CFU g^{-1}) from sod/soil in mowed and poultry manure-amended sod plots.

Treatment	Day 7	Day 14	Day 21	Day 28	Day 49	Day 70
Sod						
Never Mowed	6.5a*†	6.2a*	6.3a*	6.3a*	6.4a*	4.9a
Never Mowed control	4.8	4.7	4.3	5.1	3.8	4.6
Mowed Biweekly	6.3a*	6.1a*	6.2a*	5.9a*	3.9a*	5.4a
Mowed Biweekly control	4.0	4.8	4.3	4.3	5.1	BD
Mowed Weekly	6.6a*	6.3a*	6.3a*	6.6a*	5.9a*	4.9a
Mowed Weekly control	4.6	4.9	3.9	4.4	4.4	BD
Soil						
Never Mowed	5.0a*	5.0a*	5.0ab*	4.5a*	4.0a*	3.3a
Never Mowed control	4.1	3.8	3.3	3.1	3.1	3.2
Mowed Biweekly	5.1a*	5.3a*	5.1a*	4.5a*	3.7a	3.6a
Mowed Biweekly control	3.9	2.8	3.7	2.7	3.0	3.7
Mowed weekly	5.2a*	5.2a*	4.6b	4.5a*	4.0a*	3.3a
Mowed weekly control	4.0	4.0	3.9	3.6	3.1	3.5

† Values at each interval and sample type sharing the same letter are not significantly different (p ≥ 0.05). None of the controls were significantly different from one another. * Significantly different (p ≤ 0.05) from unmanured controls. ND- Not determined. BD - Below detection levels.

Table 2. Average fecal streptococci concentration (log CFU g^{-1}) from sod/soil in mowed and poultry manure-amended sod plots.

manure-amended plots. These results were consistent with previous rain simulation studies on bacterial survival and infiltration in frequently mowed sod plots (Gandhapudi, 2004) in which mowing did not significantly affect the fecal bacteria concentrations recovered in lysimeters pans.

Because mowing had no effect on bacteria survival, different treatments were used in the study as replicates to study fecal coliform and fecal streptococci survival in sod and soil. The fecal coliform concentration in sod increased from 7 to 14 days after manure application, suggesting net growth, and thereafter decreased slowly for the rest of the study period. In contrast, the fecal coliform concentrations in soil slowly but continuously declined after manure application, without any evidence of net growth during the first 14 days. The fecal coliforms in sod and soil had only an approximate 25-fold decrease in 49 days. However, fecal coliform concentration in sod and soil declined below the detection limits (1000 CFU g^{-1} in sod and 100 CFU g^{-1} in soil) 70 days after manure application. The difference in detection limits was due to the difference in initial dilution.

The fecal streptococci concentration in sod and soil declined very slowly after manure application for the duration of experiment (70 days). There was only an approximate 15-fold decrease in fecal streptococci concentration observed in 70 days and the fecal streptococci concentration exceeded 4 x 10^4 CFU g^{-1} in sod and 2.0 x 10^3 CFU g^{-1} in soil even 70 days after manure application. However, fecal streptococci concentrations at 70 days were not different from unmanured control plots.

4.1.1 Mortality rates

A first order die-off model was used to describe fecal coliform and fecal streptococci mortality in this study because the first order die-off model has been widely and successfully used to describe fecal bacteria mortality in bacteria survival studies (Edwards and Daniel, 1992; Reddy et al., 1981; Stoddard et al., 1998). A 35-day model (between Day 14 and Day 49), excluding the periods with net growth, was used to describe the fecal coliform mortality in sod and a 49-day model (between Day 7 and Day 49) was used to describe the fecal coliform mortality in soil. The linear regression model (log CFU g^{-1} = k Days + constant) describing mortality rates indicated that there was no difference between mortality rates in sod and soil, and that the average fecal coliform mortality rate (k) was 0.06 log cells day^{-1} (R^2= 0.57 in sod; R^2 = 0.53 in soil). Redistribution of fecal bacteria in manure during mowing can presumably have facilitated growth, but attempts were not made to calculate growth rates for individual treatments. Lack of significant differences in net mortality rates was likely due to confounding effects of growth and mortality.

A 70-day linear regression model (log CFU g^{-1} = k Days + constant) was used to describe fecal streptococci mortality in sod and soil. The average fecal streptococci mortality rates in this model were 0.02 log cells day^{-1} (R^2= 0.53) in sod and 0.03 log cells day^{-1} (R^2 = 0.69) in soil. We assume that very low fecal streptococci mortality rates in sod and soil might have been influenced by the background fecal streptococci populations. The fecal streptococci mortality rate in the control plots did not correlate with the fecal streptococci mortality rates in the manure-amended population. In unmanured controls, the fecal streptococci concentrations did not change significantly throughout the study.

Studies that used poultry litter as a soil amendment have reported mortality rates ranging from 0.06–0.29 day^{-1} for fecal coliforms and 0.06-0.357 day^{-1} for fecal streptococci (Crane et al., 1980; Zhai et al., 1995). Our mortality rates were comparable to the mortality rates reported elsewhere, although the simple first order die-off model used in this study to describe the mortality of fecal coliform and fecal streptococci in sod and soil showed a poor R^2, indicating that the model was not a good fit for the data.

Moisture, temperature, and nutrient availability are important factors that influence fecal coliform and fecal streptococci mortality in soil. Entry et al. (2000), for example, reported that decreasing soil moisture and increasing soil temperature substantially increased the mortality of total coliforms and fecal coliforms in soil. Our results suggest that fecal coliform and fecal streptococci mortality rates were also influenced by soil moisture and temperature. During the study period almost every sampling period was preceded by a rain event that substantially increased the gravimetric moisture content in the soil to 29-40% (Fig. 1). Weekly rainfall exceeded 5-year averages in 6 of 10 sample periods (Fig. 2). The average 70-day temperature during the study was 17–27 °C in sod and 22–25 °C in soil.

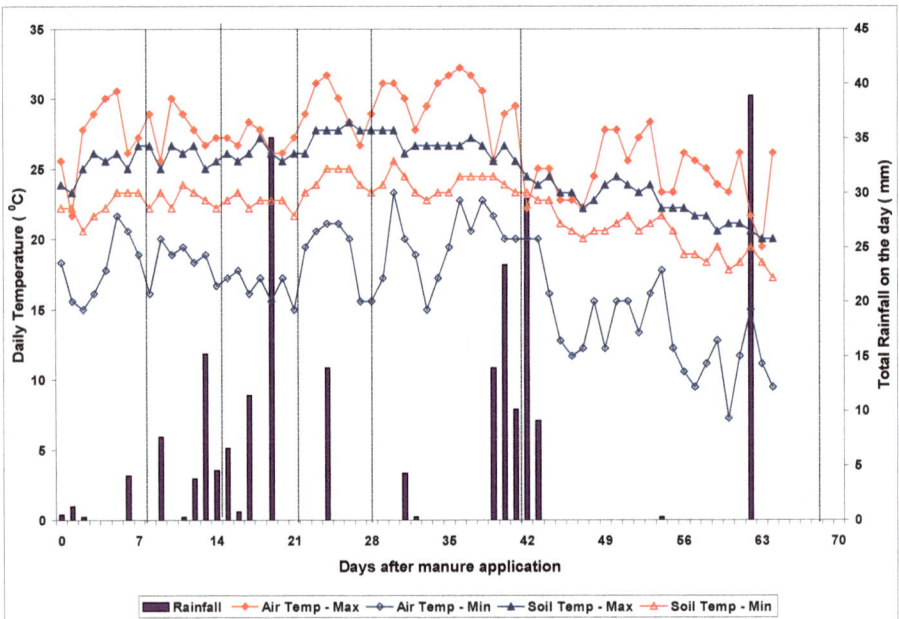

Fig. 1. Daily maximum and minimum air and soil temperatures, and total precipitation during the study period (July 2003 – October 2003) (weather data from Maine Chance Research Farm, Lexington KY). Dotted lines in the graph indicate the sampling periods during the study.

4.2 Antibiotic resistance patterns

Antibiotic resistance patterns of E. coli (EC) and fecal streptococci (FS) changed with time. The E. coli in sod and soil generally lost resistance followed by a return to initial patterns of resistance; whereas, the fecal streptococci in sod and soil generally had periods of increased resistance followed by a return to initial patterns. A summary of the significant differences of means by antibiotic and date from sod and soil for EC are shown in Table 3. A summary of the significant differences of means by antibiotic and date from sod and soil for FS are shown in Table 4.

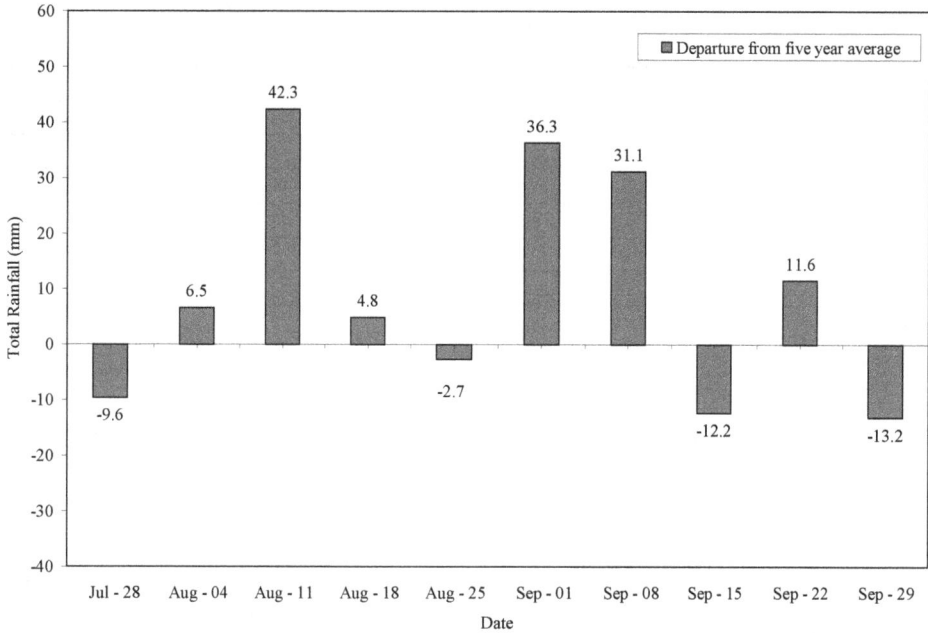

Fig. 2. Weekly rainfall departure during the study period (July – September 2003) from the past five year average (1998-2002). (Data obtained from Spindletop Research Farm Weather Station, Lexington KY).

Escherichia coli (EC) Isolates – Sod. There were five sampling dates for the sod EC isolates. The samples were collected at days 0, 7, 14, 28, and 49 after poultry application. The choice of antibiotic(s) for the study played a large role in the detection of bacterial changes with time. This was evident based on different resistance patterns among the seven antibiotics, thus providing more unique 'signatures' for each isolate. Statistical analysis of the sod data indicated that there was no significant treatment or sampling date main effect or interaction for ampicillin and cephalothin. The remaining antibiotics (i.e., erythromycin, rifampin, streptomycin, tetracycline, and trimethoprim) all produced significantly different antibiotic resistance patterns (ARPs) with sampling date. There were no significantly different date by treatment interactions or treatment main effects.

As the area surrounding the antibiotic or zone of inhibition increases, the resistance of the bacteria to the antibiotic decreases, and vice versa. The resistance of EC to erythromycin, rifampin, streptomycin, tetracycline, and trimethoprim significantly decreased with time. Generally, the bacteria showed initial changes in resistance at day 14 for all of the antibiotics that had significant date effects.

Antibiotic	Day 0	Day 7	Day 14	Day 21	Day 28	Day 49
			Sod			
Ampicillin	17a[†]	16a	17a	ns[‡]	18a	18a
Cephalothin	18a	15a	17a	ns	17a	18a
Erythromycin	9a	8a	13b	ns	16c	17c
Rifampin	9a	8a	10a	ns	13b	13b
Streptomycin	14a	15a	17b	ns	19c	18bc
Tetracycline	21a	20a	23b	ns	24b	24b
Trimethoprim	18a	23b	26b	ns	29c	28c
			Soil			
Ampicillin	18a	19a	ns	18a	19a	17a
Cephalothin	17a	16a	ns	17a	19a	17a
Erythromycin	11a	8a	ns	10a	18b	17b
Rifampin	9a	8a	ns	9a	13b	12c
Streptomycin	16a	17a	ns	17a	20b	18c
Tetracycline	20a	22ac	ns	19a	25b	24bc
Trimethoprim	23a	25ab	ns	26b	28c	28c

[†] Values at each interval and sample type sharing the same letter are not significantly different (p ≥ 0.05). [‡] ns = not sampled

Table 3. Date and mean values of antibiotic inhibition zones (mm) for *E. coli* isolates from sod and soil.

E. coli (EC) Isolates – Soil. There were five sampling dates for the soil EC isolates. The samples were collected at days 0, 7, 21, 28, and 49 after poultry application. Similar to the sod data, there was no significant treatment or date main effect or interactions with ampicillin and cephalothin. The sampling dates were significantly different from each other using erythromycin, rifampin, streptomycin, tetracycline, and trimethoprim. The EC from the soil also had decreased resistance to all of the antibiotics with time. However, the initial changes in resistance occurred at day 21 which was approximately one week later than the sod. This would suggest that migration of fecal bacteria from the sod to the soil may have occurred with time.

The treatment by sampling date interactions were significantly different for erythromycin and tetracycline. The resistance of EC decreased with time in the 'Mowed Every Week' and 'Mowed Biweekly' treatments for erythromycin, including the control plots. In the mowed treatments, the significant decrease in antibiotic resistance occurred between day 0 and day 21. However, the 'Never Mowed' treatments receiving poultry manure had increased resistance of bacteria at day 21 followed by a decrease to initial levels of resistance. The resistance of EC to trimethoprim decreased by day 28 and remained at that suppressed level until the last sampling date on day 49 for both the 'Never Mowed' and 'Mowed Every Week' treatments. Similar to the 'Never Mowed' treatment for erythromycin, the 'Mowed Biweekly' treatment for trimethoprim resulted in an increased level of resistance by day 28 and returned to initial levels for the remaining sampling dates. There were no significant changes with time in the control treatment.

Antibiotic	Day 0	Day 7	Day 14	Day21	Day 28	Day 49	Day 70
			Sod				
Ampicillin	22a†	23a	22a	ns‡	24a	21a	23a
Cephalothin	15b	10a	9a	ns	17b	14b	18b
Erythromycin	17a	11b	9b	ns	19a	20a	20a
Rifampin	16a	14ab	10b	ns	17a	18a	16a
Streptomycin	6a	7a	6a	ns	9b	10b	7a
Tetracycline	21b	11a	11a	ns	16ab	21b	23b
Trimethoprim	26a	25a	23a	ns	27a	21a	25a
			Soil				
Ampicillin	23ab	25a	24a	22ab	23ab	20b	16c
Cephalothin	16ab	9c	10c	16ab	19a	13bc	12bc
Erythromycin	18a	10b	12b	18a	17a	16a	16a
Rifampin	21a	12cd	10d	18ab	15bcd	14bcd	16abc
Streptomycin	8abc	6c	6c	9ab	10a	7bc	7bc
Tetracycline	21a	9c	13bc	17ab	16ab	20a	19a
Trimethoprim	25ab	29a	22b	24ab	20bc	23b	16c

† Values at each interval and sample type sharing the same letter are not significantly different (p ≥ 0.05). ‡ ns = not sampled

Table 4. Date and mean values of antibiotic inhibition zones (mm) for fecal streptococci isolates from sod and soil.

Fecal Streptococci (FS) Isolates – Sod. There were six collection dates for the sod FS isolates. The samples were collected at days 0, 7, 14, 28, 49, and 70 after poultry application. Trimethoprim produced no statistically significant main effects or interactions. Cephalothin, erythromycin, rifampin, streptomycin, and tetracycline produced significant date main effects. There were no significant treatment main effects for any antibiotic used in this study. The statistical analysis indicated that ampicillin and streptomycin produced significant treatment by date interactions. All of the antibiotics that had significant date effects except for streptomycin went through a phase of increased resistance at approximately day 7 with a subsequent phase at day 28 that was generally not significantly different from day 0. Streptomycin showed an opposite trend, whereby the bacterial response was a slight decrease in resistance at day 28 followed by an increase back to initial patterns of resistance at day 70. This may be an artifact of significant treatment by date interactions for streptomycin.

The most significant differences for treatment by date interactions of ampicillin occurred in the 'Mowed Biweekly' treatment when compared to the other treatments. There was a two phase cycle that was marked by increased resistance of FS to ampicillin followed by a return to initial (day 0) patterns of resistance patterns. There were two of these cycles that were documented over the 70-day sampling period. The first cycle began at day 7 and ended at day 28. The second cycle began at day 49 and ended at day 70. The 'Mowed Weekly' treatment for treatment by date interactions of streptomycin contained ARPs that indicated decreased periods of resistance occurring at day 49 and returning to day 0 patterns at day

70. The treatment by date interactions for the control treatments of ampicillin and streptomycin were also statistically significant. There were decreases in resistance to both antibiotics at day 28.

Fecal Streptococcus (FS) Isolates – Soil. There were seven collection dates for the soil FS isolates. The samples were collected at days 0, 7, 14, 21, 28, 49, and 70 days after poultry application. All seven of the antibiotics used in this study produced significant date main effects, but there were no significant treatment effects or treatment by date interactions. The results for FS in soil were the most ambiguous for this study. The results for FS in sod and EC in sod and soil had definitive resistance patterns that changed similarly with time across antibiotics within each organism and medium. However, upon evaluation of FS in soil, the data suggested an increased resistance at day 7 through day 14. This was more pronounced with cephalothin, erythromycin, rifampin, streptomycin, and tetracycline. Ampicillin and trimethoprim produced ARPs that showed progressively increasing resistance of FS throughout the sampling dates. These results, as those for EC, may be explained by a gradual migration of the organisms from sod to soil.

4.2.1 Rates of correct classification based on antibiotic resistance

The rate of correct classification or RCC for sod and soil by date was analyzed for EC and FS. The six total distinct dates used for EC were divided into two date groups, early and late, and the initial background (day 0) was excluded. The early date included 7, 14, and 21 days after poultry application. The late date included 28 and 49 days after application. The seven total distinct dates for FS were also divided into two groups, early and late, with exclusion of the initial background. The early date for FS included 7, 14, and 21 days after poultry application. The late date included 28, 49, and 70 days after application.

The RCC for EC using resubstitution analysis showed that the database correctly classified 92% of the sod isolates and 70% of the soil isolates for the early collection dates. The database correctly classified 70% of the sod isolates and 85% of the soil isolates for the late collection dates. These results coincided with the analysis of the significant differences of means by antibiotic and date from sod and soil as discussed previously. That is, the data support the idea that migration of fecal bacteria from the sod to the soil may occur with time. The correct classification of bacteria is highest for the early dates of sod while the majority of the bacteria resides in the surface or sod portion of the profile. Over time, the bacteria migrate to the lower area or the soil portion of the profile. For these dates, the RCC becomes lower for sod and higher for soil.

The RCC for FS using resubstitution analysis showed that the database correctly classified 85% of the sod isolates and 59% of the soil isolates for the early collection dates. The database correctly classified 69% of the sod isolates and 58% of the soil isolates for the late collection dates. The results for FS are more ambiguous than those reported for EC. While the RCC for sod also decrease over time, the RCC for soil remain relatively unchanged. It is worth noting that host source origin is typically classified. In this case, the medium, i.e., sod and soil, is effectively being classified with moderate success. Rates of correct classification of 60% or higher are considered useful by resource managers (Harwood et al., 2000), which makes the rates reported here of significant value.

Principle Component Analysis (PCA) was a useful tool when applied to the EC database. The variables used to compute the PCA were the seven antibiotics used for the profiles. The cumulative percent of variability accounted for by the first two axes was 72% which described most of the variability among the seven antibiotics. Axis one, which accounted for 55% of the variability, appeared to be associated with the antibiotics erythromycin, rifampin, and streptomycin. The second axis appeared to have large loadings for ampicillin and cephalothin. The graph of the PCA output for EC is shown in Figure 3 where period 1 = 0 days (background), period 2 = 7, 14, and 21 days, and period 3 = 28 and 49 days after poultry litter application. The dates were combined into early (background, period 1 = 0 days), intermediate (one to three weeks after application, period 2 = 7, 14, and 21 days), and late (anything after three weeks, period 3 = 28 and 49 days). Graphing the two axes based on period reveals grouping in the data. Period 1 data are not structured and agrees with previous findings for these are background data collected prior to poultry application. The data for period 2 resolve as two groups suggesting that a transitional period occurs between one and three weeks after poultry application as bacterial populations migrate from sod to soil. The data for period 3 are grouped together with no further changes up to 7 weeks after poultry application. The groups change relative to axis 1 which suggests that date primarily affects erythromycin, rifampin, and streptomycin antibiotic resistance patterns.

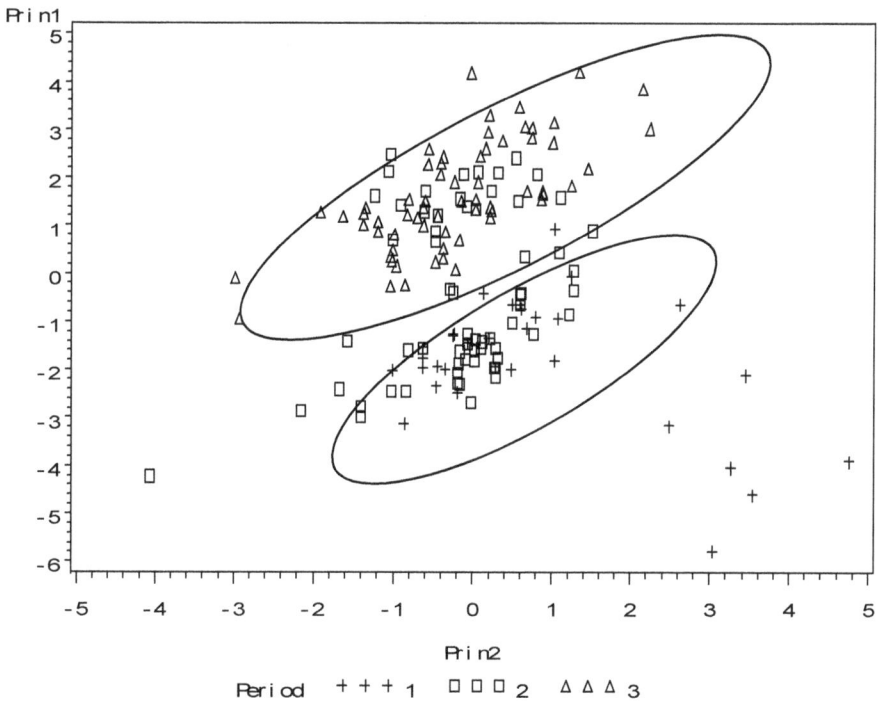

Fig. 3. Principle components analysis for *Escherichia coli* by date. Sod and soil isolates were combined in this analysis.

The graph of the PCA output for FS is shown in Figure 4. The PCA for the FS dataset showed that the cumulative percent of variability accounted for by the first two axes is 64%, which described most of the variability among the seven antibiotics. Axis one, which accounted for 43% of the variability, appeared to be associated with the antibiotics cephalothin, erythromycin, and rifampin. Axis two had large loadings for ampicillin and trimethoprim. The dates are the same as those described for EC with an addition of 70 day data added to period 3. There appeared to be no structure to the data presented in the plot, and no distinct grouping patterns.

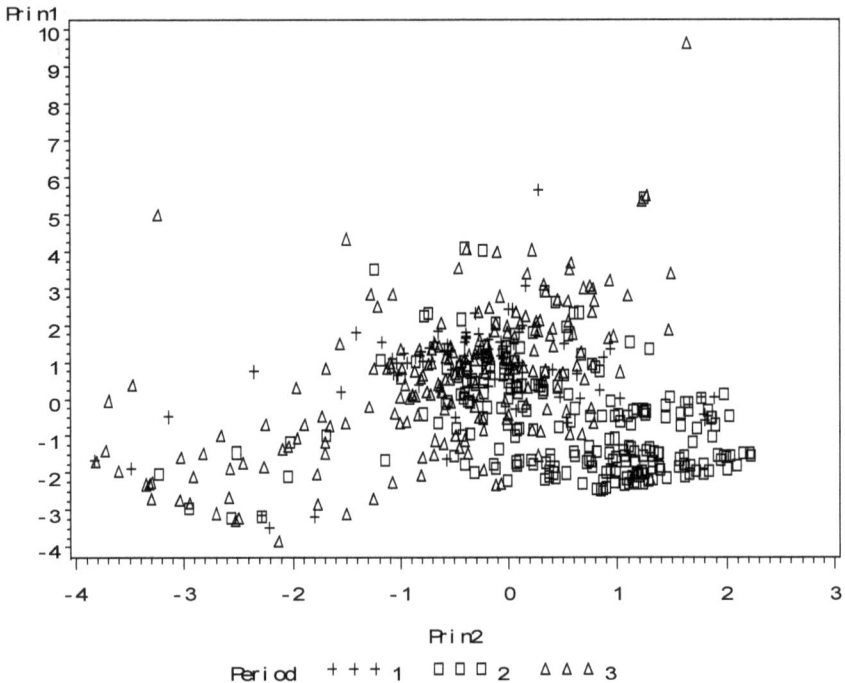

Fig. 4. Principle components analysis for fecal streptococci by date. Sod and soil isolates were combined in this analysis.

5. Conclusions

This study showed that disturbance (e.g. mowing) had little or no effect on EC and FS mortality in sod or soil in our study environment. It was suspected that the selection of mowing height, preservation of residue, and consistently wet weather combined to minimize treatment effects. The relatively prolonged survival of the fecal bacteria promoted the potential for runoff during the study, as well as potential for phenotypic variability as revealed by the MST profiles. The fecal bacteria appeared to persist in the environment for extended periods. Mowing frequency did not appear to affect the resistance profiles of *E. coli* and fecal streptococci for seven antibiotics. However, characterization of the same fecal bacterial population by means of MST was not consistent for that same time period; thereby suggesting that MST by this method was a time-dependent technique. Sampling time after our initial poultry manure application did appear to significantly affect the profiles recovered. Ampicillin and cephalothin were considered good indicators of antibiotic resistance over time for *E. coli* in sod or soil as there were no significant differences between sampling dates.

The selection of antibiotic to identify changes in microbial populations over time appears to play an important role in the effective use of MST. Based on the results from this study (Ritchey and Coyne, unpublished), ampicillin and cephalothin may be good choices to determine sources of EC in soil or sod and trimethoprim may provide useful information when studying FS in sod because there were no significant differences with time which indicates temporal stability when using these antibiotics.

6. Acknowledgement

Funding for this project was provided, in part, by a grant from the General Assembly of the Commonwealth of Kentucky – Senate Bill 271.

7. References

Berry, E.D. & Miller, D.N. (2005) Cattle feedlot soil moisture and manure content: II. Impact on *Escherichia coli* O157. *J. Environ. Qual.*, Vol. 34, No. 2, (March), pp. 656-663, ISSN 0047-2425

Carson, C.A., Shear, B.L., Ellersieck, M.R. & Asfaw, A. (2001) Identification of fecal *Escherichia coli* from humans and animal by ribotyping. *Appl. Environ. Microbiol.*, Vol. 67, No. 4, (April), pp. 1503-1507, ISSN 0099-2240

Caugant, D.A., Levin, B.R. & Selander, R.K. (1981). Genetic diversity and temporal variation in the *E. coli* population of a human host. *Genetics*, Vol. 98, No. 3, (July), pp. 467-490, ISSN 0016-6731

Collins, R. (2004) Fecal contamination of pastoral wetlands. *J. Environ. Qual.*, Vol. 33, No. 5, (September), pp. 1912-1918, ISSN 0047-2425

Crane, S.R., Westerman, P.W. & Overcash, M.R. (1980) Die-off of fecal indicator organisms following land applications of poultry manure. *J. Environ. Qual.*, Vol. 9, No. 1, (January-March), pp. 531-537, ISSN 0047-2425

Dombek, P.E., Johnson, L.K., Zimmerley, S.T. & Sadowsky, M.J. (2000) Use of repetitive DNA sequences and the PCR to differentiate *Escherichia coli* isolates from human and animal sources. *Appl. Environ. Microbiol.*, Vol. 66, No. 6, (June), pp. 2572-2577, ISSN 0099-2240

Edwards, D. R. & Daniel, T.C. (1992) Environmental impacts of on-farm poultry waste disposal – a review. *Bioresource Technology*, Vol. 41, No. 1, pp. 9-33, ISSN 0960-8524

Ellis, J.R. & McCalla, T.M. (1978) Fate of pathogens in soils receiving animal wastes – A review. *Trans. ASAE*, Vol. 21, No. 2, pp. 309-313, ISSN 0309-0313

Entry, J.A., Hubbard, R.K., Thies, J. E. & Furhmann, J.J. (2000). The influence of vegetation in riparian filterstrips on coliform bacteria: II. Survival in soils. *J. Environ. Qual.*, Vol. 29, No. 4, (July-August), pp. 1206-1214, ISSN 0047-2425

Gandhapudi, S.K. (2004) Managing fecal bacteria and nutrient contamination in poultry manure-amended sod by mowing and alum addition. M.S. Thesis, University of Kentucky, Lexington, KY.

Gordon, D.M. (2001). Geographical structure and host specificity in bacteria and the implications for tracing the source of coliform contamination. *Microbiol.*, Vol. 147, No. 5, (May), pp. 1079-1085, ISSN 1350-0872

Graves, A.K., Hagedorn, C., Teetor, A., Mahal, M., Booth, A.M. & Reneau, R.B. (2002) Antibiotic resistance profiles to determine sources of fecal contamination in a rural Virginia watershed. *J. Environ. Qual.*, Vol. 31, No. 4, (July), pp. 1300-1308, ISSN 0047-2425

Guan, S., Xu, R., Chen, S., Odumeru, J., & Gyles, C.. (2002). Development of a procedure for discriminating among *Escherichia coli* isolates from animal and human sources. *Appl. Environ. Technology*, Vol. 68, pp. 2690-2698, ISSN 1994-7887

Hagedorn, C., Robinson, S.L., Filtz, J.R., Grubbs, S.M., Angier, T.A. & Reneau, R.B. (1999). Determining sources of fecal pollution in a rural Virginia watershed with antibiotic resistance patterns in fecal streptococci. *Appl. Environ. Microbiol.*, Vol. 65, No. 12, (December), pp. 5522-5531, ISSN 0099-2240

Hartel, P.G, Summer, J.D., Hill, J.L., Collins, J.V., Entry, J.A. & Segars, W.I. (2002) Geographic variability of *Escherichia coli* ribotypes from animals in Idaho and Georgia. *J. Environ. Qual.*, Vol. 31, No. 4, (July), pp. 1273-1278, ISSN 0047-2425

Harwood, V.J., Whitlock, J. & Withington, V. (2000). Classification of antibiotic resistance patterns of indicator bacteria by discriminant analysis: Use in predicting the source of fecal contamination in subtropical waters. *Appl. Environ. Microbiol.*, Vol. 66, No. 9, (September), pp. 3698-3704, ISSN 0099-2240

Howell, J.M., Coyne, M.S. & Cornelius, P. (1995). Fecal bacteria in agricultural waters of the bluegrass region of Kentucky. *J. Environ. Qual.*, Vol. 24, No. 3, (May-June), pp. 411-419, ISSN 0047-2425

Jenkins, M.B., Hartel, P.G., Olexa, T.J. & Stuedemann, J.A. (2003). Putative temporal variability of *Escherichia coli* ribotypes from yearling steers. *J. Environ. Qual.*, Vol. 32, No. 1, (January), pp. 305-309, ISSN 0047-2425

Johnson, L.K., Brown, M.B., Carruthers, E.A., Ferguson, J.A., Dombek, P.E. & Sadowsky, M.J. (2004) Sample size, library composition, and genotype diversity among natural populations of *Escherichia coli* from different animals influence accuracy of determining sources of fecal pollution. *Appl. Environ. Microbiol.*, Vol. 70, No. 8, (August), pp. 4478-4485, ISSN 0099-2240

Kentucky Geological Survey. (2002). Kentucky landscape-astonishing beauty and hidden hazards. Available from
http://www.uky.edu/KGS/pubs/infocus.htm

Lu, Z., Lapen, D., Scott, A., Dang, A. & Topp, E. (2005) Identifying host sources of fecal pollution: Diversity of *Escherichia coli* in confined dairy and swine production systems. *Appl. Environ. Microbiol.*, Vol. 71, No. 10, (October), pp. 5992-5998, ISSN 0099-2240

McClellan, S.L., Daniels, A.D. & Salmore, A.K. (2003) Genetic characterization of *Escherichia coli* populations from host sources of fecal pollution by using DNA fingerprinting. *Appl. Environ. Microbiol.*, Vol. 69, No. 5, (May), pp. 2587-2594, ISSN 0099-2240

Reddy, K.R., Khaleel, R. & Overcash, M.R. (1981). Behavior and transport of microbial pathogens and indicator organisms in soils treated with organic wastes. *J. Environ. Qual.* Vol. 10, No. 3, (July-Sept), pp. 255-264, ISSN 0047-2425

Ritchey, S.A. and Coyne, M.S. (2009). Applying MAR analysis to identify human and non-human fecal sources in small Kentucky watersheds. *Water Air Soil Pollut*, Vol. 196, No. 1-4, (June), pp. 115-125, ISSN 0049-6979

SAS Institute. (1999). SAS/STAT user's guide version 8. Available from http://v8doc.sas.com/sashtml/

Sinton, L.W., Braithwaite, R.R., Hall, C.H. & Mackenzie, M.L. (2007) Survival of indicator and pathogenic bacteria in bovine feces on pasture. *Appl. Environ. Microbiol.*, Vol. 73, No. 24, (December), pp. 7917-7925, ISSN 0099-2240

Stoddard, C.S., Coyne, M.S. & Grove, J.H. (1998). Fecal bacteria survival and infiltration through a shallow agricultural soil: Timing and tillage effects. *J. Environ. Qual.*, Vol. 27, No. 6, (November-December), pp. 1516-1523, ISSN 0047-2425

Unc, A. & Goss, M.J. (2003) Movement of fecal bacteria through the vadose zone. *Water Air Soil Pollut.*, Vol. 149, No. 1-4, (October), pp. 327-337, ISSN 0049-6979

United States Environmental Protection Agency. (2000) National water quality inventory: 2000 report. Available from http://www.epa.gov/305b/2000report/

Wiggins, B.A., Cash, P.W., Creamer, W.S., Dart, S.E., Garcia, P.C., Gerecke, T.M., Han, J., Henry, B.L., Hoover, K.B., Johnson, E.L., Jones, K.C., McCarthy, J.G., McDonough, J.A., Mercer, S.A., Noto, M.J., Park, Phillips, M.S., Purner, S.M., Smith, B.M., Stevens, E.N. & Varner, A.K. (2003). Use of antibiotic resistance analysis for representativeness testing of multiwatershed libraries. *Appl. Environ. Microbiol.*, Vol. 69, No. 6, (June), pp. 3399-3405, ISSN 0099-2240

Wiggins, B.A., Andrews, R.W., Conway, R.A., Corr, C.L., Dobratz, E.J., Dougherty, D.P., Eppard, J.R., Knupp, S.R., Limjoco, M.C., Mettenburg, J.M., Rinehardt, J.M., Sonsino, J., Torrijos, R.L. & Zimmerman, M.E. (1999) Use of antibiotic resistance analysis to identify nonpoint sources of fecal pollution. *Appl. Environ. Microbiol.*, Vol. 65, No. 8, (August), pp. 3483-3486, ISSN 0099-2240

Wiggins, B.A. (1996) Discriminant analysis of antibiotic resistance patterns in fecal streptococci, a method to differentiate human and animal sources of fecal pollution in natural waters. *Appl. Environ. Microbiol.*, Vol. 62, No. 11, (November), pp. 3997-4002, ISSN 0099-2240

Zhai, Q., Coyne, M.S. & Barnhisel, R. I. (1995) Mortality rates of fecal bacteria in subsoil amended with poultry manure. *Bioresource Technology*, Vol. 54, No. 2, pp. 165-169, ISSN 0960-8524

5

Trends of Antibiotic Resistance (AR) in Mesophilic and Psychrotrophic Bacterial Populations During Cold Storage of Raw Milk, Produced by Organic and Conventional Farming Systems

Patricia Munsch-Alatossava[1], Vilma Ikonen[1],
Tapani Alatossava[1] and Jean-Pierre Gauchi[2]
[1]Department of Food and Environmental Sciences,
Division of Food Technology, University of Helsinki,
[2]Unité de Mathématiques et Informatique Appliquées (UR 341),
Institut National de la Recherche Agronomique, Centre de Jouy en Josas,
[1]Finland
[2]France

1. Introduction

Antibiotic resistant bacteria continually arise and their increasing prevalence constitutes one of the major public health threat. The problem, earlier mainly confined to hospitals, nowadays encircles the globe (Davies & Davies, 2010; Levy, 2002; Marshall et al., 2009). Perceived once as a consequence of use, overuse and misuse of antibiotics to prevent or treat diseases, as growth promotants for food animals, or as pesticides for agriculture, more explanations for high AR levels in bacteria were recently brought. The picture became darker when came evidences that environmental microbiota present in antibiotic free environments showed to possess an as enormous and diverse number of AR genes as present in pathogenic microbiota (Aminov, 2009). Further evidences point to micro-organisms associated with food, animals, and water as the main sources for resistance genes; commensals among them food commensals are also considered as a reservoir of AR (Knezevic & Petrovic, 2008; Straley et al., 2006), in fact according to Marshall et al. (2009) a rather underappreciated reservoir of AR. In developed countries, several parameters define a raw milk of "good quality" when it is absent of drug or antibiotics residues, when the legal limit of somatic cells per millilitre of milk is below $4x10^5$ /mL (excessive values may be indicating the presence of mastitis in the cow herd), when the bacteriological acceptance level is satisfied. In the later, the sanitation of raw milk is ensured by the determination of the standard plate count (Chambers, 2002) that aims to enumerate aerobic "total bacteria" present in milk; grade A or 1 (acceptable for industrial use) is attributed to milk that contains less than $1x10^5$ CFU/ml, determined on agar plates after 2 days incubation at 32°C, or 3 days at 30°C. After milking, numerous contamination sources raise the bacterial load along the cold chain of raw milk storage and transportation (Chambers, 2002; Cousin, 1982). The cold storage that aims to preserve food or milk from excessive bacterial development, however also selects bacterial types which have perfectly adapted to low temperatures : psychrotrophic bacteria, able to grow below 7°C, present in raw milk are well known for their spoilage features (production of various heat-stable exoenzymes) which affect raw or processed dairy products with significant economic impact. Mainly, out of some exceptions like the human pathogens (toxin producer of *B. cereus* species, or *Listeria* spp: Gray et al., 2006; Schoeni & Lee Wong, 2005), most psychrotrophic bacteria associated to raw milk of which many are Gram-negative, are generally considered as benign.

Foodstuffs are produced by either conventional (CP) or organic (OP) systems. Consumer demands for organic products generally perceived as more safe, is growing in Europe and the United States, offering increased business opportunities and wealth for rural regions (European Commission, 2008; Jacob et al., 2008). The organic food chain supply is guaranteed at the base first by producers which must adhere to strict rules: organic milk is defined by the European Commission as "milk that comes from cows, sheep and goats living in a welfare-oriented animal husbandry: outdoors in summer with access to pasture and indoors in winter when the climate is rough, with organic forage and enough space for regular exercise" (European Commission, 2008). Several principles are underlying organic production such as minimisation of the use of non-renewable resources and off-farms inputs, recycling of wastes and by-products of plant and animal origin as input in plant and livestock production, the feeding of livestock with organic feed (produced mainly at the farm), synthesized allopathic veterinary medicinal products, like antibiotics may be used with restriction on courses of treatment and withdrawal period (European Council Regulation, 2007); organic dairy cattle are treated for mastitis with the same antimicrobials as dairy cows from conventional systems. In Finland, at least 50% of the feed has to be produced by the farm; each cow can only be treated 3 times a year for independent diseases and the time for milk delivery acceptance to dairies is twice as long as for normal systems (Finnish Food Safety Authority, 2008); on a total of 2.2×10^9 L of milk delivered to dairies about 1.3% was produced by organic farming systems (Information Centre of the Ministry of Agriculture and Forestry, 2009). The use of ABs in Finland for cattle was surveyed by Thompson et al. (2008): for acute mastitis, parenteral treatments are based on benzyl penicillins (83%) and fluoroquinolones (11%); ampicillin combined with cloxacillin (36%), or cephalexin combined with streptomycin (26%) were intramammarily administered. Finland, together with Norway and Sweden, have lower ABs usage practices compared to seven other European countries (Grave et al., 2010). Considering the bacteriological quality of the milk, as well as the level of antimicrobial residues (Finnish association for milk hygiene, 2008), altogether the quality of Finnish raw milk is excellent.

While characterizing some raw milk gram-negative psychrotrophs, it was observed that besides having spoilage features (Munsch-Alatossava & Alatossava 2006), these bacteria also carried antibiotic multiresistant features: moreover, the study suggested that the AR load was higher for isolates that apparently spent a longer time in cold storage (Munsch-Alatossava & Alatossava 2007); another study, that considered bacterial raw milk psychrotrophs selected for their spoilage features, compared the AR levels of 79 bacterial isolates originating from CP (6) or OP (9) milk samples. With exception of gentamicin for which similar percentages of AR were recorded for CP and OP samples, we observed a lower prevalence of AR for OP samples; resistance levels to trimethoprim-sulfamethoxazole were 25 and 14% for CP and OP samples respectively, and resistance percentages were higher for ceftazidim and ciprofloxacin (a quinolone) for CP-originating isolates (Munsch-Alatossava, Xheng, Alatossava, unpublished data). To further answer to the question on whether AR levels may be different/lower for isolates retrieved from OP compared to CP milk samples, to follow the respective trends for mesophilic and psychrotrophic populations over time during cold storage (4 days at 4°C), the present study was undertaken: the AR to four ABs (gentamicin, ceftazidim, levofloxacin, and trimethoprim-sulfamethoxazole, representatives of 4 different classes) was evaluated for mesophilic and psychrotrophic bacteria for 12 raw milk samples (6 for each farming system); changes at the bacterial communities level during cold storage were investigated by DGGE.

2. Materials and methods

2.1 Cold storage of raw milk samples

Representative bovine raw milk samples of lorry tanks were collected into sterile bottles; samples were kept on ice until arrival at Helsinki University, at which time 100 ml were added to sterile 250 ml-bottles. Six bottles were placed on a multi-place magnetic stirrer (Variomag) and partially immersed in a refrigerated water bath (MGW Lauda MS/2) which allowed, with help of an immersion thermostat, a constant temperature to be maintained (modified from Munsch-Alatossava et al., 2010). The raw milk samples were continuously mixed at 220 rpm and kept at 4 ± 0.1 °C for 4 days.

2.2 Antibiotic resistance

The experimental procedures followed the EUCAST guidelines (2000). The microbiological analyses were performed immediately after milk samples arrived; all bacterial counts were determined from duplicate or triplicate agar cultures at day 0 (shortly after reception of the samples) and day 4 (after cold storage); 500 µl or raw milk were serially diluted in saline solution (0.85 % NaCl); 50µl of the diluted samples were spread on Mueller-Hinton (Lab M) agar plates. Four antimicrobial agents [gentamicin (Aminoglycosides), ceftazidim (β-lactams, Cephems), levofloxacin (Quinolones) and trimethoprim-sulfamethoxazole (at a ratio of 1/19, a Folate pathway inhibitor) (Sigma)] were added to agar, according to the EUCAST guidelines (EUCAST, 2000). The ABs solutions were freshly prepared by dissolving the powders in following solvents: water for G (gentamicin), 0.1M phosphate buffer (pH7) for C (ceftazidim), 0.1M NaOH for L (levofloxacin), 0.1M lactic acid for T (trimethoprim), and 95% ethanol for S (sulfamethoxazole) (EUCAST, 2000). With exception of S, all AB solutions were filter sterilized prior to the addition to adequately cooled agar. The AB concentrations were 16 mg/L for GI, 4 mg/L for GII, 32 mg/L for CI, 8 mg/L for CII, 8 mg/L for LI, 2 mg/L for LII, 8 mg/L trimethoprim with 152 mg/L sulfamethoxazole for TSI, and 4 mg/L trimethoprim with 76 mg/L sulfamethoxazole for TSII, which correspond to the MICs (GII, CII, LII and TSII) to 4-fold the MIC (GI, CI, LI), or to 2-fold the MIC (TSI) as indicated by EUCAST for pseudomonads. Agar plates were stored overnight at 4°C, and protected from light. Following the analyses, the plates were incubated for 2-3 days at 30°C, or for 10 days at 7°C to enumerate the "total" bacteria (mesophiles) and psychrotrophs, respectively.

2.3 Statistical analysis

2.3.1 Judicious remarks about ANOVA (ANalysis Of VAriance)

Usual analysis of variance is well known in the field of research and laboratories as an efficient statistical method enabling to analyse results following experimental designs, and to test for significant differences between means. Concerning milk and its microflora, also ANOVA was used (Freitas et al. 2009; Ma et al. 2003). Thanks to the Fisher-Snedecor and Student tests, ANOVA enables to detect factors, to highlight interactions of the considered factors, which both significantly impact on the response (continuous) of the studied phenomenon. However, ANOVA is not considered as robust as it is susceptible to variations of the assumptions on which this method is grounded; more precisely, the statistical tests' validity of ANOVA are "sensitive" to these variations. The validity is relying on three fundamental restrictive assumptions: A) Distribution of the residuals is normal; B) Variance of errors is constant; C) The data does not contain outliers. If one of these hypotheses is strongly violated, conclusions about significant level of the effects of the factors may be questionable or erroneous. In practice for a particular study, the hypothesis A is very difficult to be proved due to usual low amount of repetitions for a certain treatment (a combination of factors set at a certain level); in addition, if this assumption is not respected the impact on the Student test result is rather low, contrarily to the Fisher Snedecor test; however, this hypothesis has been so often checked by numerous experimental studies, that one may assume it is approximately often respected.

The hypothesis B is easily checked on the graphical analyses of "residuals"; if the hypothesis B is not respected, one common way to proceed even though not optimal consists in stabilizing variation by considering the logarithmic values of the results of the response. Also from the observation of the usual ANOVA graphics (given by standard statistics software) the hypothesis C can be checked. Mathematically it can be demonstrated that statistical tests are hampered by the presence of many outliers which may lead to erroneous conclusions. Moreover in the presence of orthogonal or almost orthogonal experimental designs, the outliers promote high levels (for example triple) of interactions of no meaning; typically one interaction AxBxC between three factors A, B, C may be declared significant, even though in the ANOVA model none of the three main effects of the three factors appears. How to overcome the harmful impact of the outliers on the significance of the ANOVA model? The elimination of extreme results due to outliers constitutes one solution, however in the presence of a limited amount of repetitions in practice this option is not applicable. Consequently it is difficult to validate the hypothesis C. To overcome this problem, no ideal method exists. Nevertheless, to compare several samples one alternative consists in the use of non parametric statistical tests like the Kruskal-Wallis test (Conover 1980) for example, which considers the ranks of the results of the response. For example, for the 6 following results of bacterial counts (expressed as CFU/ml) 0, 1.9×10^4, 1.5×10^5, 2.0×10^5, 2.4×10^5 and $1,5 \times 10^9$, the extreme values 0 and $1,5 \times 10^9$ may be badly estimated by the ANOVA model, and will generate excessive residuals. With a non parametric statistical approach, the values will be substituted for ranks, here 6, 5, 4, 3, 2, and 1.

2.3.2 RAPD definition

The data analysed in this study are bacterial counts enumerated on Petri dishes, characterized by a rather high variability, which impacted on hypothesis C, and which did not permit the straightforward use of a reliable ANOVA model. Consequently, bacterial counts were transformed into ratios, which were replaced then by ranks according to the prerequisite of the Kruskal-Wallis test, before performing the classical ANOVA. What is meant by ratio? Due to the natural microbiological variability, we considered the CFU (colony forming units) on a Petri dish (in the presence of one AB) not as an absolute value but as a relative value compared to a control plate, which implicated the introduction of a ratio. The ratio here referred to as RAPD was defined for a particular treatment X. RAPD corresponds to the ratio of the amount of bacterial colonies (as CFU/ml) enumerated under this treatment X divided by the number of bacteria enumerated on the corresponding control plates (in the absence of the AB). The treatment X was characterized itself by a combination of factors, like the sample type (milk from CP or OP systems), the population type whether psychrotrophs (P) or mesophiles (M), a sampling day D (D= 0 or 4, that will lead to RAP0 and RAP4 respectively), an AB type, and an AB concentration.

Thus RAPD constitues another way to quantify AR prevalence, while the classical quantification of AR prevalence is generally defined as the percentage of resistant bacteria considering the corresponding "total" bacteria enumerated.

2.3.3 Experimental design

The experimental design was based on the following four fixed factors: the antibiotic (AB) type (whether G, C, L or TS, as detailed above), the concentration of the AB (Dose) which corresponded to a higher level (I) or a lower level (II), the storage time of the milk (day) whether 0 (initial counts) or 4 (after 4 days cold storage), and finally the milk sample noted (ECH) which accounted for the six distinct lorry tanks samples (whether from CP or OP systems). The factor ECH was also introduced as a fixed factor in order to identify an eventual "milk collecting effect". Each treatment corresponded to a defined condition resultant from one modality of every factor (AB, Dose, ECH).

2.3.4 Refinement of ANOVA

Once the ANOVA model has been established, significant factors are identified. If one significant factor presents only 2 modalities, the interpretation is clear: a change of the modality impacts significantly on the level of the response. But if the significant factor presents more than two modalities, the interpretation is not straightforward. Further analyses of the microbiological data are requested, which are not often performed according to the microbiological literature. After the ANOVA table is established, for factors with more than two modalities, pairwise or multiple comparisons of the means of the response associated to the modalities of the factors are requested. On a statistical point of view, as this latter is the most rigorous approach, it was employed in this study. Among the available methods for multiple comparisons of means was chosen the REGW test (Einot & Gabriel, 1975; Ryan, 1959, 1960; Welsch, 1977) that is powerful and particularly adapted for our type of data. The method is available on the SAT/STAT version 8.1 software (SAS Institute, NC, USA).

2.3.5 Use of a non parametric statistical test

One major aim of this study was to compare the trend of RAPD between the two sampling days (Day 0 and Day 4), for a certain treatment. Considering the non normal distribution of the 12 values of RAP0 and RAP4, the mean comparison with a Student test was not possible. Therefore, the analyses were pursued with the use of the non parametric Wilcoxon test (as detailed in page 215 by Conover 1980), implemented in the NPAR1WAY procedure of the SAS/STAT statistical software. This test is also based on ranks: eight treatments (AB=G at dose I, AB=G at dose II.....AB=TS at dose II) were examined for each bacterial type; for both conventional and organic milk types, altogether 32 conditions were considered.

2.4 DGGE (Denaturing Gradient Gel Electrophoresis) analyses

Bacterial DNA was extracted with PathoProof™ mastitis PCR assay kit (Finnzymes, Finland). 16S rDNA sequences were amplified by nested-PCR. Firstly, a 700-bp fragment that comprises the V3 region of bacterial 16S rDNA was amplified, and served as template for the 2nd PCR reaction which yielded PCR products of about 200 bp, as described by Ogier et al. (2002). These primers flank the V3 region (that corresponds for *E.coli* to positions 436-499) which shows variability between different species. DGGE analyses were performed with the BioRad DCode ™ Universal Mutation Detection System (BioRad, USA). The samples were electrophoresed with a denaturing gradient of 35-70% urea and formamide at 70V for 21h. Gels were stained with SYBR Gold (Invitrogen, USA) and photographed on a UV transillumination table (UVItec Ltd, UK). The images were analysed with Gel Compar®II (version 5.1, Applied Maths, Belgium). The similarity between samples was calculated with Pearson's correlation coefficient and UPGMA (Unweighted pair-group method using arithmetic averages) was used as a clustering method. The maximum parsimony cluster analyses were performed with the boostrap value of 1000. The data is presented as a dendrogram of DGGE profiles from conventional (C1 to C6) and organic (O1 to O6) raw milk samples at days 0 and 4.

3. Results

3.1 Bacterial counts and percentage of psychrotrophs

Initial "total" bacterial counts, determined for the raw milk samples (C1 to C6, O1, O2, O3 and O6), were comprised between 3.4 and 4.12 log-units, indicating that the raw milks were of excellent quality (Fig. 1).

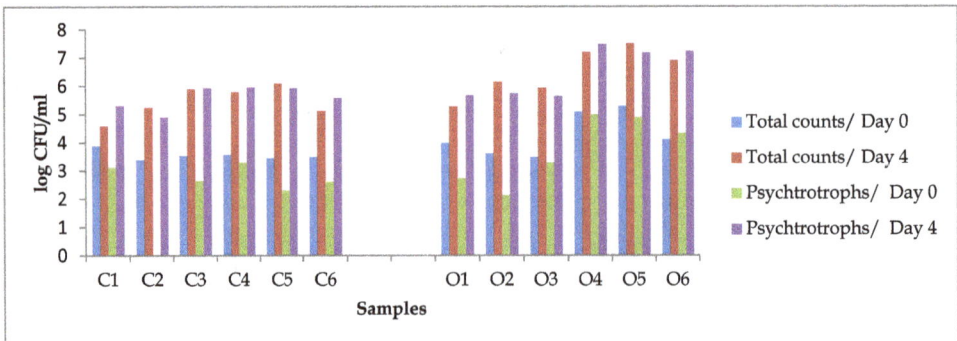

Fig. 1. Bacterial counts on Mueller Hinton agar plates expressed in log CFU/ml, determined for conventional (C1 to C6) and organic (O1 and O6) raw milk samples.

Trends of Antibiotic Resistance (AR) in Mesophilic and Psychrotrophic Bacterial Populations During
Cold Storage of Raw Milk, Produced by Organic and Conventional Farming Systems

129

For samples O4 and O5, the mesophilic bacterial counts were 5.1 and 5.3 log-units respectively, suggesting that these milks were longer cold stored prior to the analyses of these samples. At day 4, total counts exceeded 10^5 CFU/ml for all considered samples, to the exception of C1 for which the growth was only of 0.7 log-unit. With exceptions of C4, O3, O4, O5 and O6, psychrotrophic were lower than mesophilic counts for all other samples. The proportion of psychrotrophs (ratio of psychrotrophs/total bacterial counts) increased notably between the two sampling days /day 0 and day 4) for most samples: whereas, the initial proportion of psychrotrophs in samples C1, C2, C3, C5, C6, O1 and O2 was below 20%, considerable higher proportions were determined from C4 (50%), O3 (60%), O4 (80%), O5 (40%) and O6 (100%) at day 0. After 4 days storage at 4°C, psychrotrophic bacteria largely dominated in samples C1, C3, C4, C6, O1, 04, and 06 (100%), whereas the proportions ranged between 40 and 70% for C2, C5, O2, O3 and O5.

3.2 AR load evaluated by RAPD mean values

When combining all results from the different investigated ABs, following observations were made considering RAPD: for CP milk samples, the RAP0 mean values were similar for mesophilic (M) and psychrotrophic (P) populations, whereas for OP samples the RAP0 was slightly lower for mesophiles, contrarily to psychrotrophs for which it was highest (0.245) (Fig.2).

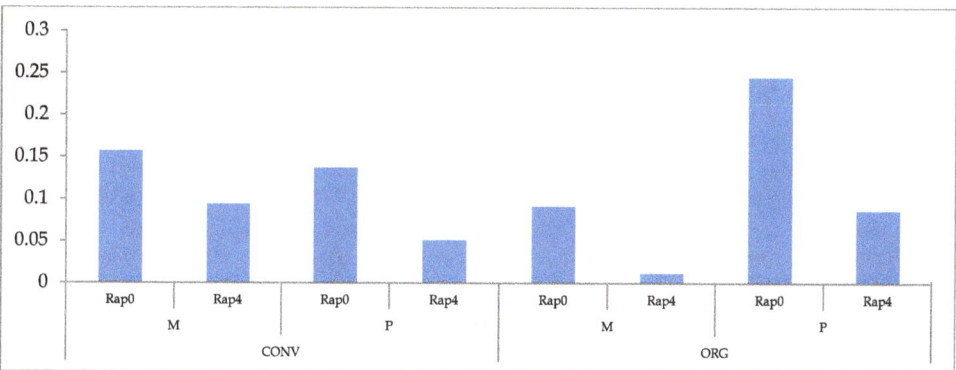

Fig. 2. Mean RAPD values from CP and OP raw milk samples at sampling days 0 or 4, determined for mesophiles (M) and psychrotrophs (P).

All RAP4 mean values were lower than the corresponding RAP0 values, irrespective of the origin of the samples or the bacterial population types. The major drop was observed for psychrotrophic populations retrieved from OP milk samples. For the mesophiles, the AR evaluated through RAPD clearly indicated a decrease for both types of samples, even though more important for bacteria retrieved from OP samples.

3.3 Comparison of RAPD mean values to evaluate the impact of cold storage

The trend of RAPDs were obtained by the results of the NPAR1WAY/REGW procedure (introduced in section 2.3.5). A typical example of the SAS-output where RAP4 was compared to RAP0 is detailed in Table 1.

| Wilcoxon Scores (Rank Sums) for Variable rep | | | | | |
| Classified by Variable day | | | | | |
Day	N	Sum of Scores	Expected Under H0	Std Dev Under H0	Mean Score
0	12	127.0	150.0	15.060747	10.583333
4	12	173.0	150.0	15.060747	14.416667
Average scores were used for ties.					

Wilcoxon Two-Sample Test	
Statistic	127.0000
Normal Approximation	
Z	-1.4939
One-Sided Pr < Z	**0.0676**
Two-Sided Pr > $|Z|$	0.1352
t Approximation	
One-Sided Pr < Z	**0.0744**
Two-Sided Pr > $|Z|$	0.1488
Z includes a continuity correction of 0.5.	

Table 1. Output obtained with the Wilcoxon test applied to mesophiles present in CP raw milk samples, for one AB (G) at concentration I. In this example, RAP0 = 10.58 and RAP4= 14.42, however the t approximation value of 0.1488 indicated that RAP0 and RAP4 were statistically equivalent.

The conclusions from each comparison are summarised in Table 2 a,b. The mean RAP4 values only exceeded the mean RAP0 values for TS (red colour), at both concentrations, for psychrotrophic (P) populations retrieved from CP samples (Table 2a); with the exception of mesophiles (M) enumerated on C-containing plates, for which the RAP4 were lower than the RAP0 values (green colour), in all other conditions (yellow colour), the relative AR levels were equivalent. On the side of the populations retrieved from OP raw milk samples, for half of the conditions, RAP4 values were lower (green colour) or equal (yellow colour) to RAP0; but RAP4 widely exceeded RAP0 for 8 conditions (red colour), mostly for psychrotrophs (Table 2b).

3.4 Mean RAP4 from OP compared to mean RAP4 from CP raw milk samples

The comparison of the mean RAP4 values indicated that for 10 cases out of 16, the AR levels were similar after 4 days storage (yellow colour), irrespective of the milk type; mesophilic populations retrieved on C-containing plates, as well as mesophiles and psychrotrophs enumerated on G-plates (lower concentration, II) from OP samples carried less AR features (green colour)(Table 3); but, psychrotrophs from OP samples, enumerated on L (II) and TS-plates (I), exhibited much superior levels of AR as compared to CP raw milk samples (red colour).

3.5 Ranking of the four considered ABs

For both CP or OP samples, the ranking of the ABs was obtained with REGW based analyses that followed ANOVA. An example is given in Table 4 (a,b).

a)

G	I	M	=
		P	=
	II	M	=
		P	=
C	I	M	<
		P	=
	II	M	<<
		P	=
L	I	M	=
		P	=
	II	M	=
		P	=
TS	I	M	=
		P	>
	II	M	=
		P	>

b)

G	I	M	>
		P	>>
	II	M	=
		P	=
C	I	M	<<
		P	=
	II	M	<<
		P	=
L	I	M	>>
		P	>
	II	M	=
		P	>>
TS	I	M	>>
		P	>>
	II	M	=
		P	>>

Table 2. Mean RAP4 values compared to the mean RAP0 values from CP (a) and OP (b) raw milk samples, for the four ABs tested at concentrations I and II (I>II) for mesophiles (M) or psychrotrophs (P). The symbols =, <, and > are meaning RAP4 equalled, or was significantly below or superior to RAP0, respectively.

G	I	M	=
		P	=
	II	M	<<
		P	<<
C	I	M	<<
		P	=
	II	M	<<
		P	=
L	I	M	=
		P	=
	II	M	=
		P	>>
TS	I	M	=
		P	>>
	II	M	=
		P	=

Table 3. Mean RAP4 values from OP compared to mean RAP4 values from CP raw milk samples, determined for each AB at concentrations I and II (I>II), for mesophiles (M) or psychrotrophs (P). The symbols =, <<, and >> are meaning that RAP4 from OP samples were significantly and respectively equal, much inferior or superior to RAP4 determined for the CP raw milk samples.

Source	DF	Sum of Squares	Mean Square	F Value	Pr > F
Model	32	61772.45833	1930.38932	10.78	<.0001
Error	63	11279.54167	179.04034		
Corrected Total	95	73052.00000			

R-Square	Coeff Var	Root MSE	RAP4 Mean
0.845596	27.58886	13.38060	48.50000

Source	DF	Type I SS	Mean Square	F Value	Pr > F
AB	3	30643.27083	10214.42361	57.05	<.0001
dose	1	7315.04167	7315.04167	40.86	<.0001
ech	5	8529.00000	1705.80000	9.53	<.0001
AB*dose	3	3033.89583	1011.29861	5.65	0.0017
AB*ech	15	9065.47917	604.36528	3.38	0.0004
dose*ech	5	3185.77083	637.15417	3.56	0.0067

a)

Alpha	0.05		
Error Degrees of Freedom	63		
Error Mean Square	179.0403		
Number of Means	2	3	4
Critical Range	8.8494249	9.2716373	10.19334

Means with the same letter are not significantly different.			
	Mean	N	AB
A	65.125	24	4
A	62.354	24	2
B	46.375	24	1
C	20.146	24	3

b)

a) Dependent Variable: RAP4 ; Values of RAP4 were replaced by ranks
b) Ryan-Einot-Gabriel-Welsch Multiple Range Test for RAP4
NOTE: This test controls the Type I experiment wise error rate.

Table 4. a) Analysis of variance of RAP4 ranks from mesophiles present in CP samples. The R-square value was equal to 0.85 and the F p-value was < 0.0001, which was indicative of a good ANOVA model. All three effects (AB, dose, sample /ech) and their interactions were influential with a predominant and significant effect of the AB. b) Output from the REGW test. For the same samples, AB4 (TS) and AB2(C) had equivalent effects, higher to AB1(G) and to AB3 (L); AB1 and AB3 were not equivalent.

No important differences distinguished CP and OP raw milk samples when considering the ranking of the four ABs according to their respective prevalence for mesophiles (M) or psychrotrophs (P) (Fig. 3a, b).

The same ranking, with a preponderant C-resistance was characteristic of day 0 and was observed for all populations types retrieved whether from CP or OP raw milk samples; a slightly higher AR for TS was observed for mesophiles from CP samples, whereas for G and L a similar ranking was noticeable for both sample types. Higher AR was recorded for psychrotrophs from OP samples compared to CP samples for C, TS and L, with the exception of G for which similar levels were observed (Fig. 3a, b). At day 4, the same

Trends of Antibiotic Resistance (AR) in Mesophilic and Psychrotrophic Bacterial Populations During
Cold Storage of Raw Milk, Produced by Organic and Conventional Farming Systems

133

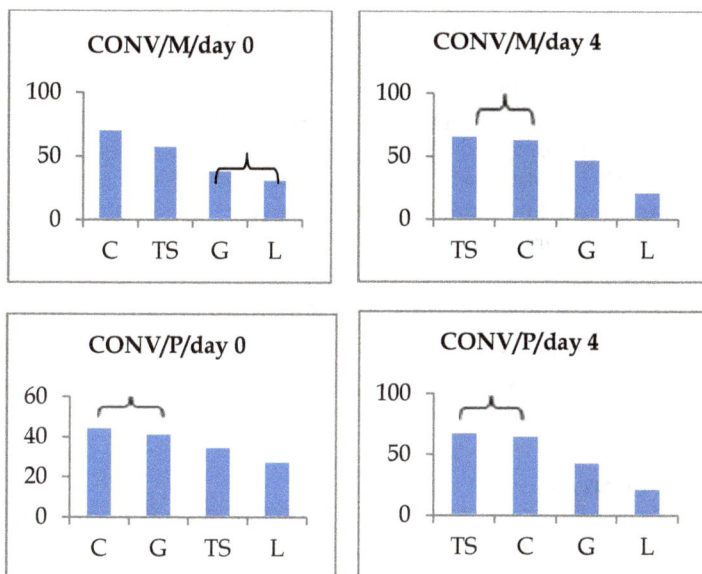

a)

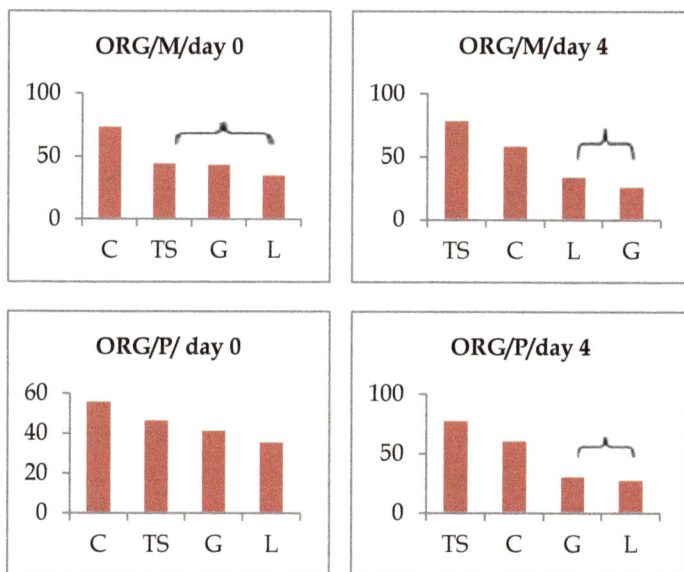

b)

Fig. 3. AR prevalence, estimated by multiple comparison of means from CP (a) and OP (b) raw milk samples over time, determined from combined results with both concentrations (I and II) of each AB. The mean values were obtained with the REGW multiple range test for RAP0 and RAP4. [Noteworthy, ABs that were similarly ranked are grouped in a bracket].

ranking of the ABs was observed for TS and C; the levels were equivalent for psychrotrophs and mesophiles from CP samples (Fig. 3a) whereas TS supplanted C for both mesophiles and psychrotrophs from OP samples (Fig. 3b). For G, similar levels of AR were recorded from CP samples for both psychrotrophs and mesophiles at days 0 and 4, in contrast to OP samples in which the AR dropped over time by about half for both types of bacterial populations (Fig. 3a,b). L-resistance was least prevalent at day 0, mostly also at day 4; a decrease of AR was recorded over time for mesophiles from CP samples and psychrotrophs from CP and OP raw milk samples.

3.6. Ranking of the milk samples according to their total AR load

At day 0, the AR levels (as means determined with the Ryan-Einot-Gabriel-Welsch multiple range test) were comprised between 38-60 and 28-50 for mesophiles and psychrotrophs from CP samples, respectively (Fig. 4a).

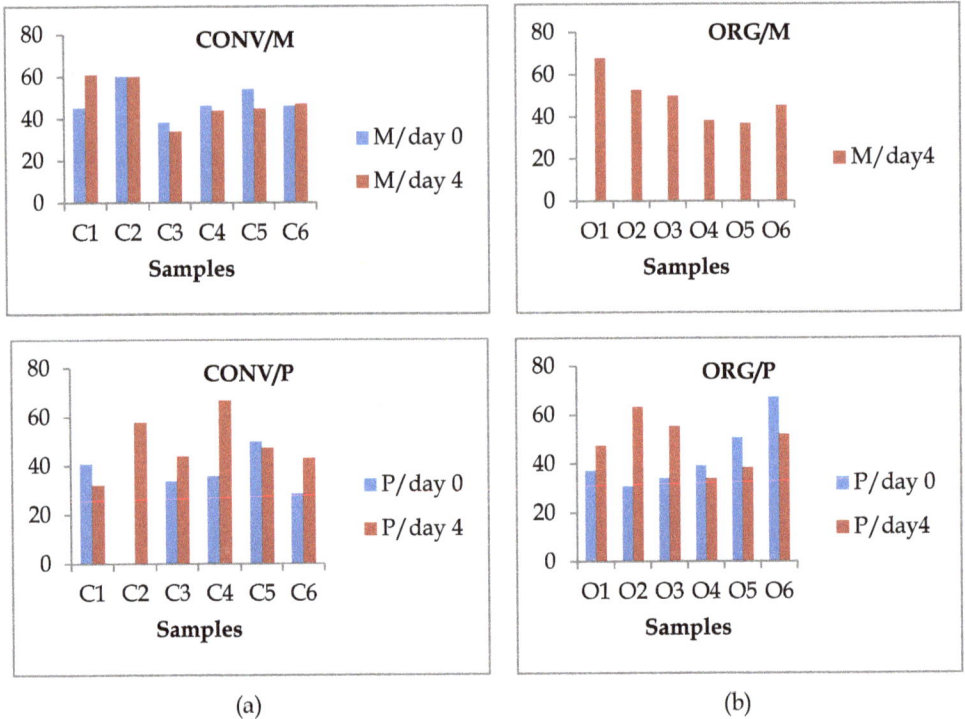

Fig. 4. AR load from multiple comparison of sample means for CP (a) and OP (b) raw milk samples at days 0 and 4 determined for mesophiles (M) and psychrotrophs (P).

At day 4, the mean values ranged between 32-60 and 32-67 for the mesophiles and psychrotrophs respectively (Fig. 4a). Mesophiles from samples C3, C4, C5 showed moderate decrease of the AR between days 0 and 4, contrarily to the psychrotrophic populations recovered from the same samples, which increased by 10 and 30 for samples C3, C4 respectively, or slightly decreased for C5 (Fig. 4a). Mesophiles from sample C2 were the highest AR carriers at days 0 and 4 whereas sample C3 was the lowest at both sampling days; sample C1 was the second lowest at day 0, and second highest at day 4. No model enabled to rank the six OP samples at day 0; however at day 4, the comparison between mesophiles and psychrotrophs showed that samples may be similarly ranked over time (like O3, O5) or not (sample O1), (Fig. 4b).

3.7 DGGE profile analyses of CP and OP raw milk samples at sampling days 0 and 4.

At day 0, the primer set yielded relatively complex fingerprints for C1, C2, C3, C4, C5, C6, O1, O2, and O3 as the PCR amplicons migrated along the whole length of the denaturing gradient gel (Fig. 5), indicative of a high variability in GC%, hence a high species diversity, irrespective of the milk type.

Based on Gel Compar TM analyses, some samples displayed profiles with as many as 27 or 26 bands for C6 and O1 respectively, whereas C4, O4, O5 displayed simpler profiles comprising only 10-11 bands. Profiles from CP samples (C1, C5, C6) that yielded the highest amount of bands clustered as well as O1, O2 and O3 from OP raw milk samples (Fig. 5), and showed similar community structure. The 4 days-cold storage implicated for most samples a simpler profile, as less bands were detected; with exception of C1, all CP raw milk samples clustered while the profiles of C5 and C6 still formed a sub-cluster. Cold storage affected O1, O2 and O3 differently: the samples O1 and O2 remained clustered despite a drop of the similarity values (77.2% to 52.3 %) between both sampling days (Fig. 5).

Samples O4, O5 and O6 were least affected by cold storage, as all three samples formed almost exact pairs at days 0 and 4 with similarity values of 75%, 88.5%, and 87.5% for O6, O5 and O4 respectively, indicative of small changes in the bacterial community between the sampling days. For most of the samples, following the cold storage (4°C for 4 days), the banding patterns were more located on the top of the gel, indicative of less bacterial diversity among communities, and domination of species with higher AT%. To some extent, CP and OP samples were distinguished by DGGE analyses.

4. Discussion

The statistical analyses of RAPD means and RAPD trends during cold storage revealed 1) a higher AR level for psychrotrophic populations present in OP compared to CP milk samples at day 0 (Fig. 2); 2) a similar drop of C-resistant mesophilic, and raise of TS-resistant psychrotrophic bacteria over time for both types of samples (Table 2a,b); 3) an increase of L-resistant (at both concentrations) and partial increase (at one concentration) of G-resistant psychrotrophs for OP samples (Table 2a,b); 4) RAP4 from OP was lower to RAP4 from CP in 4 cases of 16, was similar to RAP4 from CP in 10 other tested conditions, but exceeded RAP4 from CP in 2 cases (Table 3). All preceding observations indicate that the AR load on bacterial populations from OP samples may be as high if not higher than for CP samples. When considering the farming type practices, small or no differences in AR levels were reported by Sato et al. (2004) for *Campylobacter* spp. isolates from organic and conventional dairy herds, by Roesch et al. (2006) when the AR of udder pathogens was investigated in dairy cows, by Ray et al. (2006) for *Salmonella*, or by Garmo et al. (2010) for coagulase-negative staphylococci: the frequency of AR in organic farms was not so different from

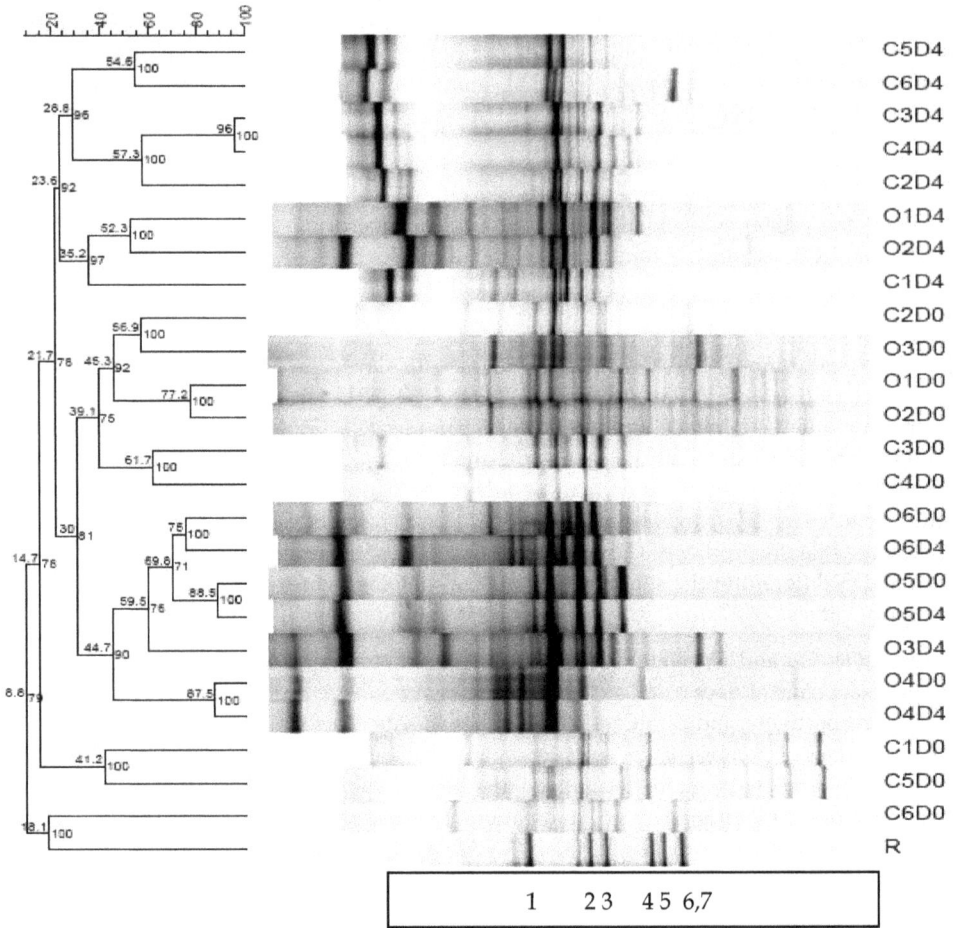

Fig. 5. Dendrogram of DGGE profiles from CP (C1 to C6) and OP (O1 to O6) raw milk samples determined at day 0 (D0) and after 4 days storage at 4°C (D4). The reference standards include the following species: 1, *Listeria innocua* CCUG 15531T (ATCC 33090) ; 2, *Acinetobacter johnsonii* HAMBI 1969 (ATCC 17909) ; 3, *Pseudomonas tolaasii* LMG 2342T (ATCC 33618); 4, *Bacillus cereus* HAMBI 250 (ATCC 10987) ; 5, *Escherichia coli* HAMBI 99 (ATCC 11775) ; 6, *Stenotrophomonas maltophilia* HAMBI 2659 (ATCC 13637) ; 7, *Burkholderia cepacia* HAMBI 1976 (ATCC 25416). [ATTC, American Type Culture Collection; CCUG, Culture Collection University of Göteborg; HAMBI, Culture Collection of the University of Helsinki; LMG, Belgian Collection of Microorganisms].

conventional farms. Also Ruimy et al. (2010) recorded similar levels of resistant Gram-negative bacteria for both organic and conventional produced fruits and vegetables. However, other studies report still higher susceptibilies to antibiotics for samples originating from organic production systems.

Trends of Antibiotic Resistance (AR) in Mesophilic and Psychrotrophic Bacterial Populations During
Cold Storage of Raw Milk, Produced by Organic and Conventional Farming Systems

137

Compared to RAP0 values obtained for 18 CP samples (analysed in a previous study), which ranged between 0.0788 and 0.1576, it appeared that the mesophylic populations from organic raw milk samples analysed here had a rather low AR load (0.092), contrarily to the psychrotrophs for which the mean RAP0 value 0.2456 was the highest so far observed for all milk samples investigated and for which the mean values ranged between (0.1378-0.158). The RAP4 value from OP samples (0.0869) was still the highest encountered for psychrotrophs among all so far investigated raw milk samples for which the RAP4 values were comprised between 0.030 and 0.051 (Fig. 2, and Munsch-Alatossava et al. 2012).

In this study, irrespective of the milk type or the investigated bacterial population types (psychrotrophs or mesophiles), C-resistance was most prevalent at day 0 (rather fresh milk) whereas TS-resistance was equivalent to C-resistance (for CP samples) or higher (for OP samples) at day 4 (after the milk underwent a longer cold storage) (Fig. 3a, b). Similar observations were made in the previous study that considered 18 raw milk samples from conventional production systems (Munsch-Alatossava et al. 2012) for which TS-resistance supplanted C-resistance in prevalence following the cold storage. To some extent, AR prevalence at day 0 does mirror AB usage: Kools et al. (2008) in an overview of published data around ABs usage in Europe, indicated the following relative proportions of total AB use for Finland: β-lactams and cephalosporins (62%), Sulfonamides and trimethoprim (16%), Aminoglycosides (2%) and fluoroquinolones/quinolones (0.6%).

By summing up the values obtained from the ranking of the four ABs according to their prevalence at each sampling day and for each population type (Fig. 3a,b), the total of the means (from the REGW test) from each AB reached 194 for mesophiles from both CP and OP raw milk samples at days 0 and 4. Also, psychrotrophs from OP samples exhibited the same level of total AR at day 4 (194), against 178 at day 0. For psychrotrophs from CP samples, the total of the means from each AB was 146 and 184 at days 0 and 4, respectively. From the analysed samples, it appeared that the multiresistant trait was as common among mesophilic bacteria whether they originated from CP or OP samples. Compared to mesophiles, multiresistance seemed to be less common among psychrotrophs at day 0; however, the cold storage permitted a significant raise of the number of multiresistant isolates (more important for CP samples), but the total AR reached a superior value for psychrotrophs from OP samples at day 4. The AB ranking revealed a notable different impact of the cold storage on the AR trend considering the investigated bacterial population types (Fig. 3a, b):

- since the total AR loads were around 194 for both milk types over time, changes at the level of mesophiles appeared to be mainly qualitative (for example, replacement of bacterial species rather resistant to C by species rather resistant to TS)
- changes at the level of psychrotrophs were both qualitative (TS resistance was more frequent than C resistance at day 4 for OP samples), but also quantitative as suggested from the increase of the AR load by respectively 38 and 16 units for psychrotrophs from CP and OP systems during cold storage; the increase may be lower in the later case due to the particular features of samples O4, O5 and O6.

Interestingly, the statistical analyses of RAPD, which enabled a sample ranking according to the "AR loads" revealed that samples may be or not similarly ranked over time following the cold storage, depending on the considered populations (whether mesophiles or psychrotrophs)(Fig. 4a,b). Noteworthy, samples O5 and O6 were ranked as highest AR carriers on the side of the psychrotrophs at day 0 whereas, at day 4, a partition into two classes considered O3, O1 and O2 as high AR carriers, and O6, O5 and O4 as lower ones. Clearly, the cold storage affected differently OP samples while for samples O1, O2 and O3 the AR, estimated as relative amounts, increased, the AR decreased for O4, O5 and O6.

The high RAP0 and RAP4 values of the six considered OP samples (Fig. 2) bring up the question on whether the AR load is the consequence of different milk production practices or may be sample dependant. Part of the answer is given by the RAP0 and RAP4 values, together with their respective variation ranges: the RAP0 and RAP4 variation ranges were comprised between 0-12 (mean 0.2456) and 0-0.996 (mean 0.0869) respectively, for psychrotrophs enumerated from OP samples. In a previous study where the AR was followed over time (at days 0, 2 and 4 of cold storage) from CP raw milk samples it was noticed that RAP2 (determined after 2 days cold storage) and the corresponding variation range largely supplanted RAP0 and RAP4 values and their corresponding variation ranges (Munsch-Alatossava et al. 2012). Moreover ANOVA performed on RAP0 and RAP4 ranks revealed significant main effect (F values from the Fischer-Snedecor test, p<0.0001 were highest) of the "AB type" for all analysed conditions (day0/day4; mesophiles/psychrotrophs; conventional/organic production systems) to the exception of psychrotrophs from organic milk samples for which the "sample" was the most important factor.

Consequently, we hypothesize that since total counts for O4 and O5 were highest at day 0 (around and slightly above 10^5 CFU/ml, Fig. 1), lower for O6 which however exhibited the highest percentage of psychrotrophs at day 0 (100%), the excessively high value of Rap0 may be due to the samples O4, O5 and O6, which were most probably longer cold stored prior to the initial analyses as compared to O1, O2 and O3. This point is reinforced by the DGGE based analyses of OP samples, as for the samples O4, O5 and O6 the profiles at day 4 were quite similar as the ones of day 0, indicative of little changes in the bacterial community over time (Fig. 5). Like for other studies, DGGE based data confirmed the potential of this approach to investigate changes in raw milk at population levels. Clearly, the cold storage (4 days at 4°C) promoted a reduction of dominant bacterial species: similar observations were made with DGGE based analyses for raw milk stored at 4°C for 24h by Lafarge et al. (2004), but also for meat (Li et al., 2006).

To some extent, results from DGGE analyses were coherent with plating results: the samples C1, C5, C6, O1 and O2 showed the highest bacterial diversity at day 0 as visible from the most complex banding patterns (Fig. 5). The same samples presented the lowest percentages of psychrotrophs in the initial microflora at day 0 (data not shown), suggesting that these samples were more fresh, and had the lowest storage history. Conversely C4 and O4, for which high percentages of psychrotrophs were recorded at day 0, yielded electrophoretic patterns with fewest bands amounts (Fig. 5).

What could explain such high if not higher AR levels in bacteria from organic compared to conventional production systems? Even though any use of antimicrobials may create the potential for AR development, at day 0, the usage patterns of ABs could somehow constitute one part of the explanation (Kools et al., 2008; Thomson et al., 2008). Manure contains substantial amounts of both antimicrobials and antimicrobial-resistant microorganisms; agricultural practices that prevail in organic production systems where chemical fertilizers are prohibited, and are replaced by antibiotic-polluted manure applications, and where at least 50% of the feed is produced on the farm may also partially explain rather high AR levels in OP compared to CP samples. As milk is the target of numerous sources of contaminations (soil, environment...), it may be not that surprising if AR levels are at least as high for OP as for CP samples .

In 2008, the European Commission launched the European Union ´s new organic farming campaign under the slogan "Organic farming, Good for nature, Good for you". At the same time, the European Food Safety Authority (2008) attempted to evaluate to which extent food serves as a source for the acquisition by human of antimicrobial-resistant bacteria and whether foodborne antimicrobial resistance constitutes a biological hazard.

The statistics applied for data treatment on ranks of RAPD which compared the AR load in milk over time as quantified through RAPD (indicative of relative amounts) suggested that the AR level, the AR trend over time may be less "milk production type" than "sample" dependant; the main determinant may be the initial microflora. Whether cold storage of raw milk promotes the raise of AR, of multiresistant traits among bacteria and whether it affects differently conventionally or organic produced milk needs still to be further investigated. The image of safer and healthier food is most often associated to organic food by consumers. Whether initial good intentions based on a more rare use of ABs (typical for organic production systems), contrarily to conventional systems with more frequent use of ABs, are diverted by microbial activity needs further clarifications.

5. Conclusion

In this study, AR was highest at day 0 for psychrotrophs present in OP samples. Even though the cold storage globally promoted a drop of RAP values (as relative amount of AR) over time, in detail the trends were more contrasted as the AR load increased for psychrotrophs from OP samples for both L and TS at both tested concentrations, during the 4 days storage at 4°C. The AR only dropped for mesophiles, from both sample types, for C at both concentrations. For OP samples, if C-resistance was most frequent at day 0 (which corresponds to rather fresh milk), TS-resistance was more common at day 4 (when the milk already underwent a certain cold storage). Based on DGGE pattern analyses, the bacterial communities fingerprints appeared to be at both sampling days "milk age" and "milk type" dependant as the clustering distinguished CP and OP raw milk samples, with different freshness e.g. more or less cold stored. Moreover the changes in bacterial populations structure, following cold storage, indicated a shift in banding patterns towards AT-rich regions, suggesting that the cold storage of raw milk promotes the dominance of AT-rich species over time, irrespective of the milk type.

6. Acknowledgments

We thank J. Rekonen for providing the raw milk samples from conventional dairy farming systems and Juva Organic Ltd for the organic raw milk samples. We are very grateful to Applied Maths (Belgium) for the 2 weeks free access to GelCompar®II.

7. References

Aminov, R.I. (2009). The role of antibiotics and antibiotic resistance in nature. *Environmental Microbiology*, Vol.11, pp. 2970-88.

Chambers, J.V. (2002). The microbiology of raw milk, In: *Dairy Microbiology Handbook,* 3rd *edition.* Edited by R. K. Robinson, New York: Wiley-Interscience, pp. 39-89.

Conover, W.J. (1980). *Practical Non Parametrics Statistics,* 2nd edition, John Wiley & Sons; New York.

Cousin, M.A. (1982). Presence and activity of psychrotrophic microorganisms in milk and dairy products: a review. *Journal of Food Protection,* Vol. 45, pp. 172-207.

Davies, J.& Davies, D. (2010). Origins and evolution of antibiotic resistance. *Microbiology and Molecular Biology Reviews,* Vol. 74, pp. 417-433.

Einot, I. & Gabriel, K.R. (1975). A study of the power of several methods of multiple comparisons. *Journal of the American Statistical Association,* Vol. 70 (351), pp. 574-583.

European Commission (2008). Organic Farming-What makes milk organic? www.organic-.farming.europa.eu.

European Committee for antimicrobial susceptibility testing (EUCAST), (2000). Determination of minimum inhibitory concentrations (MICs) of antibacterial agents by agar dilution. *CMI* Vol.6, pp.509-515.

European Council Regulation (EC) No834/2007 of June 2007 on organic production and labelling of organic products and repealing regulation (EEC) No2092/91.

European Food Safety Authority (2008). Foodborne antimicrobial resistance as a biological hazard (Question No EFSA-Q-2007-089) by the Biohaz panel (Andreoletti et al.)

Finnish association for milk hygiene. (2008) http://www.maitohygienialiitto.fi

Finnish Food safety authority (2008) http://www.evira.fi

Freitas, R.; Nero, L.A. & Carvalho, A.F. (2009). Technical note: Enumeration of mesophilic aerobes in milk: Evaluation of standard official protocols and Petrifilm aerobic count plates. *Journal of Dairy Science,* Vol. 92, pp. 3069-3073.

Garmo, R.T.; Waage, S.; Sviland, S.; Henriksen, B.F.; Østerås, O. & Reksen, O. (2010). Reproductive performance, udder health, and antibiotic health, and antibiotic resistance in mastitis bacteria isolated from Norwegian red cows in conventional and organic farming. *Acta Veterinaria Scandinavica,* Vol. 52, pp. 1-13.

Gray, M.J.; Freitag, N.E. & Boor, K.J. (2006). How the bacterial pathogen *Listeria monocytogenes* mediates the switch from environmental Dr. Jekyll to pathogenic Mr. Hyde. *Infect ion and Immunity,* Vol. 74, pp. 2505-2512.

Grave, K.; Torren-Edo, J. & Mackay, D. (2010). Comparison of the sales of veterinary antibacterial agents between 10 European countries. *Journal of Antimicrobial Chemotherapy,* Vol. 65, pp. 2037-2040.

Information Centre of the Ministry of Agriculture and Forestry (2009). Matilda tietopalvelu. Maito and kananmunat. http://www.matilda.fi.

Jacob, M.E.; Fox, J.T.; Reinstein, S.L. & Nagaraja, T.G. (2008). Antimicrobial susceptibility of foodborne pathogens in organic and natural production systems: an overview. *Foodborne Pathogens and Disease,* Vol. 5, pp. 721-730.

Knezevic, P. & Petrovic, O. (2008). Antibiotic resistance of commensal *Escherichia coli* of food-producing animals from three Vojvodinian farms, Serbia. *International Journal of Antimicrobial Agents,* Vol. 31, pp. 360-363.

Kools, S.A.E., Moltmann, J.F. & Knacker, T. (2008). Estimating the use of veterinary medicines in the European union. *Regulatory Toxicology and Pharmacology,* Vol. 50, pp. 59-65.

Lafarge, V. ; Ogier, J.-C.; Girard, V.; Maladen, V.; Leveau, J.-Y.; Gruss, A. & Delacroix-Buchet, A. (2004). Raw cow milk bacterial population shifts attributable to refrigeration. *Applied and Environmental Microbiology*, Vol. 70, pp. 5644- 5650.

Levy, S.B. (2002). Factors impacting on the problem of antibiotic resistance. *Journal of Antimicrobial Chemotherapy*, Vol. 49, pp. 25-30.

Li, M.Y; Zhou, G.H.; Xu, X.L. ; Li, C.B. & Zhu,W.Y.(2006). Changes of bacterial diversity and main flora in chilled pork during storage using PCR-DGGE. *Food Microbiology*, Vol.23, pp. 607-611.

Ma, Y.; Barbano, D.M. & Santos, M. (2003). Effect of CO_2 addition to raw milk on proteolysis and lipolysis at 4 °C. *Journal of Dairy Science*, Vol. 86, pp. 1616-1631.

Marshall, B.M.; Ochiend, D.J. & Levy, S.B. (2009). Commensals: Underappreciated reservoir of antibiotic resistance. *Microbe*, Vol. 4, pp. 231-238.

Munsch-Alatossava, P. & Alatossava, T. (2006). Phenotypic characterization of raw milk-associated psychrotrophic bacteria. *Microbiological Research*, Vol. 161, pp. 334-346.

Munsch-Alatossava, P. & Alatossava, T.(2007). Antibiotic resistance of raw-milk associated psychrotrophic bacteria. *Microbiological Research*, Vol. 162, pp. 115-123.

Munsch-Alatossava, P.; Gursoy, O. & Alatossava, T. (2010). Potential of nitrogen gas (N_2) to control psychrotrophs and mesophiles in raw milk. *Microbiological Research*, Vol. 165, pp. 122-132.

Munsch-Alatossava, P.; Gauchi, J.-P.; Chamlagain, B. & Alatossava, T. (2012). Trends of antibiotic resistance in mesophilic and psychrotrophic bacterial populations during cold storage of raw milk, ISRN Microbiology, In Press.

Ogier, J.C.; Son, O. ; Gruss, A.; Tailliez, P. & Delacroix-Buchet, A. (2002). Identification of the bacterial microflora in dairy products by temporal temperature gradient gel electrophoresis. *Applied and Environmental Microbiology*, Vol. 68, pp. 3691-3701.

Ray, K.A.; Warnick, L.D.; Mitchell, R.M.; Kaneene, J.B.; Ruegg, P.L.; Wells, S.J.; Fossier, C.P.; Halbert, L.W. & May, K. (2006). Antimicrobial susceptibility of *Salmonella* from organic and conventional dairy farms. Journal of Dairy Science, Vol. 89, pp. 2038-2050.

Roesch, M.; Perreten, V.; Doherr, M.G.; Schaeren, W.; Schällibaum, S. & Blum, J.W. (2006). Comparison of antibiotic resistance of udder pathogens in dairy cows kept on organic and on conventional farms. *Journal of Dairy Science*, Vol. 89, pp. 989-997.

Ruimy, R.; Brisabois, A.; Bernede, C.; Skurnik, D.; Barnat, S.; Arlet, G.; Momcilovic, S.; Elbaz, S.; Moury, F.; Vibet, M.-A.; Courvalin, P.; Guillemot, D. & Andremont, A. (2010). Organic and conventional fruits and vegetables contain equivalent counts of Gram-negative bacteria expressing resistance to antibacterial agents. *Environmental Microbiology*, Vol. 12, No.3, pp. 608-615.

Ryan, T.A. (1959). Multiple comparisons in psychological research. *Psychological Bulletin*, Vol. 56, pp. 26-47.

Ryan, T.A. (1960). Significant tests for multiple comparisons of proportions, variances and other statistics. *Psychological Bulletin*, Vol. 57, pp. 318-328.

Sato, K.; Bartlett, P.C.; Kaneene, J.B. & Downes, F.P. (2004). Comparison of prevalence and antimicrobial susceptibilities of *Campylobacter* spp. isolates from organic and conventional dairy herds in Wisconsin. *Applied and Environmental Microbiology*, Vol. 70, pp. 1442-1447.

Schoeni, J.L.& Lee Wong, A.C. (2005). *Bacillus cereus* food poisoning and its toxins (Review). *Journal of Food Protection*, Vol. 68, pp. 636-648.

Straley, B.A.; Donaldson, S.C.; Hedge, N.V.; Sawant, A.A.; Srinivasan, V.; Oliver, S.P. & Jayarao, B.M.(2006). Public health significance of antimicrobial- resistant gram-negative bacteria in raw bulk tank milk. *Foodborne Pathogens and Disease*, Vol. 3, pp. 222-233.

Thompson, K.; Rantala, M.; Hautala, M.; Pyörälä, S. & Kaartinen, L. (2008). Cross-sectional prospective survey to study indication-based usage of antimicrobials in animals: Results of use in cattle. *BMC Veterinary Research*, Vol. 4, pp. 15-21.

Welsch, R.E. (1977). Stepwise multiple comparison procedures. *Journal of the American Statistical Association*, Vol. 72 (359), pp. 566-575.

6

Emergence of Antibiotic Resistant Bacteria from Coastal Environment – A Review

K.C.A. Jalal[1], B. Akbar John[1], B.Y. Kamaruzzaman[1] and K. Kathiresan[2]
*[1]Department of Biotechnology, Kulliyyah of Science,
International Islamic University Malaysia,
[2]Centre of Advanced Studies in Marine Biology,
Annamalai University,
[1]Malaysia
[2]India*

1. Introduction

Antibiotic resistance in microbes is a growing issue of human health. The extraordinary ability of microbes to develop resistance to various antibiotics attracted evolutionary scientists and environmental biologists in recent years. Historically, the use of antimicrobial agents started in 1904 with the discovery of Tripan red by Ehrlich and Shiga (Browning & Gulbransen, 1936). In 1929, penicillin was discovered by Alexander Fleming when his group found that the fungus *Penicilium notatum* produces a very selective inhibitor for *Staphylococcus* sp. Fleming's discovery showed that not only synthetic agents like Ehrlich's "Magic Bullet" but also a microbial product can be an effective antimicrobial drug (Hare, 1970). In 1943, Waksman started to use the word "antibiotics" when he discovered streptomycin (Wainwright, 1988). After the initial age of discovery and since the 1970s many antimicrobial agents have been developed together with the discoveries of new antibiotics. It is well documented that the evolution of antibiotic resistance in bacterial strains is a direct consequence of natural selection applied by widespread use of antibiotic drugs (Benveniste & Davies, 1973). The providential experiment by Fleming demonstrated the production of antibiotics (Penicillin) which eventually led to its large-scale production from mold *Penicillium notatum* in the 1940s. As early as the late 1940s resistant strains of bacteria began to appear due to their extraordinary ability in gaining resistance towards any particular antibiotics with elapsing generation (Shoemaker et al., 2001; Chopra & Roberts et al., 2001; Doern et al., 2001). In 1980 it was estimated that 3–5% of *S. pneumoniae* were penicillin-resistant and by 1998, 34% of the *S. pneumoniae* sampled were resistant to penicillin. Currently, it is estimated that more than 70% of the bacteria that cause hospital-acquired infections are resistant to at least one of the antibiotics used to treat them (NIAID, 2006).

Antibiotics are defined as a chemical substance derived from microorganisms, which have the capacity to inhibit growth, and even destroying other microorganisms in a dilute solution (ICON, 2003). Antibiotics are low-molecular-mass (<1500 kDa), products of secondary metabolism and nonessential for the growth of producing organisms, but are very important for human health. They have unusual structures and are most often formed during the late growth phase of the producing microorganisms. These secondary metabolites have exerted a major impact on the control of infectious diseases and other medical conditions, and the development of pharmaceutical industry. Their use has contributed to an increase in the average life expectancy in the USA, which increased from 47 years in 1900 to 74 years (in men) and 80 years (in women) in 2000 (Reynolds, 2010). Probably, the most important use of secondary metabolites has been as anti-infective drugs. In 2000, the market for such anti-infectives was US$55 billion and in 2007 it was US$66 billion, with the estimated global antibiotic consumption of between 100,000 and 200,000 tonnes per year (Demain & Sanchez, 2009).

Coastal environment plays a very important role as habitat to a number of plants and animals. They serve as breeding and nursery grounds, shelters, sources of food for various marine lives. In the recent times, pollution of coastal areas represents one of the most important environmental problems because it causes economic and tourism damages as well as affects health quality. It was noted that antibiotics released into the aquatic environment are of great concern for the three important reasons: (1) Contamination of water used for drinking, irrigation and recreation, (2) Widespread occurrence of bacterial resistance to antibiotics, and (3) Negative effect on microbes which play vital role in nutrient cycling (e.g. nitrogen cycle) and regeneration of nutrients in aquatic ecosystems (Costanzo et al., 2005). The use of antibiotics is the main treatment applied to control bacterial illness in fish farms (Castro et al., 2008). Due to the use of a wide variety of antibiotics, aquaculture has been implicated as potential environment to the development and selection of resistant bacteria and a source of these pathogens to other animals and humans (Hatha et al., 2005; Serrano, 2005). It has also been noted that sediment samples containing microorganisms with antibiotic resistance alter the production of β-lactamase in the human defence system (Lu, et al., 2010). The issue of antibiotic resistance was extensively addressed in the scientific literature describing the presence of antibiotics in the environment (e.g. Nygaard et al., 1992; Samuelsen et al., 1992). But, a comprehensive review on the emergence of antibiotic resistance strains from the aquatic habitat is still scanty.

3. Antibiotic resistance an ecological perspective

Although antibiotics have been used in large quantities for some decades, until recently the existence of these substances in the environment has received little attention. It is only in recent years that a more complex investigation of antibiotic substances has been undertaken in order to permit an assessment of the environmental risks (Kümmerer, 2009a & b). Within the last decade, an increasing number of studies covering antibiotic input, occurrence, fate and effects have been published (Kümmerer, 2009 b; Björkman et al., 2000; Alanis, 2005). Antibiotic resistance is one of the major challenges for human medicine and veterinary medicine. However, there is still a lack of understanding and knowledge about sources, presence and significance of resistance of bacteria against antibiotics in the aquatic environment despite the numerous studies performed (Kümmerer, 2009b).

Antibiotic resistance can reach the environment with the potential of adversely affecting aquatic and terrestrial organisms which eventually might reach humans through drinking water and food chain (Edquist & Pedersen, 2001; Prior, 2008; Aarestrup et al., 2008). The history of resistance due to the use of antibiotics has only recently been described in more detail (Edquist & Pedersen, 2001; Prior, 2008). In general, the emergence of resistance is a highly complex process which is not yet fully understood with respect to the significance of the interaction of bacterial populations and antibiotics, even in a medicinal environment (Björkman et al., 2000; Martinez & Baquero, 2000; Alanis, 2005). The transfer of resistant bacteria to humans could occur via water or food if plants are watered with surface water or sewage sludge, if manure is used as a fertilizer, or if resistant bacteria are present in meat (Perreten et al., 1997; Khachatourians, 1998; Dolliver & Gupta, 2008). The significance of the transfer of antibiotic resistance from animals to humans is not clearly understood. However, to minimize this route and the unwanted intake of antibiotics, the antibiotic content of fishery products is monitored by authorities in many countries (WHO, 2003; IM, 1989; FAAIR, 2002).

Many bacterial species multiply rapidly enough to double their numbers every 20-30 minutes, therefore, their ability to adapt to changes in the environment and survive unfavorable conditions often results in the development of mutations that enable the species to survive in changing external conditions (Ferenci, 2008). Research on the use of antibiotics in aquaculture shows similar results with the medical use of antibiotics (Weston, 1996). The important research findings in this regard are: (1) The use of one antibacterial agent can increase levels of resistance not only to that specific drug but also to many others, even those using very different modes of antibacterial action (cross-resistance). (2) Antibacterial resistance does not always respond in a predictable fashion correlating with the amount of drugs used or with the concentrations of residues in the environment (Hernando et al., 2006).

3.1 Coastal environment

Coastal Environment plays a very important role as habitat to a number of microbes, plants and animals. They serve as breeding grounds, shelters, sources of food for marine life, and are home to a number of endangered species (Kuijper, 2003). Over half of the current global population lives within 200 km of the coastline. For the future, the Centre for Climate Systems Research (CCSR) of the Earth Institute at Columbia University estimates a strong growth of coastal population by 2025. The coastal zone contains natural systems that provide more than half of the global ecosystem goods (e.g., fish, oil, minerals) and services (e.g., natural protection from storms and tidal waves, recreation). In addition, 14 of the world's 17 largest megacities are located along coasts and most of them are located in Asia's fastest growing economies (www.loicz.org). The overcrowding of beaches has led to large-scale destruction of some of these habitats and has reduced their ability to adapt to drastic environmental changes. Development, climate change, and commercialization have all contributed a major part in increasing the pressure on beach ecosystems. Besides this fact, anthropogenic input of various pollutants especially antibiotics into the aquatic environment has increased the resistant capacity of the bacterial strains. In general, bacterial load is higher in the sediments compared to the overlying water body. Hence, more investigations were carried out on surface soil samples (Jensen et al., 2001; Tolls, 2001; Marengo et al., 1997. It has been noted that persistence of antibiotics in soil depends on many factors including soil type, climate, and class of antibiotics (Bonaventura, 2004). Most antibiotics are recycled in soils through natural cycles but some of them have a long half-life (Kumar et al., 2005; Kümmerer, 2009a). According to Marengo et al. (1997), less than 1% of sarafloxacin, an antibiotic used widely in poultry production, degrades in the soil after 80 days of incubation. These antibiotics may leach to ground water or move to surface waters via surface runoff. Olapade et al., (2006) have reported that these antibiotics find their way to the coastal and marine environment.

Antibiotics have both quantitative and qualitative effects on the native microbial communities in soil environment (Nygaard et al., 1992). Although antibiotic concentrations in most soils are not at therapeutic levels to cause inhibitory effects on bacterial population, it may still influence the selection of antibiotic resistant bacteria in the niche (USEPA, 2002). Jensen et al. (2001) have recorded an increased antibiotic resistance among *Pseudomonas* sp. and *Bacillus cereus* after exposure to soil sediments. Many antibiotics have a strong tendency to bind with soil particles (Tolls, 2001; Kummerer et al., 2003). Distribution coefficients ($K_{d,solid}$) as high as 2300, 6310, and 128 L kg^{-1} have been reported for tetracycline, enrofloxacin, and tylosin, respectively (Kummerer et al., 2003). Our research team has earlier shown that the bacterial isolates from the tropical mangrove sediments are 100% resistant against β - lactam antibiotics (ampicillin, amoxicillin and penicillin). Bacterial isolated from mangrove sediment soil have exhibited 66.7 and 77.8% resistance against chloramphenicol and streptomycin, respectively, suggesting that the lipid composition may play a key role in preventing the entrance or binding of antibiotics to the cell (Jalal et al., 2010). Interestingly, All the isolates are susceptible to ciprofloxacin since it inhibits the enzyme topoisomerase II that causes the negative super-coil in DNA strands and thus permits transcription or replication. All the bacterial isolates display Multi Antibiotic Resistance (MAR) index higher than 0.2 indicating the high-risk sources of contamination in the environment (Jalal et al., 2010).

3.2 Aquaculture

In aquaculture fields, high loads of antibiotics in sediments at concentrations potent enough to inhibit the growth of bacteria have been reported (Costanzo et al., 2005; Hatha et al., 2005; Hirsch et al., 1999; Holmström et al., 2003; Kümmerer, 2009a &b). Resistant bacteria may be present in sediments because of the application of antibiotics in fish farming or because of selection through the antibiotics present in the sediments. The fact that the exposure is highly concentrated must also be considered to be critical. The substances used in fish farming can enter sediments directly from water without undergoing any kind of purification process. Some investigations have demonstrated the presence and persistence of antibiotics applied extensively in fish farming in sediments beneath fish farms (Kümmerer, 2003). Fluoroquinolones, sulphonamides and tetracyclines are strongly adsorbed (Kümmerer, 2009b) and therefore, they can readily accumulate in the sediments. It is not clearly known as to what degree and under what circumstances the compounds are effective after sorption or whether they are released to contribute to resistance. Antimicrobials can have qualitative and quantitative effects upon the resident microbial community in sediments. In the fish farming sector (aquaculture, mariculture, etc.), the widespread use of antibiotics for treating bacterial diseases is associated with the development of antibiotic resistance in *Aeromonas hydrophila, Aeromonas salmonicida, Edwardsiella tarda, Edwardsiella icttaluri, Vibrio anguillarum, Vibrio salmonicida, Pasteurella piscida* and *Yersinia ruckeri* (Serrano, 2005). Bacteria resistant against these compounds have been detected in sediments. Increased antibacterial resistance in sedimentary bacteria is often the most sensitive environmental indicator of past antibacterial use (Kümmerer, 2003). Various patterns of resistance among strains were isolated from very close geographical areas during the same year, suggesting diverse patterns of drug resistance in environmental bacteria within this area. In addition, the cross-resistance patterns have suggested that the resistance determinants among *Vibrio* spp. are acquired differently within sediment and seawater environments (Neela et al., 2007).

As far as intensive shrimp culture goes, a large amount of shrimp food and antibiotics have been used to increase production and to protect shrimp from diseases (EJF, 2003). Consequently, a large portion of feeds and antibiotics enters the water as wastes, causing water pollution (Le et al., 2003). Several studies have demonstrated the presence of antibacterial residues in fish farms (Weston, 1996; Capone et al., 1996; Herwig et al., 1997). Recent studies have shown that many antibiotics persist in the sediment and in the aquatic environment for several months following administration (Bjorklund et al., 1991; Lai et al., 1995; Pouliquen & Le, 1996; Hirsch et al., 1999; Miranda & Zemelman, 2002).The residues of antibacterial agents may affect the sedimentary microbial community and introduce antibiotic resistance in the bacteria (Hektoen et al., 1995; Tendencia & Dela Pena, 2002). Mc Phearson et al. (1991) have observed that individual and multiple antibiotic resistances are associated with antimicrobial use. A study in Thailand has indicated that the pattern of antibiotic use among the farms can cause the risk of the development of resistant bacteria strains (Holmostro"m et al., 2003). Little is known about the occurrence of antibiotic resistant bacteria in marine sediments near fish farms (Schmidt et al., 2000; Tendencia & DelaPena, 2001).

4. Antibiotic resistance in sea food

Sea foods are often susceptible to spoilage by putrefactive microorganisms. Sea foods usually spoil much more rapidly than meats obtained from warm blooded animals when stored at ordinary refrigerator temperatures, and the reason for this is almost certainly because of the marine products that are invariably contaminated with psychrophilic bacteria (Witter, 1961). These organisms not only multiply quite rapidly at refrigerator temperatures, but spoil fish about twice as fast at 37^0 F as at 30^0 F (Bluhm et al., 1956). Though proper vessel and fish plant sanitation are obviously highly desirable for production of high quality fish, it is quite possible to prepare fish of excellent bacteriological quality in quite primitive premises. In other words, the maintenance of high sanitary standards on fishing vessels and at shore plants does not necessarily insure good quality fish, though from an aesthetic stand point alone such conditions are highly desirable. It is the actual handling and treatment of the fish themselves which is of prime importance in determining their quality.

Reviews and original articles dealing with antibiotics in fish or shellfish preservation have been published from other laboratories (Tomiyama et al., 1955; Ingram et al., 1956). Antibiotics have been commonly used to preserve the fish from bacterial contamination. In 1943 penicillic acid was prepared and tested as a possible preservative for fish with poor success (Tarr, 1944). Later penicillin and streptomycin were examined with similar disappointing results (Tarr, 1948). In the spring of 1950, a number of the newer antibiotics were studied and the findings were much more encouraging since Aureomycin, Terramycin and Chloromycetin all gave quite significant preservation in comparatively low concentration (Boyd & Tarr, 1956). Further experiments proved that of 14 antibiotics examined, Aureomycin (chlortetracycline, CTC) was found most effective (Tarr et al., 1954) and it is with this antibiotic that all applied studies have been conducted (Gillespie et al., 1955; Steiner and Tarr, 1955; antibiotics as food preservatives; Tarr et al., 1954).

Effect of several new antibiotics and furan derivatives on growth of bacteria in fish products have been studied and they are: (1) Antibiotics: Aureomycin (Lederle Laboratories), Amphomycin, Etamycin, Bryamycin (Bristol Laboratories, Inc.); and (2) Furan derivatives: Furoxone, Furadantin, Nitrofurazone (Furacin), and N. F. 56 (N-5-nitro-2 furfurylidene-l-aminoguanidine sulphate) (Eaton Laboratories, Inc.) (**Table 1**). The technique is similar to that employed in previous studies with ground flesh (Tarr et al., 1950).

Compound	concentration (µg/g)	Bacterial counts (colony forming units × 10^6/g) at temperature			
		1°C		5°C	
		6	8	6	6
None		27	>600	600	130
Aureomycin (CTC)	2.5	1.3	0.5	7	19
Amphomycin	5			450	
Bryamycin	5				98
	10	92	340		
	20	19	470		
Etamycin	5		910		
	10		380		
Furoxone	2.5				32
Furadantin	2.5				85
Nitrofurazone	2.5				114
	10	37	>900		
	25	57	310		
	50	19	900		
NF-56	2.5				63
	25	157	837		
	50	76	367		
CTC+ Bryamycin	5				
	10	2.7	8		
CTC+ Bryamycin	2.5				
	5	4	1		
NF-56+ Bryamycin	25		>900		
	10				
Nitrofurazone+ Bryamycin	25				
	10	18	400		

Table 1. Effect of various antibiotics and Furan derivatives on growth of bacteria in Minced Lingod muscle at 0⁰ and 4⁰C (Boyd et al., 1955).

The search for antibiotics or other substances which could prove valuable in preventing microbiological spoilage of fish or fish waste products is continuing, and the results of trials with several new antibiotics and furan derivatives are presented. It has been argued that suppression of natural bacterial flora of fish by introduction of CTC might create favorable conditions for the growth of food poisoning microorganisms.

5. Antimicrobial resistance in drug development

5.1 Mechanism of antibiotic resistance in bacteria

A key factor in the development of antibiotic resistance is the ability of infectious organisms to adapt quickly to new environmental conditions. Bacteria are single-celled organisms that, compared with higher life forms, have small numbers of genes. Therefore, even a single random genetic mutation can greatly affect their ability to cause disease. And because most microbes reproduce by dividing every few hours, bacteria can evolve rapidly. A mutation that helps a microbe surviving to an antibiotic exposure will quickly become dominant throughout the microbial population. Microbes also often acquire resistance genes from each other through horizontal gene transfer mechanism which might enable them to be a multiple antibiotic resistant strain. It is also noted that the specificity of the interactions between antibiotics and various protein sequences within a bacterium resultse in significantly high ratio of mutations in its genome which leads to antibiotic resistance. There is also a relatively high possibility that a particular mutation in a certain target sequence will result in antibiotic resistance.

Antibiotics generally target a variety of essential bacterial functions. For instance, the β-lactam antibiotics and vancomycin interrupte cell wall synthesis of pathogens, whereas macrolides and tetracyclines disrupt the protein synthesis at ribosomal level. Bacteria may develop their antibiotic properties by a variety of mechanisms. According to a study by Nicolaou (2001), one mechanism of resistance is by degrading the antibiotic in a step by step process. This degradation starts when bacterial β-lactamases hydrolyzes the β-lactam ring thus rendering these antibiotics ineffective. A secondary resistance mechanism is then triggered when the antibiotic target is altered. As the next step, bacteria may block the entry of antibiotic to the site of action, resulting in decreased absorption, which in turn results in bacteria with decreased sensitivity to vancomycin due to thicker cell walls. Finally, bacteria may develop efflux pumps that actively pump antibiotics out of the cell so that they do not reach their target. Nicolaou also tested the findings experimentally with macrolides and has found that if the ribosomal binding site for macrolides changes so that these antibiotics bind with decreased affinity, then protein synthesis will not be disrupted.

5.2 Drug discovery

When bacteria contact with chemical substances, they show a positive or negative chemotaxis. If the substrates are acceptable for bacteria or can support bacterial growth, they show a positive chemotaxis and utilize the substrate as an organic source. If toxic, they respond by escaping from the chemical(s). Antibiotics selectively inhibit bacteria based on targeting a specific structure or function of bacteria, which means antibiotics act as toxins to bacteria. Mostly the targets of antibiotics are prokaryote-specific mechanisms and structures, which are not present in eukaryotes or they have different characteristics from those of eukaryotic cells. However, bacteria inherently have potential drug resistance mechanisms or they can acquire exogenous genes conferring drug resistance. Drug resistance therefore, occurs by such mechanisms. At present, four main categories of drug resistance mechanisms are known (Li & Nikadio, 2009). They are: (1) Drug inactivation or modification: for example, enzymatic deactivation of *Penicillin* G in some penicillin-resistant bacteria through the production of β-lactamases, (2) Alteration of target site: for example, alteration of PBP — the binding target site of penicillins — in MRSA and other penicillin-resistant bacteria, (3) Alteration of metabolic pathway: for example, some sulfonamide-resistant bacteria do not require para-aminobenzoic acid (PABA), an important precursor for the synthesis of folic acid and nucleic acids in bacteria inhibited by sulfonamides. Instead, like mammalian cells, they turn to utilizing preformed folic acid, and (4) Reduced drug accumulation: by decreasing drug permeability and/or increasing active efflux (pumping out) of the drugs across the cell surface (Li & Nikadio, 2009) .Some of these mechanisms have been well studied at the molecular level (Walsh, 2003).

The integrated approaches for maximizing the diversity of microbes in drug discovery programs have been reviewed recently, with selective isolation of novel microorganisms (Knight et al., 2003; Zhang et al., 2005; Bian et al., 2008; Wagner-Dobler et al., 2002). Recently Cubist Pharmaceuticals has constructed a multi-drug resistant *E. coli* strain, which carries resistance markers for 17 of the most frequently produced antibiotics. Thus, a comparison of extract activities against sensitive and resistant *E. coli* strains will allow researchers to rapidly discovering novel and specific active compounds that can be used as effective drugs against pathogenic strains (Baltz, 2008). From these studies, it is strongly anticipated that metagenomic libraries of the drug resistant microbial strains will drive drug discovery process now and in the future. Hence, undoubtedly, metagenome analysis technology combined with high throughput screening will bring innovation to the drug discovery.

6. Impact of antibiotic resistance on human health

It has been widely understood that the bacteria and other microorganisms that often cause infections are known to be remarkably resilient and have the ability to develop ways for surviving drugs that are meant to kill or weaken them. Recent scientific evidence suggests that during the last decade, antibiotic resistance by various mechanisms has increased worldwide in bacterial pathogens leading to treatment failures in human and animal infections (Singer et al., 2003). However, the resistance against different types of biocides (including disinfectants, antiseptics, preservatives, sterilants) has been studied and characterized (Russell, 1990 & 1995). Only limited sound scientific evidence to correctly assess the risks of antibiotic resistance induced by resistance to biocides is available (SCENIHR, 2009). Furthermore, research indicates that biocides and antibiotics may share some common behaviour and properties in their respective activity and in the resistance mechanisms developed by bacteria (Russell, 2003, Sheldon 2005).

Although antibiotic usage has clearly benefited the animal industry and helped providing affordable animal protein to the growing human population, the use of antibiotics in food production has also contributed to the emergence and spread of antibiotic multiple resistance (AMR). Along with antibiotics used for human medicine, the use of antibiotics for animal treatment, prophylaxis and growth promotion exerts an inestimable amount of selective pressure toward the emergence and propagation of resistant bacterial strains.

Animals can serve as mediators, reservoirs and disseminators of resistant bacterial strains and/or AMR genes. Consequently, imprudent use of antimicrobials in animals may eventually result in increased human morbidity, increased human mortality, reduced efficacy of related antibiotics used for human medicine, increased healthcare costs, increased potential for carriage and dissemination of pathogens within human populations and facilitated emergence of resistant human pathogens (**Figure 1**).

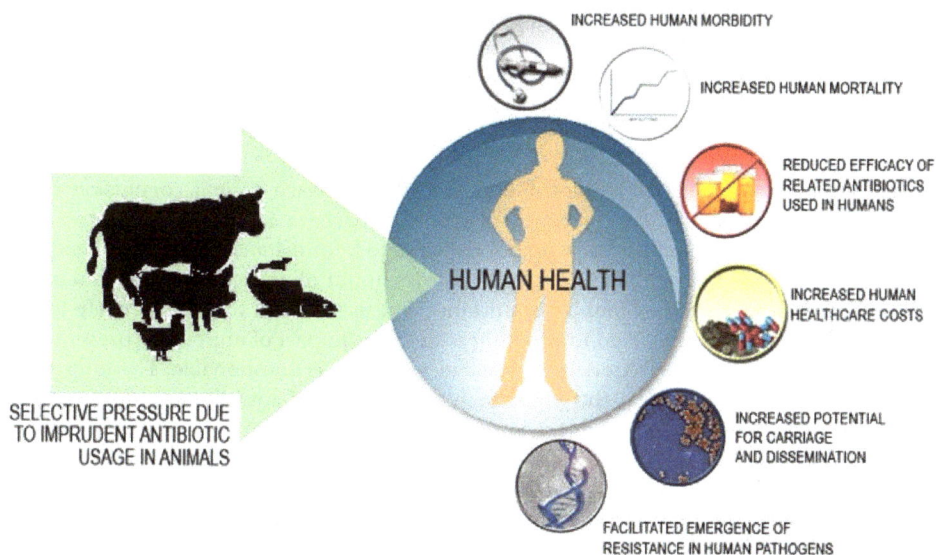

INCREASED HUMAN MORBIDITY

INCREASED HUMAN MORTALITY

REDUCED EFFICACY OF RELATED ANTIBIOTICS USED IN HUMANS

INCREASED HUMAN HEALTHCARE COSTS

INCREASED POTENTIAL FOR CARRIAGE AND DISSEMINATION

FACILITATED EMERGENCE OF RESISTANCE IN HUMAN PATHOGENS

HUMAN HEALTH

SELECTIVE PRESSURE DUE TO IMPRUDENT ANTIBIOTIC USAGE IN ANIMALS

Fig. 1. The Human Health Impact of Antimicrobial Resistance in Animal Populations

According to Helms et al., (2002), the patients infected with pansusceptible *Sal*monella typhimurium are 2.3 times more likely to die within 2 years after infection than persons in the general Danish population, and that patient infected with strains resistant to amplicillin, chloramphenicol, streptomycin, suldonamide and tetracycline are 4.8 times (95% CI 2.2 to 10.2) more likely to die within 2 years. Furthermore, they have established that quinolone resistance in this organism is associated with a mortality rate 10.3 times higher than the general population.

It has been well documented that antimicrobial resistance due to a particular antibiotic used in food animals may result in reduced efficacy of most or all members of that same antibiotic class, some of which may be extremely important for human medicine (McDonald et al., 2001). The current pharmaceutical era faces multi resistant infectious disease organisms that are difficult and, sometimes, impossible to treat successfully. When there is an increase in numbers of bacteria that are resistant to antibiotics, it will be more difficult and more expensive to treat human bacterial infections. According to a study published by the Centers for Disease Control and Prevention (CDC), up to date, there are more than 100 antibiotics approved by the US Food and Drug Administration for human use. As antibiotics fail to treat recurring infections, the consequences include frequent visits to the doctor, hospitalization or even a need for a more expensive medication as a replacement for the existing ineffective ones (Levy, 2002). Increased healthcare costs are another important consequence of antimicrobial resistance. Increased costs are due to the need for additional antibiotic treatments, longer hospitalization, more diagnostic tests, higher professional costs and more pain management. In 1998, the Institute of Medicine estimated the annual cost of infections caused by antibiotic-resistant bacteria at US$ 4 to 5 million per year (McGowan, 2001). This occurrence of antibiotic resistance is found all over the world and has become a very serious problem in the treatment of diseases. The US Office of Technology Assessment report has attributed a cost of $1.3 billion per year for antibiotic-resistant infections in US hospitals. The fiscal cost of treating antibiotic resistant infections worldwide has been estimated to be many billions of dollars per year.

7. Conclusion

At present, there is insufficient information available to reach a final conclusion on the significance and impact of the presence of resistant bacteria in the environment which would allow the assessment of the potential risks related, for instance, to human health and ecosystem functions. Currently, it is thought that the input of antibiotics in general as well as from hospitals seems to be of minor importance, at least in terms of resistance. Up to now, antibiotics have not been detected in drinking water. The impact of antibiotics present in the aquatic environment on the frequency of resistance transfer is questionable. The information available to date suggests that the input of resistant bacteria into the environment from different sources seems to be the most important source of resistance in the environment. Therefore, the prudent use of antibiotics and disinfectants will significantly reduce the risk for the general public and for the environment. This not only means limiting the duration of selective pressure by reducing the treatment period and the continuous use of sub-therapeutical concentrations, but also includes controlling the dissemination of antibiotics being used, as well as prudent monitoring of resistance. However, a full environmental risk assessment cannot be performed on the basis of the data available; the availability of such data is a prerequisite if proper risk assessment and risk management programs for both humans and the environment are to be undertaken. Therefore, the careful use of antibiotics and the restriction of their input into the aquatic environment are the matters of necessity.

8. References

Aarestrup, F.M.,. Wegener, H.C., & Collignon, P. 2008. Resistance in bacteria of the food chain: epidemiology and control strategies. Expert Review of Anti-Infective Therapy. 6(5): p. 733-50.

Alanis, A.J. 2005. Resistance to Antibiotics: Are We in the Post-Antibiotic Era? Archives of Medical Research 36, 697-705.

Baltz, R. H. 2008. Renaissance in antibacterial discovery from actinomycetes. Current Opinion in Pharmacology. 8, 557–563.

Benveniste R, & Davies J. 1973. Mechanisms of antibiotic resistance in bacteria. Annual Review of Biochemistry. 42:471-506.

Bian, J., Song, F. & Zhang, L. 2008. Strategies on the construction of high-quality microbial natural product library. A review. Wei Sheng Wu Xue Bao 48, 1132–1137.

Bjorklund, H, Bergh, R.B., CMI, & Bylund, G. 1991. Residues of oxolinicacid and oxytetracycline in fish and sediments from fish farms. Thesis, Bjdrklund, H.

Oxytetracycline and oxolinic acid as antibacterials in aquaculture analysis, pharmacokinetics and environmental impacts. Department of Biology, Abe Akademi University, Finland.

Björkman, J., Nagaev, I., Berg, O.G., Hughes, D., & Andersson, D.I. 2000. Effects of Environment on Compensatory Mutations to Ameliorate Costs of Antibiotic Resistance. Science 287, 1479-1482.

Bluhm, H.M., Boyd, J.W., Muirhead, C.R., Tarr, H.L. 1956. Use of antibiotics for the preservation of fish and sea foods. American Journal of Public Health Nations Health. 46(12):1531-9.

Bonaventura, C., & Johnson, F.M. 2004. Healthy Environments for Healthy People. EHPS. Vol 1/105. Environmental Health Perspectives.

Boyd, J.W., & Tarr, H.L.A., 1956. Effect of chlortetracycline and storage temperatures on quality of shucked oysters. fishery research. Bd. Canada, Prog. Rep. Pacific coast stas., No. 105: 12-13.

Boyd, J.W., Bissett, H.M., & Tarr, H.L.A., 1955. Further observations on the distribution of chlortetracycline throughout ice blocks. Ibid. No. 102-14-15.

Browning, C.H., & Gulbransen, R., 1936. Immunity following cure of experimental Trypanosoma brucei infection by a chemotherapeutic agent. The Journal of Pathology and Bacteriology 43, 479-486.

Capone, D.G., Weston, D.P., Miller, V., & Shoemaker, C., 1996. Antibacterial residues in marine sediments and invertebrates following chemotherapy in aquaculture. Aquaculture 145, 55-75.

Castro, S.B.R., Leal, C.A.G., Freire, F.R., Carvalho, D.A., Oliveira, D.F., & Figueiredo, H.C.P. 2008. Antibacterial activity of plant extracts from Brazil against fish pathogenic bacteria. Brazilian Journal of Microbiology.39. No. 4. doi: 10.1590/S1517-83822008000400030

Chopra, I., & Roberts, M., 2001. Tetracycline Antibiotics: Mode of Action, Applications, Molecular Biology, and Epidemiology of Bacterial Resistance. Microbiology and Molecular Biology Reviews. 65, 232-260.

Costanzo, S.D., Murby, J., & Bates, J. 2005. Ecosystem response to antibiotics entering the aquatic environment. Marine Pollution Bulletin 51, 218-223.

Demain, A.L., & Sanchez, S., 2009. Microbial drug discovery: 80 years of progress. Journal of Antibiotics. 62, 5-16.

Doern, G.V., Heilmann, K.P., Huynh, H.K., Rhomberg, P.R., Coffman, S.L., & Brueggemann, A.B., 2001. Antimicrobial Resistance among Clinical Isolates of Streptococcus pneumoniae in the United States during 1999-2000, Including a Comparison of Resistance Rates since 1994-1995. Antimicrobial Agents Chemotheraphy. 45, 1721-1729.

Dolliver, H.A., & Gupta, S.C., 2008. Antibiotic losses from unprotected manure stockpiles. Journal of Environmental Quality. 37, 1238-1244.

Edquist, L.E., & Pedersen, K.B. 2001. Antimicrobials as growth promoters: resistance to common sense. In: Harremoës, P. (Chairman), Gee, D. (EEA Ed.), MacGarvin, M. (Executive Ed.), Stirling, A., Keys, J., Wynne, B., Guedes Vas, S. (Eds.), Late lesson From Early Warnings: The Precautionary Principle 1896–2000. Environmental Issue Report No. 22, European Environment Agency, Copenhagen, pp. 93–109.

EJF. 2003. Risky Business: Vietnamese Shrimp Aquaculture — Impacts and Improvements. London, UK7 Environmental Justice Foundation. pp. 44.

FAAIR, Policy recommendations. Clinical Infectious Diseases, 2002. 34 Suppl 3: p. 76-87.

Ferenci T. 2008. Bacterial physiology, regulation and mutational adaptation in a chemostat environment. Advances in Microbial Physiology. 53:169-229.

Gillespie, D.C., Boyd, J.W., Bissett, H.M., & Tarr, H.L.A., 1955. Ices containing chlortetracycline in experimental fish preservation. Ibid. 9:296-300.

Hare, R. 1970. The Birth of Penicillin, Allen & Unwin, London.

Hatha, M., Vivekanandhan, A.A., Julie Joice, G., & Christol, 2005. Antibiotic resistance pattern of motile aeromonads from farm raised fresh water fish. International Journal of Food Microbiology 98, 131-134.

Hektoen, H., Berge, J.A., Hormazabal, V., & Yndestad, M., 1995. Persistence of antibacterial agents in marine sediments. Aquaculture 133, 175-184.

Helms, M., Vastrup, P., Gerner-Smidt, P., & Molbak, K. 2002. Excess Mortality Associated with Antimicrobial Drug-Resistant SalmonellaTyphimurium. Emerging Infectious Diseases. 8(5):490-495.

Hernando, M.D., Mezcua, M., Fernández-Alba, A.R., & Barceló, D., 2006. Environmental risk assessment of pharmaceutical residues in wastewater effluents, surface waters and sediments. Talanta 69, 334-342.

Herwig, R.P., Gray, J.P., & Weston, D.P., 1997. Antibacterial resistant bacteria in surficial sediments near salmon net-cage farms in Puget Sound, Washington. Aquaculture 149, 263-283.

Hirsch, R., Ternes, T., Haberer, K., & Kratz, K.L., 1999. Occurrence of antibiotics in the aquatic environment. The Science of The Total Environment 225, 109-118.

Holmström, K., Gräslund, S., Wahlström, A., Poungshompoo, S., Bengtsson, B.E., & Kautsky, N., 2003. Antibiotic use in shrimp farming and implications for environmental impacts and human health. International Journal of Food Science & Technology 38, 255-266.

ICON, 2003. Antibiotics: A Medical Dictionary, Bibliography, and Annotated Research Guide to Internet References. San Diego, CA: ICON Health Publications, 2003. http://www.answers.com/topic/antibiotic#ixzz1SzZAoJuz

IM, 1989. Institute of Medicine. Human health risks with the subtherapeutic use of penicillin or tetracyclines in animal feed. 1989. Washington, D.C.: National Academy Press.

Ingram, M., Barnes,E., & Shewan, J.M., 1956. Problems in the use of antibiotics for preserving meat and fish. Food science abstracts 28: 121-136.

Jalal, K.C.A., Fatin, Mardiana, Akbar John, B., Kamaruzzaman, Y.B., & Mohd. Nor. 2010. Antibiotic Resistance Microbes in Tropical Mangrove Sediments, East Coast Peninsular Malaysia. African Journal of Microbiology Research Vol. 4 (8), pp. 640-645

Jensen, L.B., Baloda, S., Boye, M., & Aarestrup, F.M., 2001. Antimicrobial resistance among Pseudomonas spp. and the Bacillus cereus group isolated from Danish agricultural soil. Environment International 26, 581-587.

Khachatourians, G.G., 1998. Agricultural use of antibiotics and the evolution and transfer of antibiotic-resistant bacteria. Canadian Medical Association Journal 159, 1129-1136.

Knight, V., Sanglier, J.J., DiTullio, D., Braccili, S., Bonner, P., Waters, J., Hughes, D., & Zhang, L., 2003. Diversifying microbial natural products for drug discovery. Applied Microbiology and Biotechnology 62, 446-458.

Kuijper, M.W.M., 2003. Marine and coastal environmental awareness building within the context of UNESCO's activities in Asia and the Pacific. Marine Pollution Bulletin 47, 265-272.

Kumar, K., Gupta, S., Chander, Y., Singh, A.K., 2005. Antibiotic Use in Agriculture and Its Impact on the Terrestrial Environment, in: Donald, L.S. (Ed.), Advances in Agronomy. Academic Press, pp. 1-54.

Kümmerer, K., 2003. Significance of antibiotics in the environment. Journal of Antimicrobial Chemotherapy 52, 5-7.

Kümmerer, K., 2009a. Antibiotics in the aquatic environment - A review - Part I. Chemosphere 75, 417-434.

Kümmerer, K., 2009b. Antibiotics in the aquatic environment - A review - Part II. Chemosphere 75, 435-441.

Lai, H.T., Liu, S.M. & Chieln, Y.H. 1995. Transformation of chloramphenicol and oxytetracycline in aquaculture pond sediments. Journal of Environmental Science and Health, Part A. Toxic / Hazardous Substances and Environmental Engineering. A30:1987–1993.

Le Tuan Xuan, Munekage Yukihiro, Phan Dao Anh Thi, Quan Dao & Quynh Thi. 2003. The environmental quality of shrimp ponds in mangrove areas. Proceedings of the Thirteenth (2003) International Offshore and Polar Engineering Conference Honolulu, HI, USA, May25 – 30; ISSN: 1098-6189 (set) 1-880653-60-5 (set). p. 255–262.

Levy, S. B. 2002. The antibiotic paradox: How the misuse of antibiotics destroys their curative powers. Cambridge: Perseus Publishing.

Li, X, & Nikadio H. 2009. Efflux-mediated drug resistance in bacteria: an update. Drug 69 (12): 1555–623.

Lu, S.Y., Zhang, Y.L., Geng, S.N., Li, T.Y., Ye, Z. M., Zhang, D.S., Zou, F., & Zhou, H.W., 2010. High Diversity of Extended-Spectrum Beta-Lactamase-Producing Bacteria in an Urban River Sediment Habitat. Applied Environmental Microbiology. 76, 5972-5976.

Marengo, J.R., Kok, R.A., O'Brien, K., Velagaleti, R.R., & Stamm, J.M., 1997. Aerobic biodegradation of (14C)-sarafloxacin hydrochloride in soil. Environmental Toxicology and Chemistry 16, 462-471.

Martinez, J.L., & Baquero, F., 2000. Mutation Frequencies and Antibiotic Resistance. Antimicrobial Agents Chemotheraphy. 44, 1771-1777.

McDonald, L.C., Rossiter, S., Mackinson, C., Wang, Y.Y., Johnson, S., Sullivan, M., Sokolow, R., DeBess, E., Gilbert, L., Benson, J.A., Hill, B. & Angulo, F.J. 2001. Quinupristin-Dalfopristin resistant *Enterococcus faecium* on chicken and in human stool specimens. New England Journal of Medicine. 345(16):1155-60.

McGowan Jr, J.E. 2001. Economic Impact of Antimicrobial Resistance. Emerging Infectious Diseases. 7(2):286-292.

McPhearson, R.M., DePaola, A., Zywno, S.R., Motes Jr, M.L., & Guarino, A.M., 1991. Antibiotic resistance in Gram-negative bacteria from cultured catfish and aquaculture ponds. Aquaculture 99, 203-211.

Miranda, C.D., & Zemelman, R., 2002. Bacterial resistance to oxytetracycline in Chilean salmon farming. Aquaculture 212, 31-47.

Neela, F., Nonaka, L., Rahman, M., & Suzuki, S., 2009. Transfer of the chromosomally encoded tetracycline resistance gene *tet* (M) from marine bacteria to; *Escherichia coli* and; *Enterococcus faecalis*. World Journal of Microbiology and Biotechnology 25, 1095-1101.

NIAID, 2006. The problem of antimicrobial resistance. National Institute of Allergy and Infectious Diseases, Division of Microbiology and Infectious Diseases, www.niaid.nih.gov/dmid/antimicrob

Nicolaou, K.C. 2001. A close look at the inner workings of microbes in the era of escalating antibiotic resistance is offering new strategies for designing drugs. Scientific American 2001; Vol 284: p 54-61.

Nygaard, K., Lunestad, B.T., Hektoen, H., Berge, J.A., & Hormazabal, V., 1992. Resistance to oxytetracycline, oxolinic acid and furazolidone in bacteria from marine sediments. Aquaculture 104, 31-36.

Olapade, O.A., Depas, M.M., Jensen, E.T., & McLellan, S.L., 2006. Microbial Communities and Fecal Indicator Bacteria Associated with Cladophora Mats on Beach Sites along Lake Michigan Shores. Applied Environmental Microbiology. 72, 1932-1938.

Perreten, V., Schwarz, F., Cresta, L., Boeglin, M., Dasen, G., & Teuber, M., 1997. Antibiotic resistance spread in food. Nature. 389, 801-802.

Pouliquen, H., & Le Bris, H., 1996. Sorption of oxolinic acid and oxytetracycline to marine sediments. Chemosphere 33, 801-815.

Prior, L.S.O.S., 2008. The 2008 Garrod Lecture: Antimicrobial resistance—animals and the environment. Journal of Antimicrobial Chemotherapy 62, 229-233.

Reynolds, D., 2010. Modern Medicine and The Overuse Of Antibiotics. http://www.healthytheory.com/modern-medicine-and-the-overuse-of-antibiotics

Russell, A.D. 2003. Biocide use and antibiotic resistance: the relevance of laboratory findings to clinical environmental situations. Lancet Infectious Disease. 3:794-803.

Russell, A.D., 1990. Mechanisms of bacterial resistance to biocides. International Biodeterioration 26, 101-110.

Russell, A.D., 1995. Mechanisms of bacterial resistance to biocides. International Biodeterioration & Biodegradation 36, 247-265.

Samuelsen, O.B., Torsvik, V., & Ervik, A., 1992. Long-range changes in oxytetracycline concentration and bacterial resistance towards oxytetracycline in a fish farm sediment after medication. Science of The Total Environment 114, 25-36.

SCENIHR, 2009. Scientific Committee on Emerging and Newly Identified Health Risks. Assessment of the Antibiotic Resistance Effects of Biocides. European Commission. pp.1-87.

Schmidt, A.S., Bruun, M.S., Dalsgaard, I., Pedersen, K., & Larsen, J.L., 2000. Occurrence of Antimicrobial Resistance in Fish-Pathogenic and Environmental Bacteria Associated with Four Danish Rainbow Trout Farms. Applied Environmental Microbiology. 66, 4908-4915.

Serrano, P.H. 2005.. Responsible use of antibiotics in aquaculture. In: Food and Agriculture Organization (FAO) Fisheries Technical Paper, 469, Roma, 97 p.

Sheldon, A.T. Jr. 2005.Antiseptic "resistance": real or perceived threat? Clinical Infectious Diseases. 40:1650-6.

Shoemaker, N.B., Vlamakis, H., Hayes, K., & Salyers, A.A., 2001. Evidence for Extensive Resistance Gene Transfer among Bacteroides spp. and among Bacteroides and Other Genera in the Human Colon. Applied Environmental Microbiology. 67, 561-568.

Singer, R.S., Finch, R., Wegener, H.C., Bywater, R., Walters, J., Lipsitch, M., 2003. Antibiotic resistance--the interplay between antibiotic use in animals and human beings. The Lancet Infectious Diseases 3, 47-51.

Steiner, G., & Tarr, H.L.A., 1955. Transport and storage of fish in refrigerated sea water: II. Bacterial spoilage of blue black salmon in refrigerated sea water and in ice, with and without assed chlortetracycline. Fish research Bd. Canada, Prog. Rep. pacific coast sras, No: 104: 7-8.

Tarr, H.L.A., & Deas, C.P., 1948. Action of sulpha compounds, antibiotics and nitrite on growth of bacteria in fish and flesh. Journal of fishery research. Bd. Canada. 7: 221-223.

Tarr, H.L.A., 1944. Chemical Inhibition of Growth of Fish Spoilage Bacteria. Journal of the Fisheries Research Board of Canada 6c, 257-266.

Tarr, H.L.A., Boyd, J.W., & Bissett, H.M., 1954. Antibiotics in food processing. Experimental preservation of fish and beef with antibiotiocs. Journal of Agriculture Food chemistry. 2: 372-375.

Tarr, H.L.A., Southcott, B.A., & Bissett, H.M., 1950. Effect of several antibiotics and food preservatives in retarding bacterial spoilage of fish. Fish. Res. Bd, Canada, Prog. Rep. pacific coast stas. No. 83:35-38.

Tendencia, E.A., & Dela Peña, L.D., 2002. Level and percentage recovery of resistance to oxytetracycline and oxolinic acid of bacteria from shrimp ponds. Aquaculture 213, 1-13.

Tolls, J., 2001. Sorption of Veterinary Pharmaceuticals in Soils: A Review. Environmental Science & Technology 35, 3397-3406.

Tomiyama, T., Nomura, M., & Kuroki,S. 1955. Effectiveness of aureomycin on keeping quality of sardine. Bulletin of Japanese society of scientific fisheries. 21: 262-266.

USEPA, 2002. Environmental and Economic Benefit Analysis of Final Revisions to the National Pollutant Discharge Elimination System Regulation and the Effluent Guidelines for Concentrated Animal Feeding Operations. EPA 821-R-03-003. USEPA Office of Water, Washington, DC.

Wagner-Döbler, I., Beil, W., Lang, S., Meiners, M., Laatsch, H., 2002. Integrated Approach To Explore the Potential of Marine Microorganisms for the Production of Bioactive Metabolites, in: Schügerl, K., Zeng, A.P., Aunins, J., Bader, A., Bell, W., Biebl, H., Biselli, M., Carrondo, M., Castilho, L., Chang, H., Cruz, P., Fuchs, C., Han, S., Han, M.R., Heinzle, E., Hitzmann, B., Köster, D., Jasmund, I., Jelinek, N., Lang, S., Laatsch, H., Lee, J., Miirkl, H., Maranga, L., Medronho, R., Meiners, M., Nath, S., Noll, T., Scheper, T., Schmidt, S., Schüigerl, K., Stäirk, E., Tholey, A., Wagner-Döbler, I., Wandrey, C., Wittmann, C., & Yim, S.C. (Eds.), Tools and Applications of Biochemical Engineering Science. Springer Berlin / Heidelberg, pp. 207-238.

Wainwright, M. 1988. Selman A.Waksman and the streptomycin controversy. Soc.gen. Microbial. Quarterly, 15: 90-92

Walsh, C. 2003. Antibiotics – Action, Origin, Resistance. ASM Press, Washington, D.C.

Weston, D.P. 1996. Environmental considerations in the use of antibacterial drugs in aquaculture. In: Baird D, Beveridge M, Kelly L,Muir J, editors. Aquaculture and Water Resources Management. Black-well Science; 140–65.

Witter, L.D., 1961. Psychrophilic Bacteria--A Review. Journal of Dairy Science 44, 983-1015.

World Health Organization 2003. Dept. of Communicable Disease Prevention Control and Eradication., Danish Veterinary Institute., and Danmarks jordbrugs forskning, Impacts of antimicrobial growth promoter termination in Denmark : the WHO international review panel' s evaluation of the termination of the use of antimicrobial growth promoters in Denmark : Foulum, Denmark 6-9, Geneva: World Health Organization. 57 p.

Zhang, L., An, R., Wang, J., Sun, N., Zhang, S., Hu, J., & Kuai, J., 2005. Exploring novel bioactive compounds from marine microbes. Current Opinion in Microbiology 8, 276-281.

7

Biofilms: A Survival and Resistance Mechanism of Microorganisms

Castrillón Rivera Laura Estela and Palma Ramos Alejandro
Universidad Autónoma Metropolitana, Departamento de Sistemas Biológicos,
México

1. Introduction

Biofilms are microbial monoespecie or multispecie (consortium) communities that are the most successful colonization among microorganisms, are ubiquitous in nature and responsible for many diseases. They are considered growing communities of microorganisms embedded in a self-produced exopolysaccharide matrix and are attached to an inert surface or living tissue (Castrillón et al., 2010).

It is believed that this organization represents the mode of cell growth that allows cells to survive in hostile environments, disperse to form new niches and gives them significant advantages in protection against environmental fluctuations such as humidity, temperature, pH, the concentration of nutrients and waste removal (Costerton et al., 1987, Hall-Stoodley et al., 2004).

There is an association between the presence of biofilm-grown microorganisms with delayed wound healing and various diseases such as endocarditis, otitis media, chronic prostatitis, cystic fibrosis, periodontitis, and related infections medical devices and implants responsible for nosocomial infections (Castrillón et al., 2011, Donlan & Costerton, 2002). The latter share common features, although the causative organism and the site of infection are very different, they all evade host defenses and resist treatment with antimicrobials. In general, bacteria in biofilms tolerate high levels of antibiotics compared with planktonic cells (free). The ability of biofilm formation is not restricted to any specific group of bacteria or fungus and is now considered that under ideal conditions all microorganisms can form biofilms (Lasa et al., 2005).

2. Stages of development of biofilms

The main experimental models for studying bacterial biofilms are four: *Escherichia coli, Psedomonas aeruginosa, Bacillus subtilis and Staphylococcus aureus* (Lopez et al., 2010) and fungi *Candida albicans* and *Aspergillus fumigatus* (Kumamoto, 2002, Müller et al. 2011). In these works describes the development of a biofilm which begins with planktonic bacteria (free) that bind irreversibly to a surface in a continuous process in accordance with various stages of development are:, b) adhesion, c) synthesis of extracellular matrix, d) maturation and e) dispersion, which leads to the formation of a uniform structure of deposits and accumulations of viscous and homogeneous material surrounding the cells by a polymer matrix with open channels for water movement (Figure 1).

Any natural or synthetic surface is covered by the constituents of the local environment, electrolytes, water and organic materials form a film before the arrival of the organism which neutralize the charge over the surface (conditioning) that prevents the aproximation between bacterial cells fungi and so begins adherence, these organic compounds can serve as nutrients for these microorganisms.

Free (or planktonic) cells form a layer that is adsorbed to the surface for short periods by electrostatic attraction forces and released from it by reversible adsorption (Bos et al., 1999). In this phase the microorganisms are still susceptible to action of antibiotics.

The microorganisms in suspension are aggregated and cell adhesion occurs with same or different cells (co-aggregation) to the surface conditioned, this process is favored by several bacterial components involved in this process by overcoming the repulsive forces such as pili or flagella, and surface polymers such as lipopolysaccharide in Gram-negative bacteria and mycolic acid in Gram-positive. The expression of these microbial structures may change depending on the environment in which they are and thus change the phase of biofilm formation. Mutants no-mobile fail to form monolayers and their union as microcolonies therefore mobility structures play an important role in the initiation of biofilm (Stickler, 1999).

The physicochemical properties of the surface can exert a strong influence on the degree and extention of adherence, the germs adhere more readily to hydrophobic surfaces, non-polarized and plastics such as Teflon, compared to hydrophilic metals such as glass or metal.

Once irreversible adhesion is achieved, the cells divide and colonize the surface and when the local concentration of chemical signals produced by microbial metabolism reaches a threshold level, suggesting that the microbial population density has reached a minimum, this determines the start of phenotypic changes in the community.

The process in which a microbial cell senses the proximity of other cells reaching a critical number in a limited space in the environment, chemical signals are generated corresponding to secondary metabolites, known as *quorum sensing*, this fact results in the autoinduction in the synthesis of the extracellular matrix or exopolysaccharide (composed of polysaccharides, proteins, nucleic acids and lipids), and thus gets to the maturation of biofilm formation with subsequent three-dimensional structure, generated by water channels that serve as the microcirculation in colonies. When the message is large enough, the organism responds like a mass and behaves as a group (Keller & Surette, 2006). The composition of the exopolysaccharide or glycocalyx is different for each bacteria and fungus, and varies depending on culture conditions, medium and substrates which are: alginate in *P. aeruginosa*, cellulose in *S. typhimurium*, rich in galactose in *V. cholerae* and poly-N-acetylglucosamine in *S. aureus* (Whitehead et al., 2001, Sutherland 1997). This matrix allows the interconnection of immobilized cells and acts as a digestive system that keeps external extracellular enzymes close to the cells and enables them to metabolize biopolymers and colloidal solids (Sauer et al., 2002, Flemming & Wingender, 2010).

The detachment may be seen as another stage of the life cycle of the biofilm, which can be reached or not depending on environmental conditions such as nutrient availability, oxygenation, pH and specific compounds because at some point the high density cell can result in severe, dynamic gradients of nutrients and toxic metabolic sub-products, then some cells are released from the matrix to colonize other surfaces closing the process of formation and development of biofilms, this process may be the result of several factors such as are: mechanical forces as the flow of blood vessel, cessation of production of exopolysaccharides and detachment factors such as enzymes that destroy the matrix or surfactants.

Fragments of biofilm with viable cells can be dispersed in liquids or aerosols. The scattering process is of interest for their potential to promote the spread of bacteria or fungi in the ambient or their ability to exploit these processes to combat infections (Hall-Stoodley & Stoodley, 2005).

For the development cycle of *Candida albicans* biofilms has shown that scattered cells show a distinct phenotype associated with increased virulence (Uppuluri et al., 2010). When the extracellular medium accumulates enough of these molecules activate specific receptors that alter gene expression and affect different phenotypes that produce virulence factors such as enzymes and toxins or rhamnolipid of *P. aeruginosa* cell that are protective of fagocytosis, the *quorum sensing* determines tolerance to antibiotics and innate inflammatory response dependent on polymorphonuclear cells.

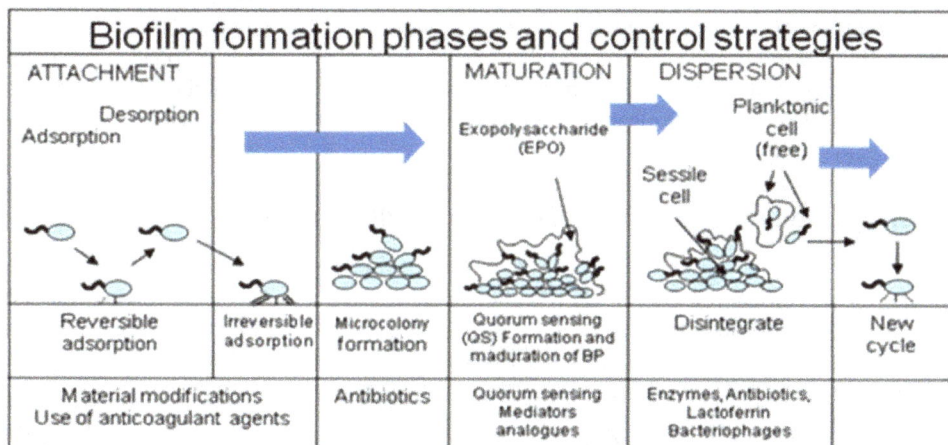

Biofilm formation phases and control strategies

ATTACHMENT			MATURATION	DISPERSION	
Reversible adsorption	Irreversible adsorption	Microcolony formation	Quorum sensing (QS) Formation and maduration of BP	Disintegrate	New cycle
Material modifications Use of anticoagulant agents		Antibiotics	Quorum sensing Mediators analogues	Enzymes, Antibiotics, Lactoferrin Bacteriophages	

Biofilm formation occurs as a series of sequential events that depend on the interaction of microorganisms on inert surfaces or living, by overcoming the repulsive forces to achieve irreversible adsorption followed by the formation of a microcolony. Upon reaching a certain population density, induce the synthesis of secondary metabolites (*quorum sensing*) that produces an exopolysaccharide formation until maturation of the biofilm. Disintegration allows the formation of a new colony or elimination. It shows the treatment options for different stages of biofilm development.

Fig. 1. Phases of biofilm formation and dispersal strategies.

The main characteristic that best distinguishes chronic infections associated with biofilm to acute infections is their response to treatment with antibiotics, in general biofilm microorganisms tolerate high levels of antibiotics compared to planktonic cells and cause recurrent episodes. In the case of acute infections these are eliminated after a short treatment. In addition, acute infections are more aggressive than those associated with chronic infections or implants as the latter persist for months or years and progress through periods of rest alternating with exacerbations.

3. Host resistance to biofilm

Biofilms cause chronic infections characterized by persistent inflammation and tissue damage despite treatment with antibiotics and innate and adaptive immune responses of the host.

Planktonic cells that are released directly from the biofilm was removed by the action of antibiotics and phagocytic cells activated, but the organization as a biofilm is considered as a very efficient defensive strategy adopted since these microorganisms grow slowly and are protected mechanisms of host resistance through various strategies among which are a) inability of antibodies, complement and lysozyme to penetrate these organizations multicellular b) production of catalase bacteria that prevents the action of hydrogen peroxide produced by oxidative mechanisms of phagocytic cells c) inhibition of host immune function such as chemotaxis, opsonization and bactericidal potential exopolysaccharide (Lasa et al., 2005).

A study has demonstrated inability of the immune system clearance sessile cells that persist for weeks and months was observed when the peritoneal cavity of rabbits were inoculated mature biofilms of *P. aeruginosa* in immunocompetent animals, the penetration of phagocytic cells in the biofilm was detected, however, these cells were unable to phagocytose the bacteria (Ward et al., 1992). A similar response was described with the inoculation of fragments of the same biofilm bacteria trapped in agar beads and introduced into the lung (Woods et al., 1980).

4. Identification tests and antibiotic susceptibility in biofilms

In clinical samples, a biofilm is difficult to detect in routine diagnosis but may be recognized by light microscopy and accurate identification of bacteria in a biofilm can only be done by techniques of hybridization, fluorescein staining, the molecular probe 16SRNA domain eubacteria (EUB 338), determining live cell / dead BacLight staining or by identifying the matrix components by specialized staining techniques (Veeh et al., 2003).

Routine microbial cultures provide misleading results because they do not reflect the increasing resistance of bacteria growing in biofilms. The minimum inhibitory concentration (MIC) of bacteria grown as biofilm is 100 to 1000 times higher compared to planktonic cells despite antibiotic susceptibility in the laboratory (Costerton et al., 1999).

There are no standardized methods to date used routinely to determine the antibiotic sensitivity of bacteria grown as biofilms. When sampling swab and plating growth obtained in cultures performed standardized susceptibility testing, these same antibiotics fail to solve conventional bacterial infections This is because bacteria grow attached and the surface as a biofilm. However, in many cases it is not possible to recover the bacteria by traditional culture methods. This has been reported in infections where *Staphyococcus* biofilms emerging vascular grafts stimulate the production of antibodies against biofilms initiated within 10 days of colonization, however, cells were never recovered by conventional techniques of microbial culture (Costerton al ., 2003), another case is related to infections in medical devices where antibiograms shown susceptibility against some microorganisms but the infection fails to be eliminated by these antibiotics (Fux et al., 2005).

It is very important to point out that the systems sensitivity to antibiotics were traditionally performed on cells in suspension, which is equivalent to the population of planktonic cells, for this reason, is necessary to design new laboratory techniques that reveal the sensitivity of these substances directly on biofilms, this idea has been reported that antibiotics active against stationary phase bacteria *in vitro* are successful in removing biofilms *in vitro* infections (Zimmerli et al., 1998).

This information is important to consider that when it is mentioned that biofilm infection has hematogenous dissemination must specify if they are planktonic cells or biofilm fragments because there are differences in their ability to resist antibiotics, adherence and host response resistance.

5. Horizontal gene transfer

Mobile elements such as plasmids and transposons, have proven important in the transfer of antibiotic resistance is enhanced when the cell density increases and competition genetic, hence that biofilms are an ideal state to promote the horizontal transfer of genes (Ghigo, 2001). However, there is evidence that when bacteria of a biofilm is dispersed is rapidly becoming susceptible so their resistance is not the result of mutations and mobile elements (Stewart & Costerton, 2001, Stewart, 2002).

Increasing resistance to beta-lactams, aminoglycosides and fluoroquinolones has been correlated to the frequency of mutations in bacteria that grow as biofilms (Hoiby et al., 2010). These facts lead to rapid and global spread of genes in natural environments and in hospitals favoring nosocomial infections associated with biofilms.

6. Mechanisms of resistance associated with biofilms

The conventional mechanisms of resistance to antibiotics and biocides fall into four categories: direct inactivation of the active molecule, altering the body's sensitivity by changing its target of action, reducing the concentration of the drug reaches its target unchanged its chemical composition and efflux systems (Hogan & Kolter, 2002, Poole 2002). However, most information comes from studies that were performed in suspension cultures and in general, bacteria in biofilms tolerate high levels of antibiotics compared to what their planktonic cells. In different settings, the level of antibiotic resistance may vary and the factors causing this increase may differ.

The primary evidence indicates that conventional mechanisms do not explain the high resistance to antimicrobial agents associated with biofilms, although this evidence does not exclude the possibility of resistance in the growth of adherent cells. This suggests that the development of resistance in bacteria that are aggregated on surfaces or biofilm has its own intrinsic mechanisms are different and are responsible for those conventional antibiotic resistance, and although currently no single accepted mechanism, we have explored several potential candidates as responsible for this high resistance characteristic of biofilms among which are: Diffusion limited, neutralizing enzymatic, functional heterogeneity, slow growth, persistent cells and biofilm phenotype corresponding to adaptive mechanisms to stress such as efflux pumps and alterations in membrane. (Figure 2).

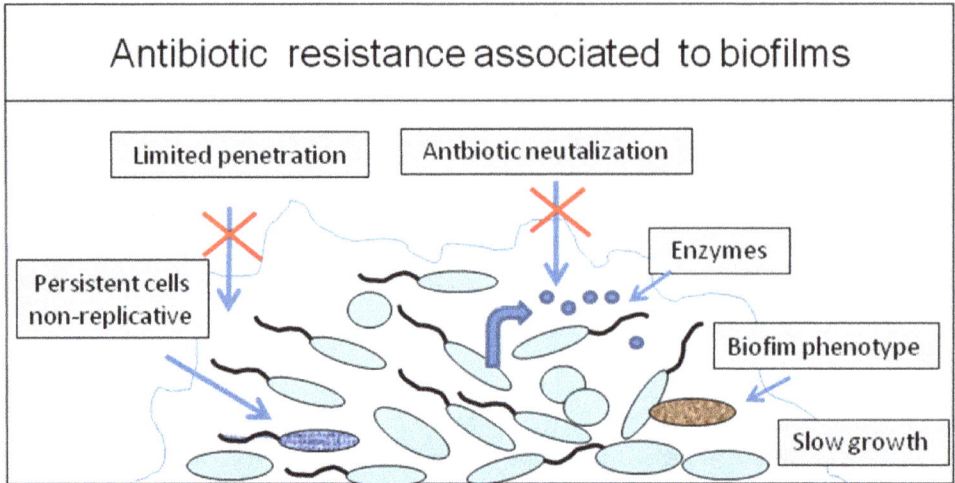

The antibiotic may be retained by interactions with the extracellular matrix or be neutralized by the production of enzymes that modify it. The metabolic heterogeneity may alter the growth preventing antibiotic action if its molecular target requires active metabolic pathways, or the oxygenation or pH gradients inhibit the action of the antimicrobial. The appearance of persistent or phenotype within biofilm makes it insensitive to the antibiotic

Fig. 2. Antibiotic resistance associate to biofilms.

6.1 Low penetration

Antibiotics can diffuse through the biofilm matrix, to inactivate the cells trapped, but this exopolysaccharide behaves as a physical barrier affecting its spread to deeper layers by direct interaction of these molecules to modify their transport to the interior, causes resistance to these antimicrobials, as well as high molecular weight molecules with cytotoxic properties as lysozyme and complement. So, while planktonic cells are quickly exposed to high concentrations of antibiotics, the microorganisms in deep layers are gradually exposed to increasing the concentration of antibiotics.

Bacteria that are deficient in polysaccharide synthesis and therefore of produce biofilm, escape from the biofilm and are susceptible to attack by immunocompetent cells. An antibiotic may be inactivated or sequestered by binding to the extracellular matrix as in the case of the alginate exopolysaccharide of *P. aeruginosa* which is anionic nature. Which explains why the fluoroquinolones and aminoglycosides penetrate slowly rapidly since the latter positively charged bind to the matrix has a negative charge, but this mechanism can be saturated if repeated doses are administrated (Lewis, 2001, Gordon et al. , 1988, Mah & O'Toole, 2001).

The penetration of chlorine does not reach concentrations greater than 20% in mixed cultures of *K. pneumoniae* and *P. aeruginosa* biofilms. In case of biofilms of *S. epidermidis* vancomycin reaches deep layers but not rifampin (Mah & O'Toole, 2001).

Has also been observed that the thickness of the biofilm is important for the penetration of hydrogen peroxide was allowed in layers with 3.5 log CFU *P. aeuroginosa* and not diffusion when the layer was 7.6 log CFU, however, the absence of catalase gene (kata) makes it easy access even if the biofilm is thick (Stewart et al., 2000).

The dissemination and death from alkaline hypochlorite (pH 11) and chlorosulphamate (pH 5.5) was evaluated on biofilms of *P. aeruginosa*. The chlorosulfamate transport was not affected unlike hypochlorite delaying their penetration, however both biocides enter to the biofilm and fail to kill cells suggesting an alternative mechanism to explain the resistance to these substances (Stewart et al., 2001).

Other explanations for the failure to altering the penetration of antimicrobial agents in biofilms *K. pneumoniae* are that the cells are stacked or is the result of problems of bioavailability of the drug (Smith, 2005).

Reduced mobility of an antibiotic is not an impenetrable barrier and is not sufficient to explain the resistance, it is assumed that other mechanisms must be involved. Recently it has been suggested that the delay in permeability through the biofilm allows the bacteria have enough time to implement adaptive responses to stress.

6.2 Neutralization

If an antibiotic penetrates the biofilm enzyme production by microorganisms can degrade or modify are synthesized by enzymes that selectively destroy the activity of antibiotics. These enzymes are a series of proteins that use multiple adaptive strategies to confer resistance such as hydrolysis (β-lactams, macrolide esterases epoxidase) and modification of antibiotics by acyltransferases, phosphorylation, glycosylation, nucleotidilación, ribosylation and transfer of thiol groups (Wright, 2005, Castrillón et al., 2003, Gallant et al., 2005, Martinez-Suarez et al., 1985). These enzymes accumulate in the glycocalyx as a result of its secretion or cell lysis (by action of the antibiotic on the microorganisms from the biofilm surface or planktonic).

Neutralization acts synergistically with delayed diffusion and degradation of the antimicrobial into the biofilm. An important mechanism of resistance in cystic fibrosis by *P. aeruginosa* is due to the overproduction of cephalosporinase AmpC enzymes which is its main mechanism of resistance to beta lactam in the presence of high levels of carbapenems such as imipenem which is a strong inducer in contrast with ceftazidime is weak probably due to its inactivation in the biofilm (Del Valle, 2009, Giwercman, 1991).

The filters impregnated with antibiotics and its direct action on biofilms *K. pneumoniae* has shown that the antibiotic diffuses only in the presence of mutant cells β-lactamases but growth is observed, suggesting that another mechanism of resistance must be considered (Anderl et al., 2000).

6.3 Heterogeneity

To determine the rate of microbial growth within a biofilm microelectrodes were used with probes for direct measurement of oxygen in different areas of the biofilm, and the use of acridine orange to identify fast-growing cells (stained orange) or slow (stained yellow/ green) according to their relative concentration of RNA / DNA. (Mah & O'Toole 2001). These studies demonstrate that biofilms are structurally and metabolically heterogeneous in which aerobic and anaerobic processes occur simultaneously and display areas so that metabolically inactive antimicrobial response may vary depending on the location of an individual cell within the community and that the high level of activity on the surface and limited or absent growth inside reduces the susceptibility to antibiotics.

These studies have shown that biofilms are heterogeneous structures with three chemical patterns that correspond to differences in concentration gradients from outside to inside the biofilm. The pattern of metabolic substrate induces a higher concentration on the outside and less inside, the metabolic product pattern is reversed to the previous and the pattern of metabolic intermediates shows a greater concentration between the boundary of the biofilm in the aqueous phase (Stewart & Franklin , 2008). These patterns bring the result that within these structures are established differences in pH gradients and oxygenation as it has been shown that the penetration of oxygen as high as 25% in the depth of the biofilm (Borriello et al., 2004). These facts are installed microbial populations aerobic or facultative anaerobes within the different layers of the biofilm, allowing us to understand the differences in susceptibility to treatment with antibiotics, which is different from the response to the free forms (plankton) that the attached (sessile).

Deprivation of oxygen and anaerobic growth of microorganisms affects the action of aminoglycosides which is modulated by the availability of oxygen and pH gradients (Wimpenny, 2000).

6.4 Slow growth

When an organism is limited nutrients, slow growing and may cause resistance to antibiotics. Cells within biofilms are under a gradient of nutrients resulting in metabolically active cells with access to these nutrients in the surface layer or on the periphery of the biofilm, in contrast, metabolically inactive cells are found within its interior. These different areas of metabolic activity correspond to different areas of antimicrobial susceptibility

The decrease in growth rate and low metabolic activities decrease the cell permeability and therefore the access of antimicrobial substances, metabolic inactivity can also reach a level where the bacteria are viable but have lost their ability to be cultivated this state of non-culturable viable cells is the main reason for the low detection of biofilm infections by standardized culture methods.

The cytotoxic action of many antibiotics is dependent on the growth of microorganisms such as penicillins that are active are active only in growing cells, many antibiotics are targeting some kind of molecular synthesis and have no effect on bacteria where this synthesis has stopped, and cells in the interior might be protected from the cytotoxic action of these substances (Brown and Allison, 1988). Penicillin and ampicillin do not attack cells that are not growing and its action is proportional to its activity, other antibiotics such as β-lactams, cephalosporins, aminoglycosides and fluoroquinolones attack stationary phase cells, but are more active in dividing cells (Costerton et al., 1999). It has been determined resistance to cetrimide on *E. coli*, ciprofloxacin on *S. epidermidis*, tobramycin and piperacillin in *P. aeruginosa*, this effect is associated with decrease in growth rate (Donlan & Costerton, 2002).

Antimicrobial peptides are natural products produced as part of the arsenal of protection in the host innate responses and target microbial membrane (Castrillón et al., 2007). Colestine peptide (polymyxin E) has been used in the treatment of multidrug-resistant cancer patients and cystic fibrosis by *P. aeruginosa* (Hachem et al., 2007), this antibiotic is the only antimicrobial activity against the central part of biofilms *in vitro*, while the metabolically active at the surface become tolerant due to the regulation system *pmr* operon genes and the MexAB-OprM. Ciprofloxacin and tetracycline are able to clear metabolically active cells so it is suggested that combination therapy with these antibiotics colistin for early eradication of *P. aeruginosa* in patients with cystic fibrosis (Pamp et al., 2008).

6.5 Persistent cells

A small percentage of the cell population remains viable after prolonged exposure (or overdoses) to antibiotics known as persistent, and gives (or not) their resistance to progeny once the selective pressure is removed. This susceptibility to the threshold of growth varies depending on the mode of action of antibiotic used.

Persistent cells are cells that temporarily quit the replication for the survival of the community and their strategy is different from the stress-related adaptive responses in which the population expresses resistance proteins in response to potential environmental damage. Persistent cells survive doses of antibiotics that kill normal cells and increase in number when there is a high cell density reached the highest number in the stationary phase suggesting that their main role is to ensure the survival of cells that are not growing (Lewis 2008).

These cells are different from the antibiotic-resistant mutants do not produce offspring resistant to the antibiotic in his absence and can grow in the presence of the antibiotic while maintaining the same minimum inhibitory concentration (MIC) in contrast to the mutants.

The main evidence of the existence of persistent cells in biofilms are: a) there is a biphasic dimension in biofilms wich means that much of the population is attacked fast and another is not affected even with a prolonged course of antibiotics, b) description of gene of persistence (*hip*) that act as regulatory circuits that allow them to enter and leave this state as a protective response, c) bacteriostatic antibiotics inhibit the growth of sensitive cells are those that contribute to persistent cell growth and preservation of biofilm d) when therapy is withdrawn biofilm again reshape (Herrera 2004).

The production of persistent cells in biofilms in bacteria is highest during the stationary phase in planktonic culture of the biofilm, however, in the case of *Candida albicans* their formation occurs only when growth occurs as a biofilm (Spoering & Lewis, 2001).

Although the date is unknown the basics of the physiology of these persistent cells, several genes involved has been described for their generation, including locus have identified three hip (high-level-persistence): A, B and AB control the frequency of this phenotype. The identification of genes and their products may be targets for developing new therapies (Keren et al., 2004).

All *hip* mutant cells produce a thousand times more cells persistent than the wild variant (Moyed & Broderick 1986). The importance of the appearance of these cells determines the success of treatment with antimicrobial use as the minimum bactericidal concentration would kill 99.9% of cells in biofilms, and the remaining would be eliminated by the immune system, without however, the presence of persistent cells limits the removal of the population of microbial cells or in the case of a dysfunction in the patient's immune response may be the cause of recurrent infections.

6.6 Biofilm phenotype

Nutritional starvation and high cell density in a limited space are important features in in the physiology of planktonic cultures reaching stationary phase. Hence the formation of a biofilm represents this natural phase of bacterial growth by increasing production of secondary metabolites such as antibiotics, pigments and other molecules, which act as signaling molecules to form (or inhibition of growth of other microorganisms) of biofilms (Lopez et al., 2010).

The response to environmental stresses such as heat shock, pH changes, oxygen and chemicals among others, cause physiological changes that act as protective antagonizing the harmful effects by inducing protective mechanisms such as efflux pumps of antibiotics, changes membrane level or phase variation.

In biofilms in response to treatment with antibiotics, appear subpopulations with different phenotypes that vary in their gene expression but not in their genetic material (Fux et al, 2005). This was confirmed when performing subcultures in fresh medium in which not only provide nutrients but also dilutes the cell-cell signaling, the cells regain susceptibility to the antibiotic, demonstrating the absence of mutations.

The gene expression patterns in biofilms of *P. aeruginosa* produce different phenotypes that differ from their planktonic counterparts (Sauer et al., 2002) and a small proportion of cells develop a protective phenotype that coexists with the cells sensitive to antibiotics and has been suggested by some authors that corresponds to that expressed by a spore (Stewart & Costerton, 2001).

A biofilm community that shows resistance to treatment by antibiotics and develops a characteristic phenotype such as biofilm growth has been called "biofilm phenotype" and have come to propose the existence of specific genes and reference to their therapeutic targets, however , DNA microarrays and gene expression in *Bacillus subtilis* biofilms differ only 6% compared to their planktonic cells and only 1% in *Pseudomonas aeruginosa*. At present, the differential expression of these genes has not proven useful for this purpose (Fux et al., 2005).

6.6.1 Efflux pumps

Accumulation of antibiotics in the periplasmic space inside the bacteria is antagonized by efflux pumps that are resistant to several classes of antibiotics including tetracyclines, macrolides, fluoroquinolones, β-lactam and reducing their concentration at sub-toxic level (Van Bambeke et al ., 2003).

Efflux pumps are protein structures that are able to expel from the bacterial cytoplasm and periplasm for bacteria toxic compounds such as antibiotics. The expression of these pumps can be permanent (constitutive expression) or intermittent (expression can be induced). These pumps may be specific to a substrate or similar compounds can be transported and may be associated with multidrug resistance (MDR). (Sánchez-Suarez et al., 2006, Grkovic et al., 2002).

In prokaryotes there are five families of efflux transporters: MF (major facilitator), MATE (multidrug and toxic efflux), RND (resistance-nodulation-division), SMR (small multidrug resistance) and ABC (ATP binding cassette). All of them require proton motive power and power supply.

The main systems reported in bacteria of interest in the clinic are: *Campylobacter jejuni* (CmeABC), *E. coli* (AcrAB-TolC, TolC-AcrEF, EmrB, EmrD), *Pseudomonas aeruginosa* (MexXY-OprM, MexCD-OprJ, and OprN MexEF Mex-XY-OprM), *Streptococcus pneumoniae* (PmrA), *Salmonella typhimurium* (AcrB) and *Staphylococcus aureus* (NorA) and *Candida albicans* (MRD1, CDR1 and CDR2) (Webber & Piddock, 2003).

It has been speculated the possibility of antibiotic resistance in biofilms of *P. aeruginosa* by the expression (or overexpression) of these pumps, however, none of the four efflux pumps in the genome of this bacterium contributes to the resistance (De Kievit et al., 2001). In contrast to these results, resistance to azithromycin is associated pumps MexAB-OprM and MexCD-OprJ to biofilm resistance mechanisms in *P. aeruginosa* (Gillis et al., 2005) and PA1874-1887 pump that is expressed at high level in both biofilms and planktonic cells (Zhang & Mah, 2008). Although the results are still inconclusive, have proposed the use of anti-inhibitor drugs efflux pumps (EPI) as potential anti-biofilm treatment have been well tolerated in humans (Kvist et al., 2008).

When cells bind to a surface, expressed a different phenotype to the planktonic cells and may be expressed as a resistance mechanism multidrug efflux pump as reported in *Escherichia coli* (AcrAB operon *mar*). When *mar* expression was evaluated in a bioreactor and as growth in biofilm, the results support the idea that *mar* operon was expressed in biofilms where the lowest level was detected compared with the equivalent in stationary phase fermenter cultures (Maira Litrán et al., 2000a). The loss of acrAB *mar* did not affect the growth as biofilms of *E. coli* and resistance to ciprofloxacin is not dependent on the regulation of *mar* operons or acrAB (Maira Litrán et al., 2000b).

In the case of *Candida albicans* pumps for azoles was noted that in mutants *cdr* planktonic cells and *mdr* were hypersusceptible to fluconazole in contrast to cells that were resistant biofilm showing that resistance is a complex phenomenon that can not be explained by a single mechanism (Ramage et al., 2002).

6.6.2 Alterations in membrane proteins

The diffusion of any antibiotic depends on the permeability of its outer membrane that allows its diffusion of different routes to the periplasmic space. Porins are channel proteins of the outer membrane of Gram-negative bacteria involved in the transport of hydrophilic molecules from the external environment to the periplasmic space.

The genes encoding porins can mutate and produce nonfunctional or altered proteins can decrease their expression. Both processes give rise to mutant bacteria deficient in porins, which have low permeability to hydrophobic molecules pass (Hancock, 1997).

A quick change of balance in the expression of porins in response to antibiotic therapy confers an advantage to the pathogen compared with the commensal microflora that is susceptible to β–lactams (Pagés et al., 2008). In the case of *P. aeruginosa porin* OprD is used for the dissemination of imipenem and resistance is associated with its three-dimensional disturbance.

Porins in *E. coli* are OmpF and OmpC operated in response to changes in osmolarity. Mutations in ompB (regulator of OmpF and OmpC) increase resistance to β-lactam antibiotics, the mutants lacking OmpF are resistant to chloramphenicol and tetracycline.

The genes encoding porins are differentially expressed in biofilms and may contribute to antibiotic resistance. The expression of ompC and three other osmotically regulated genes are increased when the bacteria grow as biofilms in the environment a protective mechanism (Mah & O'Toole 2001).

6.6.3 Phase variation

In biofilm there is capacity development of subpopulations of bacteria or fungi to switch to the dormant metabolic state as small-colony known variants (SCVs) in which they are less susceptible to growth-dependent antibiotic killing, have a defective catalase activity interfere with oxidative metabolism and uptake of aminoglycoside modifying its minimum inhibitory concentration of 8 to 16 times compared with large colonies and normal as in the case of *Enterobacter aerogenes* (Neut et al., 2007, Rusthoven al., 1979).

The phase variation plays an integral role in the formation of diverse phenotypes within biofilms and is largely responsible for the recalcitrance of infections caused by biofilms, the increase in the reversal phase coincides with the antibiotic treatment. This phenomenon has been reported for several genera and species, including *Staphylococcus* and *Pseudomonas* genus, and certain species of Enterobacteriaceae and fungi. (Costerton et al., 1999).

The phase variation causes detectable changes in colonial morphology, the small colony variants of phase variant (SCVs) in biofilms develop properties hyperadherence, autoaggregation, increased hydrophobicity and reduced motility, it has been suggested that tolerate a wide variety of aggressive environmental conditions so that this process is considered a survival mechanism.

It was considered that the phase variation is a process of cellular internal rearrangement, however recently it has been considered to occur by interactions with genetic elements outside the cell as an internal bacteriophage genetic rearrangement by suggesting a model where mobile genetic elements generate the phase variation through a collective mechanism (Chia et al., 2008).

In *Pseudomonas aeruginosa* has shown that under different environmental pressures will favor the appearance of morphological variants that relate to the phenotype of biofilm among which are the small-colony variants (SCVs), rough small-colony variant (RSCVs), wrinkled variants, and rugose colonies autoaggregating cells. The phenotypes RSCVs and SCVs play a critical role in the colonization in cystic fibrosis and mutations in the *psl* locus in variants RSCVs lose their hyperadherence and autoaggregation abilities (β Häubler et al, 2003, Kirisits et al., 2005).

The SCVs of *S. aureus* differ from normal phenotype in size as they are ten times smaller than the wild colonies and are deficient in electron transport by auxotrophism to hemin / menadione, thiamine or thymidine. Their colonies are non-pigmented on agar plates and reduced coagulase production increases resistance to aminoglycosides and cell-wall active antibiotics. The specific role of the SCVs of *S. aureus* resistance to antibiotics in biofilms is still unknown (Proctor & Peters, 1998) although its presence in mixed biofilms with *Pseudomonas* has proven to be a survival mechanism against the attack of the exotoxins of *Pseudomonas* for which its wild form is sensitive (Biswas et al., 2009).

In staphylococcal biofilm formation requires intercellular adhesin (PIA) is a polymer whose main component is N-acetylglucosamine and is synthesized by several enzymes encoded by intercellular adhesion cluster (*ica*), the presence of these genes correlated with the morphology colonial and the ability to form biofilms, so the net growth in Congo red agar form black colonies when the adhesin is present and red in its absence (Ziebuhr et al., 1997). The *ica* operon is constituted by a group of four structural genes icaA, icaB, icaC and a regulatory component icaR (Diemond & Miranda, 2007). Adhesin negative mutants do not produce biofilms due to an IS256 transposon in the gene icaC (Cho et al., 2002).

It has recently been reported in strains of methicillin resistant *Staphylococcus aureus* (MRSA) that the presence of *ica* locus does not guarantee that its expression and does not directly reflect the ability of biofilm formation. Has been evaluated the participation of three regulatory genes *agr* and *sar*A and as well as the alternative transcription sigma factor *sig*B latter being responsible for the variation of biofilm (Jong-Hyun et al., 2008, Eftekhar & Dadaei T, 2011).

In *S. pneumoniae* have described two variants of colonial morphology between colonies spontaneously switched between transparent and opaque, the latter capable of forming two to six times the capsule, with limited bonding capacity and the possibility of evasion of host immune system, this variation observed both in planktonic growth conditions and in biofilm. Other variants described in aged biofilms are small and not mucoid without capsule (SCVs) with capacity to form hyperadherent biofilms, in contrast to the large and mucoid variants that appear late in the biofilm adhere poorly to surfaces forming flat structures unable to form biofilms. The SCVs of *S. pneumoniae* correlated with reduced capsule production and an increase in initial attachment instead to the opaque and transparent colonies, the SCV non capsule cells are not reversible due to a deletion in the capsule operon cps3DSU (Allegrucci & Sauer, 2007).

In *Candida parapsilosis* was previously thought that it was not able to form true filaments and biofilms, we now know they are not as large as those of *Candida albicans* and concentric phenotype forms quantitatively more biofilm in contrast to the smooth phenotype as it does in lesser extent and does not invade the agar (Laffey & Butler, 2005).

The coexistence of microorganisms in biofilms may lead to the emergence of phenotypic variants as in the case of *Pseudomonas putida* and *Acinetobacter* strain C6 where the excretion of benzoate by *Acinetobacter* as a result of the metabolism of benzyl alcohol, induces phase variation in *Pseudomonas* as rough colony (Kirkelund et al., 2007).

The importance of knowledge and isolation of these slow-growing variants (SCVs) are often misdiagnosed by routine microbiological analysis due to its unusual morphology and biochemical reactions which complicates eradication by failures in the antibiotic treatment

7. Biofilm control

Biofilms can be reformed if: a) there is growth of fragments, followed by debridement and cleaning, b) planktonic bacteria is spread, released from the biofilm residual, c) there is new growth of microorganisms in the biofilm (Cooper & Okhiria, 2010) .

Antibiofilms actions can be divided in two: 1) Prevention of formation. and 2) removal or destruction of biofilms. Among the prevention strategies for catheter-related infections that have developed protocols aqre aseptic filtered air in operating rooms which has reduced the incidence of these infections and are based on the correct implementation of the measures of asepsis during insertion and maintenance of vascular pathways. The formation and training of staff on the recommendations of the indication, insertion and maintenance of intravascular devices are the backbone of the prevention of catheter-associated infections.

The methods for controlling biofilms are basically: prevent adhesion (material handling, use of antibiotics or anticoagulants) to prevent bacterial differentiation and congregation (quorum sensing antagonists or use of lactoferrin), matrix elimination (enzymes) and recently the administration of specific bacteriophages (Figure 1).

Many of catheter-related infections due to microorganisms present in the skin are acquired when the catheters are inserted so that alternative strategies anti-colonization are being explored. Other alternatives would be to coat catheters or medical devices with antimicrobial agents (antibiotics, antiseptics and silver) incorporated into the implant material, with limited success. This is due to several reasons among which are the fact that biofilm infections are chronic and the half-life of these substances is shorter on the other hand the incorporation of these drugs can damage the implanted material or incompatibility with the host.

The coating of catheters with antibiotics or biocides such as rifampin and minocycline or cefazolin, chlorex, silver sulfadiazine and silver impregnation decreases the possibility of colonization, has also proved successful when the catheter is used for short periods and as a prophylactic measure, but counterproductive in the long term the huge problem of resistance (Lewis, 2001, Raad & Hanna, 1999).

The coating material with enzymes may be another option to prevent infections resulting from medical devices, recently reported peroxidase titanium coating which can generate antimicrobial hypothiocyanite hypoiodite or to form hydrogen peroxide or thiocyanate. This coated material and a liquid environment with substrates of the enzyme has been shown to limit the formation of biofilms of *Candida albicans* (Ahariz & Courtois, 2010).

Recently have proposed new alternatives for delivery of antibiotics into the biofilm with the use of liposomes or biodegradable complexes that allow the drug concentration at the interfaces of the biofilm (Smith, 2005).

The discovery of bacterial communication systems (*quorum sensing*) as a temporary facility during the infectious process has given an opportunity to decrease the bacterial infection by means other than growth inhibition. Because many bacteria use this communication system and control of virulence, *quorum sensing* mediators are the new targets for drug design (Hentzer & Givskov, 2003). These substances are known as quorum sensing inhibitors (QSI), which have been identified in nature and analogs have been synthesized by modifying its structure and assessed its activity in experimental systems *in vivo* and *in vitro*. QSI resistance occurs only in bacterial mutations.

In the case of gram-negative bacteria depends on the communication mechanism of the synthesis of N-acyl homoserinlactones (AHL), so they have developed analogs of this substance that are aimed at inhibiting biofilm formation by several mechanisms: a) inhibition of AHL signal generation, b) inhibiting the spread of the intracellular signal and c) inhibiting the reception of AHL. In Gram-positive bacteria that use peptides as signaling molecules of *quorum sensing*. A synthetic peptide called RIP interferes with the reception of these signals in *Staphylococcus aureus*, is active in its ability to inhibit biofilm formation in animal models (Balaban et al., 2007).

Substances that interfere in the formation of exopolysaccharide as xylitol and gallium have been used in formulations of oral biofilms management and iron chelating agents such as lactoferrin, deferoxamine and EDTA are candidates for use in controlling biofilms. Recently it was shown that lactoferrin, a ubiquitous and abundant substance in secretions, stimulates the disintegration of biofilms depends on its ability chelator of iron, essential for bacterial growth, and stability of the links necessary for the extracellular matrix biofilms. Their use encourages the release of planktonic cells rather than their aggregation and biofilm (Castrillón 2010, Rodríguez-Franco et al., 2005).

Endogenous production of enzymes allows degradation of exopolysaccharides of the biofilm to achieve dispersion of microorganisms for the generation of a new colony once the biofilm is mature and begin a new cycle of development, this allows us to propose the use of different enzymes for removal, however, due to the heterogeneity of extracellular polysaccharide, it is necessary to use a mixture enzymes for degradation. Among the most commonly used are dispersin D alginase, phage depolimerase, proteases, glycosidases: pectinase arabanase, cellulase, hemicellulase, beta-glucanase, xylanase, glucose oxidase and lactoperoxidase (Johansen et al., 1997, White, 2006, Kaplan et al., 2004).

A different approach for the treatment of biofilms is the use of bacteriophages, viruses that are specific for the bacteria to replicate inside and kill them. It has been demonstrating its effectiveness with the use of bacteriophage T4, which can infect and replicate in *Escherichia coli* breaking up the morphology of the biofilm and killing the bacteria, or in the case of phage 456 on *S. epidermidis*. (Curtin & Donlan, 2006). A bacteriophage expressing enzymes that degrade the biofilm matrix has been designed and simultaneously attack the bacterial cells of *Escherichia coli*. This design eliminates the need to express, purify and deliver large doses of enzymes to specific sites of infection that impede access by the presence of the extracellular matrix (Lu & Collins, 2007).

Pretreatment of catheters with hydrogel with a hydrolyzate of bacteriophage *P. aeruginosa* M4 reached lower cell density in biofilms after bacterial inoculation suggesting its potential use to prevent biofilm formation (Fu et al., 2010).

8. Conclusions and perspectives

The organization of the microorganisms to grow as a biofilm has been shown to have their own intrinsic mechanisms of resistance differ from those described stop the growth of microorganisms in free form. Therefore, these strategies should be considered resistance to explain therapeutic failure in the treatment of patients for whom laboratory results provide suitable sensitivity patterns.

Growth as a biofilm is a risk factor for the spread of resistance to antibiotics and biocides as a long-term treatment with a microorganism determines their survival by developing a biofilm phenotype.

Therapy in the future against biofilm-related infections should be considered as a priority to have standardized methods of diagnosis (still non-existent at the routine level) to determine differential management strategies of these infections.

As biofilms are heterogeneous in nature, antibiotics are useful to control those who are active in cells with low metabolic activity or non-actively growing cells so requires the search for new antibiotics that fit this profile.

The main strategy for controlling these infections is the use of agents that prevent biofilm formation as (*quorum sensing* inhibitors, inhibitors of synthesis of exopolysaccharides or material handling to prevent sticking) and its growth has been kept as planktonic cells to be susceptible to the action of antibiotics and host immune system. Other possible control strategies for mature biofilm consisting of dispersal of the organism by specific enzymes responsible or bacteriophage that allow differential lysis.

In conclusion, biofilm growth as a major advantage for microorganisms because of the variety of strategies developed by them not only to ensure their survival in hostile environments but to evade the antibiotics, so knowledge of the process and the mediators involved will allow us to direct them to our benefit.

9. References

Ahariz M, Courtois P. (2010). *Candida albicans* biofilm on titanium: effect of perodxidase precoating. *Medical devices: evidence and research*.Vol.3 pp. 33-40.

Allegrucci M & Sauer K (2007) Characterization of colony morphology variants isolated from *Streptococcus pneumoniae* biofilms. *J Bacteriol.* Vol. 189 pp. 2030-2038.

Anderl JN, Franlin JM, Stewart SP. (2000). Role of antibiotic penetration limitation in *Klebsiella pneumoniae* biofilm resistance to ampicillin and ciprofloxacin. *Antimicrob Agents Chemother.* Vol. 44 pp. 1818-1824.

Balaban N, Cirioni O, Giacometti A, Ghiselli R, Braunstein BJ, Silvestri C, Mocchegiani F, Saba V, Scalise G. (2007) Treatment of *Staphylococcus aureus* biofilm infection by the Quorum-sensing inhibitor RIP. *Antimicrob Agents Chemother.* Vol. 51 pp. 2226- 2229.

Biswas L, Biswas R, Schlag M, Bertram R, Götz F. (2009). Small-colony variant selection as a survival strategy for *Staphylococcus aureus* in the presence of *Pseudomonas aeruginosa*. *Appl Environ Microbiol.* Vol. 75 pp. 6910-6912.

Borriello G, Werner E, Roe F, Kim AM, Ehrlich GD, Stewart PS. (2004). Oxygen limitation contributes to antibiotic tolerance of *Psedomonas aeruginosa* biofilms. *Antimicrob Agents Chemother.* Vol.4 pp. 2659-2666.

Brown MR Allison DG, Gilbert P .(1988). Resistance of bacterial biofilms to antibiotics: a growth-rate related effect? *J Antimicrob Chemother.* Vol. 22 pp. 777-780.

Bos R, van der Mei CH, Busscher JH. (1999). Physico-chemistry of initial microbial adhesive interactions. Its mechanisms and methods for study. *FEMS Microbiol Rev.* Vol. 23 pp. 179-230.

Castrillon RLE, Palma RA, Desgarennes PC. (2003) Aminoglucósidos: una revisión reciente. *Dermatología Rev Mex.* Vol. 47 pp. 178-193.

Castrillón RLE, Palma RA, Desgarennes PC. (2007). Péptidos antimicrobianos: antibióticos naturales de la piel. *Dermatología Rev Mex.* Vol. 51 pp. 57-67.

Castrillón RLE, Palma RA, Desgarennes PMC.(2010). Importancia de las biopelículas en la práctica médica. *Dermatología Rev Mex* Vol. 54 pp. 14-24

Castrillón RLE, Palma RA, Padilla DMC. (2011) Interferencia de las biopelículas en el proceso de curación de heridas. *Dermatología Rev Mex.* Vol. 55 pp. 127-139.

Chia N, Woese CR, Goldenfeld N (2008) A collective mechanism for phase variation in biofilms. *PNAS* Vol 105 pp. 14597-14602.

Cho SH, Naber K, Hacker J, Zibuhr W. (2002) Detection of the *ica*ADBC gene cluster and biofilm formation in *Staphylococcus epidermidis* isolates from catheter-related urinary tract infections. *Int J Antimicrob Agents.* Vol. 19 pp. 570-575.

Cooper R., Okhiria O. (2010) Biofilms, wound infection and the issue control. *Wounds UK.* Vol. 6 pp. 84-90

Costerton JW, Cheng KJ, Geesey GG, Ladd TI,, Nickel JC, Dasgupta M, Marrie TJ. (1987). Bacterial biofilms in nature and disease. *Ann Rev Microbiol.* Vol. 987 pp. 435-464.

Costerton JW, Stewart PS, Greenberg EP. (1999) Bacterial biofilms: a common cause of persistent infections. *Science.* Vol. 284 pp. 1318-1322.

Costerton W, Veeh R, Shirfliff M, Pasmore M, Post Ch, Ehrlich G. (2003). The applications of biofilm science to the study and control of chronic bacterial infections. *J Clin Invest.* Vol. 112 pp. 1466-1477.

Curtin JJ, Donlan RM.(2006). Using bacteriophages to reduce formation of catheter-associated biofilms by *Staphylococcus epidermidis. Antimicrob Agents Chemother.* Vol.50 pp. 1268-1275.

De Kievit TR, Parkins MD, Gillis RJ, Srikumar H, Ceri H, Poole BH, Iglewski DG, Storey DG. (2001). Multidrug efflux pumps: expression patterns and contribution to antibiotic resistance in *Pseudomonas aeruginosa* biofilms, *Amtimicrob Agents Chemother.* Vol. 45 pp. 1761-1770.

Del Valle Martínez Rojas D. (2009) Betalactamasas tipo AmpC: generalidades y métodos para su detección fenotípica. *Rev Soc Venezolana Microbiol.* Vol. 29 pp. 78-83.

Diemond HJB, Miranda NG. (2007) Biofilm: ¿amenaza latente o factor de protección? Estado del arte. *Enf Inf Microbiol.* Vol. 27 pp. 22-28.

Donlan MR, Costerton W. (2002). Biofilms: survival mechanisms of clinically relevant microorganisms. *Clin Microb Rev.* Vol.15 pp. 167-193.

Eftekhar F, Dadaei T. (2011). Biofilm formation of *Ica*AB genes in clinical isolates of methicillin resistant *Staphylococcus aureus. Iranian J Basic Med Sci.* Vol. 14 pp. 132-136.

Flemming HC, Wingender J. (2010). The biofilm matrix. *Nature Rev Microbiol.* Vol. 8 pp. 623-633.

Fu W, Forster T, Mayer O, Curtin JJ, Lehman MS, Donlan MR (2010) Bacteriophage cocktail for the prevention of biofilm formation by *Pseudomonas aeruginosa* on catheters *in vitro* model. *Antimicrob Agents Chemother.* Vol 54 pp. 397-404

Fux CA, Costerton JW, Stewart PS, Stoodley P.(2005). Survival strategies of infectious biofilms. *Trends Microbiol.* Vol. 13 pp. 34-40.

Gallant VC, Daniels C, Leung MJ, Ghosh SA, Young DK, Kotra LP, Burrows LL.(2005). Common beta-lactamases inhibit bacterial biofilm formation. *Mol Microbiol.* Vol.58 pp. 1012-1024.

Ghigo JM. (2001). Natural conjugative plasmids induce biofilm development. *Nature.* Vol. 412 pp. 442-445.

Gillis, R., K. White, K. Choi, V. Wagner, H. Schweizer, and B. Iglewski. (2005) Molecular basis of azithromycin-resistant *Pseudomonas aeruginosa* biofilms. *Antimicrob. Agents Chemother.* Vol. 49 pp. 3858–3867.

Giwercman B, Jensen ETT, Hoiby N.. (1991) Induction of β–lactamase production in *Pseudomonas aeruginosa* biofilm. *Antimicrob Agents Chemother.* Vol.35 pp. 1008-1010.

Grkovi S, Brown MH,m Skurray RA. (2002). Regulation of bacterial drug export systems. *Microbiol Mol Biol Rev.* Vol. 66 pp. 671-701.

Gordon CA, Hodges NA, Marriott C. (1988). Antibiotic interaction and diffusion through alginate and exopolysaccharide of cystic fibrosis-derived *Pseudomonas aeruginosa. J Antimicrob Chemother* Vol. 22 pp. 667-674.

Hachem YR, Chemaly FR, Ahmar AC, Jiang Y, Boktour RM, Rjaili AG, Bodey PG, Raad II. (2007). Colistin is effective in treatment of infectious caused by multidrug-resistant *Pseudomonas aeuroginosa* in cancer patients. *Antimicrob Agents Chemother.* Vol. 51 pp. 1905-1911.

Hall-Stoodley L, Costerton WJ, Stoodley P. (2004). Bacterial biofilms: from the natural environment to infectious diseases. *Nat Rev Microbiol* Vol. 2 pp. 95-108.

Hall-Stoodley, L. & Stoodley, P. (2005). Biofilm formation and dispersal and the transmission of human pathogens. *Trends Microbiol.* Vol. 13. pp. 7-10.

Hancock RE. (1997). The bacterial outer membrane as a drug barrier. *Trends Microbiol.* Vol. 5 pp. 37-42.

Häubler S, Ziegler I, Löttel A, Götz F Rhode M, Wehmhöhner D, Saravanamuthu S, Tümmler B, Steinmetz I. (2003). Highly adherent small-colony variants of *Pseudomonas aeruginosa* in cystic fibrosis lung infection. *J Med Microbiol.* Vol. 52 pp. 295-301.

Hentzer M, Givskov M. (2003). Pharmacological inhibition of quorum sensing for the treatment of chronic bacterial infections. *J Clin Invest.* Vol 112. pp 1300-1307.

Herrera Mendoza MT. (2004). El papel del biofilm e el proceso infeccioso y la resistencia. *Nova Publicación científica.* Vol. 2 pp. 71-80.

Hogan D, Kolter R. (2002). Why are bacteria refractory to antimicrobials? *Curr Opin Microbiol.* Vol. 5 pp. 472-477.

Hoiby N, Bjarnsholt T, Givskov M, Molin S, Ciofu O. (2010). Antibiotic resistance of bacterial biofilms. *Int J Antimicrob Agents* Vol. 35 pp. 322-332.

Johansen Ch, Falholt P, Gram L.(1997). Enzymatic removal and disinfection of bacterial biofilms. *Appl Environ Microbiol,* Vol. 63 pp. 3724-3728.

Jong-Hyum K, Kim Ch, Hacker J, Ziebuhr W, Lee KB, Cho SH. (2008). Molecular characterization of regulatory genes associated with biofilm variation in a *Staphylococcus aureus* strain. *J Microbiol Biotechnol.* Vol. 18 pp. 28-34.

Kaplan BJ, Ragunath C, Velliyagounder K, Fine HD, Ramasubbu N. (2004). Enzymatic detachment of *Staphylococcus epidermidis* biofilms. *Antimicrob Agents Chemother.* Vol. 48 pp. 2633-2636.

Keller L, Surette GM. (2006). Communication in bacteria: an ecological and evolutionary perspective. *Nat Rev Microbiol.* Vol. 4 pp. 249-258.

Keren I, Shah D, Spoering A, Wang Y, Lewis I. (2004). Specialized persister cells and the mechanism of multidrug tolerance in *Escherichia coli. J Bacteriol.* Vol. 186 pp. 8172-8180.

Kirisits MJ, Prost L, Starkey M, Parsek RM (2005) Characterization of colony morphology variants isolated from *Pseudomonas aeruginosa* biofilms *Appl Environ Microbiol.* Vol 71 pp. 4809-4821.

Kikerlund HS, Haagensen AJJ, Gjrmansen M, Jorgensen MT, Tolker-Nielsen T, Molin S. (2007). Characterization of *Pseudomonas putida* rough variant evolved in a mixed-species biofim with *Acinetobacter* sp. Strain C6. *J Bacteriol.* Vol. 189 pp. 4932-4943.

Kumamoto AC. (2002). Candida biofilms. *Curr Opin Microbiol.* Vol. 5 pp. 608-611.

Kvist M, Hancock V, Klemm P. (2008). Inactivation of efflux pumps abolishes bacterial biofilm formation. *App Environ Microbiol.* Vol. 74 pp. 7376-7382.

Laffey S, Butler G (2005) Phenotype switching affects biofilm formation by *Candida parapsilosis. Microbiology* Vol 151 pp. 1073-1081.

Lasa I, del Pozo JL, Penadés JR, Leiva J. (2005). Biofilms bacterianos e infección. *An Sist Sanit Navar.* Vol. 28 pp. 163-175.

Lewis K. (2001). Riddle of biofilm resistance. *Antimicrob Agents Chemother.* Vol. 45 pp. 999-1007.

Lewis K. (2008). Multidrug tolerance of biofilms and persister cells. *Curr Topics Microbiol Immunol.* Vol. 322 pp. 107-131.

López D, Vlamakis H, Kolter R. (2010). Biofilms. *Cold Spring Harb Perspect Biol.* Vol. 2 pp. 1-11.

Lu TK, Collins JJ. (2007). Dispersing biofilms with engineered enzymatic bacteriophage. *PNAS* Vol.104 pp. 11197-11202.

Mah TFC, O'Toole GA. (2001). Mechanisms of biofilm resistance to antimicrobial agents. *Trends Microbiol.* Vol. 9. pp. 4-39.

Maira-Litrán T, Allison DG, Gilbert P. (2000a). Expression of the multiple antibiotic resistance operon (*mar*) during growth of *Escherichia coli* as a biofilm. *J Appl Microbiol.* Vol. 88 pp. 243-247.

Maira-Litrán T, Allison GD, Gilbert P. (2000b). An evaluation of the potential of the multiple antibiotic resistance operon (mar) and the multidrug efflux pump acrAB to moderate resistance towards ciprofloxacin en *Escherichia coli* biofilms. *J Antimicrob Chemother.* Vol. 45 pp. 789-795.

Martínez-Suárez VJ, Baquero F, Reig M, Pérez-Díaz JC. (1985). Transferable plasmid-linked chloramphenicol acetytransferase conferring high-lvel resistance in Bacteroides uniformis. *Antimicrob Agents Chemother.* Vol. 28 pp. 113-117.

Moyed HS, Broderick SH. (1986). Molecular cloning and expression of *hip* A, gene of *Escherichia coli* K-12 that affects frequency of persistence after inhibition of murein synthesis. *J Bacteriol.* Vol. 166 pp. 399-403.

Müller CFM, Seider M, Beauvais A. (2011). *Aspergillus fumigatus* biofilms in the clinical setting. *Medical Micology* Vol. 49(Suppl. 1)pp S96-S100.

Neut D, van der Mei H, Bulstra KS, Busscher JH. (2007). The role of small-colony variants in failure to diagnose and treat biofilm infections in orthopedics. *Acta Orthopaedica* Vol. 78 pp. 299-308.

Pagés JM, James ECh. Winterhalter M. (2008). The porin and the permeating antibiotic: a selective diffusion barrier in Gram-negative bacteria. *Nat Rev Microbiol.* Vol. 6 pp. 893-903.

Pamp JS, Gjermansen M, Johansen KH, Tolker-Nielsen T. (2008). Tolerance to the antimicrobial peptide colistin in *Pseudomonas aeruginosa* biofilms in linked to metabolically active cells, and depends on the pmr and mexAB-oprM genes. *Mol Microbiol.* Vol. 68 pp. 223-240.

Poole K. (2002). Mechanisms of bacterial biocide and antibiotic resistance. *J Appl Microbiol.* Vol. 92 pp. 55S-64S.

Proctor RA, Peters G. (1998). Small colony variants in staphylococcal infections: diagnostic and therapeutic implications. *Clin Infect Dis.* Vol. 27 pp. 419-423.

Raad I, Hanna H.(1999). Intravascular catheters impregnated with antimicrobial agents: a milestone in the prevention of bloodstream infections. *Support Care Cancer.* Vol. 7 pp. 386-390.

Ramage G, Bachmann S, Patterson FT, Wickes LB, López-Ribot JL. (2002). Investigation of multidrug efflux pumps in relation to fluconazole resistance in *Candida albicans* biofilms. *J Antimicrob Chemother.* Vol. 49 pp. 973-980.

Rodríguez-Franco DA, Vázquez-Moreno L, Ramos-Clamont, Monfort G. (2005). Actividad antimicrobiana de la lactoferrina: Mecanismos y aplicaciones clínicas potenciales. *Rev Latinoam Microbiol.* Vol. 47 pp. 102-111.

Rusthoven JJ, Davis TA, Lerner SA. (1979). Clinical isolation and characterization of aminoglucoside-resistant small colony variants of *Enterobacter aerogenes. Am J Med.* Vol. 67 pp. 702-706.

Sánchez-Suárez P, Bentiez-Bibriesca L. (2006) Procesos biomoleculares de la Resistencia a drogas. *Cancerología* Vol 1 pp. 187-199.

Sauer K, Camper AK, Ehrlich GD, Costerton JW, Davies DG. (2002). *Pseudomonas aeruginosa* displays multiple phenotypes during development as a biofilm. *J Bacteriol.* Vol. 184 pp. 1140-1154.

Smith WA. (2005). Biofilms and antibiotic therqapy: Is there a role for combating bacterial resistance by the use of novel drug delivery system? *Adv Drug Delivery Rev.* Vol. 57 pp. 1539-1550.

Stewart SP, Roe F, Rayner J, Eldins GJ, Lewandowski Z, Oschsner AU, Hassett JD. (2000). Effect of catalase on hydrogen peroxide penetration into *Pseudomonas aeruginosa* biofilms. *Appl Environ Microbiol.* Vol. 66 pp. 836-838.

Stewart SP, Costerton WJ. (2001) Antibiotic resistance of bacterial biofilms. *Lancet* Vol. 358 pp. 135-138.

Stewart SP. (2002). Mechanism of antibiotic resistance in bacterial biofilms. *Int J Med Microbiol.* Vol. 292 pp. 107-113.

Stewart SP, Franklin JM. (2008). Physiological heterogeneity in biofilms. *Nat Rev Microbiol.* Vol.6 pp. 199-210.

Stickler D., (1999). Biofilms. *Curr Opin Microbiol.* Vol. 2 pp. 270-275.

Spoering AL, Lewis K. (2001). Biofilms and planktonic cells of *Pseudomonas aeruginosa* have similar resistance to killing by antimicrobials. *J Bacteriol.* Vol. 183 pp. 6746-6751.

Sutherland WI. (1997). Microbial exopolysaccharides-structural subtleties and their consequences. *Pure & Appl Chem.* Vol. 69 pp. 1911-1917.

Uppuluri P., Ashok K. Chaturvedi KA, Srinivasan A, Banerjee M, Ramasubramaniam KA, Köhler RJ, David Kadosh D, Lopez-Ribot J. (2010). Dispersion as an important step in the *Candida albicans* biofilm developmental cycle. *PLoSPatog.* Vol. 6 pp. 1-13.

Van Bambeke F., Glupczynski Y., P. Plésiat P., J. C. Pechère JC., P. M. Tulkens PM. (2003). Antibiotic efflux pumps in prokaryotic cells: occurrence, impact on resistance and strategies for the future of antimicrobial therapy. *J Antimicrob. Chemother.* Vol. 51 pp. 1055-1065.

Veeh RH, Shirtliff EM, Petik RJ, Flood AJ, Davis CC, Seymor LJ, Hansmann AM, Kerr MK, Pasmore EM, Costerton WJ. (2003). Detection of *Staphylococcus aureus* biofilm on tampons and menses components. *J Infect Dis.* Vol. 188 pp. 519-530.

Ward KH, Olson ME, Lam K, Costerton JW. (1992). Mechanism of persistent infection with peritoneal implants. *J Med Micro.* Vol. 36 pp. 406-413.

Webber MA, Piddock LJV. (2003) The importance of efflux pumps in bacterial antibiotic resistance. *J Antimicrob Chemother.* Vol 51 pp.9-11.

White R. (2006). Flaminal®: a novel approach to wound bioburden control. *Wounds.* Vol. 2 pp. 64-77.

Whitehead AN, Barnard MLA, Slater H, Simpson JLN, Salmond PCG. (2001). Quorum-sensing in Gram-negative bacteria. *FEMS Microbiol Rev.* Vol. 25 pp. 365-404.

Wimpenny J, Manz W, Szewzyk U. (2000). Heterogeneity in biofilms. *FEMS Microbiol Rev.* Vol. 24 pp. 661-671.

Woods DE, Bass JA, Johanson WG. (1980). Role of adherence in the pathogenesis of *Pseudomonas aeruginosa* lung infection in cystic fibrosis patients. *Infect Immun.* Vol. 30 pp. 784-790.

Wright DG. (2005). Bacterial resistance to antibiotics: Enzymatic degradation and modification. *Adv Drug Deliv.* Vol. 57 pp. 1451-1450.

Zhang, L., & T.-F. Mah.. (2008). Involvement of a novel efflux system in biofilm-specific resistance to antibiotics. *J Bacteriol.* Vol. 190 pp. 4447–4452.

Ziebuhr W, Heilmann Ch, Götz F, Meyer P, Wils K, Straube E, Hacker J. (1997). Detection of the intercellular adhesion gene cluster (ica) and phase variation in *Staphylococcus epidermidis* blood culture strains and mucosal isolates. *Infect Immun.* Vol. 65 pp. 890-896.

Zimmerli W, Widmer FA, Blatter M, Frei R, Ochnsner EP. (1998). Role of rifampin for treatment of orthopedic implant-related stapylococcal infections: a randomized controlled trial. Foreign-body infection (FBI) Study Group. *JAMA.* Vol. 279 pp. 1537-1541.

8

Antibiotic Resistance, Biofilms and Quorum Sensing in *Acinetobacter* Species

K. Prashanth*, T. Vasanth, R. Saranathan,
Abhijith R. Makki and Sudhakar Pagal
Laboratory No. 6, Department of Biotechnology, Pondicherry University,
India

1. Introduction

Acinetobacter is a Gram-negative coccobacillus that is strictly aerobic, nonmotile, catalase positive and oxidase negative. It is ubiquitous in nature, being found in soil and water. Members of the genus *Acinetobacter* have now clearly emerged as opportunistic nosocomial pathogens (Forster et al., 1998). Bacteremia, pneumonia, meningitis, urinary tract and surgical wound infections are the most common infections caused by this organism (Cisneros et al., 2002; Dijkshoorn et al., 2007). The taxonomy of the genus *Acinetobacter* has undergone extensive revision during the last two decades, and at least 31 named and unnamed species have now been described (Dijkshoorn et al., 2007). Of these, *Acinetobacter baumannii* and the closely related unnamed genomic species 3 and 13 sensu Tjernberg and Ursing (13TU) species were the most clinically relevant. In recent years, multidrug-resistant (MDR) *A. baumannii* are increasingly held responsible for nosocomial infections and MDR *A. baumannii* clones are spreading into new geographic areas with increasing number of strains acquiring many resistance genes (Navon venezia et al., 2005). Unfortunately, newer extended-spectrum β-lactamases and different carbapenemases are emerging fast, leading to pan-resistant strains of *A. baumannii*.

A. baumannii appears to have the propensity for developing multiple antimicrobial resistances extremely rapidly. This bacterium has shown a remarkable tendency to develop resistance to virtually every antibiotic class (Henwood et al., 2002). The emergence and quick dissemination of multiple drug resistant (MDR) *A. baumannii* and its genetic potential to carry and transfer diverse antibiotic resistance determinants pose a major threat in hospitals world-wide. The complex interplay of MDR clones, its rapid spread, their persistence through biofilm formation, their regulation by quorum sensing (QS), transfer of resistance elements and other interactions are contributing to the increasing woes and creating additional difficulties in treating infections caused by these organisms. This review article mainly focus on antibiotic resistance in *Acinetobacter*, the current understanding of biofilm production and its correlation with antibiotic resistance as well the quorum sensing mechanisms in *Acinetobacter* species.

---

* Corresponding Author

2. Antibiotic resistance in *Acinetobacter* spp.

A. baumannii is considered the paradigm of multi-resistant bacteria as the organism has an ever-increasing list of resistance determinants that can rapidly nullify most of the therapeutic armamentarium. Both acquired and intrinsic resistance mechanisms can contribute this multi-resistance. The ability to acquire such resistance for multiple drugs may be due to either the acquisition of genetic elements carrying multiple resistant determinants or mutations affecting the expression of porins and/or efflux pump(s), which can minimize the activity of unrelated antimicrobial agents (Vila, 2007). It is also indicated that the outer membrane of *Acinetobacter* spp. acts as a substantial barrier against the penetration of these antibiotics. The results of one of the earliest studies suggest that one of the causes for the high antibiotic resistance of *Acinetobacter* is attributable to the presence of a small number of small-sized porins (Sato et al., 1991). Apart from this, it was also shown earlier that the amount of *Acinetobacter* porin was less than 5% of the Total outer membrane proteins (OMP), while that of *E. coli* it was reported to be about 60% (Rosenbusch, 1974) that contributes to reduced permeability. The most widespread β-lactamases with carbapenemase activity in *A. baumannii* are carbapenem hydrolysing class D β-lactamases mediated by OXA genes that are most specific for this species. In addition, metallo-β-lactamases have now been reported worldwide that confer resistance to all β-lactams except aztreonam (Dijkshoorn et al., 2007). Resistance to aminoglycosides in *A. baumannii* is mediated principally by aminoglycoside-modifying enzymes (AME's). Further, multidrug efflux pump such as AdeABC may have a role in aminoglycoside resistance (Wieczorek et al., 2008). Quinolone resistance is often caused by modifications in the structure of DNA gyrase secondary to mutations in the quinolone resistance determining regions of the *gyrA* and *parC* genes.

The main underlying resistance mechanisms to multiple antibiotics in *Acinetobacter* sp. can be summarily outlined as follows (i) production of hydrolysing enzymes for e.g. β-lactam hydrolysis by different kinds of β-lactamases (Class A to D β-lactamases), (ii) changes in penicillin-binding proteins (PBPs) that prevent action of β-lactams, (iii) alterations in the structure and number of porin proteins that result in decreased permeability to antibiotics through the outer membrane of the bacterial cell and (iv) the activity of efflux pumps that further decrease the concentration of antibiotics within the bacterial cell. But, among these β-lactamases, OXA- and metallo-carbapenemases seem to be more significant with their increasing incidence when compared to other β-lactamases (Livermore et al., 2006).

2.1 Resistance to β-lactam antibiotics

Resistance for β-lactams in *Acinetobacter* is been associated with the production of β-lactamases.

2.1.1 β-lactamases

Resistance due to the expression of hydrolysing enzymes such as cephalophorinases and amber class A–D β-lactamases remains as one of the extensively studied and skilful resistance mechanism among the species of *Acinetobacter*. These enzymes to some extent hydrolyze carbapenems along with other β-lactams. The most common carbapenemases detected in *A. baumannii* were either Class B β- lactamases such as metallo β- lactamases

(MBL) or class D β- lactamases (also referred as carbapenem hydrolyzing oxicillinases (CHDLs)) (Livermore, 2007). While class A carbapenemases have been frequently detected in bacteria belonging to *Enterobacteraceae* family, they were not usually found in *Acinetobacter* spp. However, *A. baumannii* producing extended-spectrum β-lactamases (ESBLs) have been reported, though it is not a common phenomenon (Livermore & Woodford, 2006). As there are emerging reports of arrival of newer broad spectrum β- lactamases such as New Delhi metallo-beta lactamase -1 (NDM-1) (Karthikeyan et al., 2010) among Gram-negative pathogens including *Acinetobacter* and their progressing hydrolysing abilities makes this group of Gram-negative bacterial pathogens as superbugs by assisting them to survive in extreme conditions. The genes that code for multiple resistances are reported to be plasmid as well as chromosomally encoded.

2.1.2 A- Class

A. baumannii, like *Pseudomonas aeruginosa*, produces a naturally occurring AmpC β-lactamase, together with a naturally occurring oxacillinase with carbapenemase properties. ESBLs are plasmid-mediated β-lactamases of predominant class A. ESBLs are capable of efficiently hydrolyzing penicillin, cephalosporin, the oxyimino group containing cephalosporins (cefotaxime, ceftazidime) and monobactams (aztreonam). β-lactamase inhibitors (clavulanic acid, sulbactam and tazobactam) generally inhibit ESBL producing strains. A wide range of class A ESBLs have been reported in *Acinetobacter* sp. such as TEM, SHV, CTX-M, GES, SCO, PER and VEB. However, these resistant determinants are not universally present in *Acinetobacter*, as there are only isolated reports of them. Some of the documented ESBLs world-wide are PER-1 from Turkey, Korea, Russia, Romania, Belgium and France; VEB-1 from France and Belgium; TEM-116 and SHV-12 from China and The Netherlands; CTX-M-2 from Korea; *bla* Shv-5 –EBSL, TEM -92 from Italy and VEB -1 from Northern France and Belgium (Naiemi et al., 2005; Nass et al., 2006, 2007; Endimiani et al., 2007). Nevertheless, they were not as common as MBL and CHDL in *Acinetobacter* species.

2.1.3 B- Class

Carbapenemases are the most versatile of all β-lactamases and many of them recognize almost all hydrolysable β-lactams. The most common hydrolyzing enzyme carbapenemases found in *A. baumannii* belong to either the class B family of beta-lactamases such as MBLs (IMP/VIM) or the OXA class D family of serine β-lactamases (Poirel, 2006). Class B β-lactamases are also referred as MBLs has the highest level of carbapenem-hydrolyzing activity among the three classes of carbapenemases. MBLs have been identified in many Gram-negative bacteria including *Acinetobacter* genomic species 13 TU and *A. baumannii* and are resistant to the commercially available β-lactamase inhibitors but susceptible to inhibition by metal ion chelators. Potent class B metallo-carbapenemases of the IMP, VIM, SIM and NDM type have been found in *A. baumannii*.

There are numerous existing reports on IMP type of MBL in *Acinetobacter* spp (Lee et al., 2003; Livermore, 2007). In *A. baumannii*, six IMP variants belonging to three different phylogroups have been identified and reported namely IMP-1 in Italy, Japan and South Korea; IMP-2 in Italy and Japan; IMP-4 in Hong Kong; IMP-5 in Portugal; IMP-6 in Brazil and IMP-11 in Japan (Poirel and Nordmann, 2006). In addition, IMP-4 has been identified in clinical isolates of *Acinetobacter junii* in Australia (Peleg et al., 2006). On the contrary, there are only few studies that have documented MBL VIM type in *Acinetobacter*. In fact more than 100 clinical isolates screened by our group showed non-existence of VIM in this part of world. Surprisingly, *P. aeruginosa* isolates collected from the same hospital in our region showed the presence of VIM type of MBL and there was no cross transmission observed (Unpublished data). VIM-2-producing *Acinetobacter* spp. have been isolated in the Far East (Lee, et al., 2003) and in Germany (Toleman, 2004), while the VIM-1 determinant has been reported only in Greece (Tsakris 2006). One study recently identified VIM-4, which is nothing but a point mutant of VIM-1 and that has been previously identified only in *Enterobacteriaceae* (Luzzaro et al., 2008) and *Pseudomonas* spp. (Pournaras et al., 2003). This report on MBL VIM-4 determinant in *Acinetobacter* spp., emphasizes the fact that CHDLs are not the solitary factor for emergence of resistance to carbapenems in this genus. Interestingly, *bla*VIM-4 was identified in a non-*A. baumannii* isolate, thereby indicating that clinically insignificant Gram-negative bacterial species may also be reservoirs for MBL-encoding genes. It is also noteworthy that the occurrence of VIM-4 in *Acinetobacter* in a country that has reported VIM-4 in *P. aeruginosa* previously (Pournaras et al., 2003). Concurrently, it was also observed in Greece that *bla*VIM-1 which is widespread in *P. aeruginosa* had apparently crossed the species barrier to reach *Acinetobacter* spp. Such examples might be yet another example of resistance genes crossing genus barrier (Tsakris et al., 2006).

A small number of reports are available on other MBL types such as SIM-1, NDM-1 encountered in *Acinetobacter* spp (Lee et al., 2005, Karthikeyan et al., 2010). Recently, a novel acquired MBL gene namely *bla*SIM-1 was detected in clinical isolates of *A. baumannii* from Korea (Lee et al., 2005). This SIM-1 is encoded by a class 1 integron-borne gene cassette and is more closely related to IMP-type enzymes than to other MBLs. Very recently new β-lactamase such as NDM-1 has been reported in *A. baumannii* (Karthikeyan et al., 2010). Interestingly, in this report NDM-1–positive isolate was also positive for both OXA-23 and IMP. The *bla*NDM-1– positive strain was more resistant to antibiotics than the strains that were harbouring both OXA-23 and IMP. Fortunately, it was found that this *bla*NDM-1–positive *A. baumannii* strain was susceptible to several fluoroquinolone antibiotics and to polymyxin B (Chen et al., 2011).

2.1.4 D- Class

The most common carbapenemases detected in *Acinetobacter* are CHDLs that are also referred as Class-D oxacillinases. Among the nine clusters of carbapenem hydrolysing oxacillinases, four have been identified to date in *A. baumannii*. These included members of OXA-23, -24, -51, and -58 families. In addition, recently a novel class D enzyme named OXA-143 has been reported from Germany. OXA-58 oxacillinase was the first enzyme to be identified in an *A. baumannii* isolate in France and subsequently this has been reported among *A. baumannii* isolates in several countries (Coelo et al., 2006). Contrary to many workers, one investigation opined that the carriage of OXA-58 but not of OXA-51 β-lactamase gene correlates with carbapenem resistance in *A. baumannii* (Tsakris, 2007). In one of the studies, epidemiologically unrelated *Acinetobacter* isolates that were positive for the presence *bla*OXA-51- and *bla*OXA-58-like carbapenemase genes was also shown to carry the *bla*VIM-1 in a class 1 integron, which is of much concern (Tsakris, 2008).

Recently, a new OXA class D β–lactamase Oxa-97 has been reported in Tunisia which belongs to Oxa58-like (subgroup) in Africa (Poirel et al., 2008). In one instance, a novel Oxa-

143- CHDL in *A. baumannii* (Higgins et al., 2009) which is not associated with insertion sequence (IS) elements or integron features has been reported, which is bracketed by 2 replicase genes and its incorporation was shown to be by homologous recombination. Oxa-143 is a class D carbapenemase is similar to OXA-66/OXA-51-like enzyme that contributes to imipenem resistance, which was first reported from Taiwan. Off late, OXA-72 oxacillinase has been also reported in several carbapenem resistant *A. baumannii* isolates in Taiwan (Lu et al., 2009).

It has also been discovered that *bla*OXA-51-like genes may be associated with carbapenem resistance in isolates with an adjacent copy of insertion sequence (IS) ISAbA1 (Turton et al., 2006). IS elements presumed to enhance β-lactamase gene expression by providing additional promoters. Repeated observations such as ISAba1, ISAba2, ISAba3, ISAba4 IS elements being often found upstream of the different β- lactamases genes in *A. baumannii* can be taken as evidence for such assumption (Chen et al., 2008; Poirel 2006a. 2006b & 2008). In addition, one recent work demonstrated that a plasmid-borne CHDL with appropriate upstream ISs was enough to confer a high level of carbapenem resistance in *A. baumannii*. Moreover, a *bla*OXA-58 gene with an upstream insertion of a truncated ISAba3 and IS1008 was detected on a plasmid obtained from a clinical carbapenem resistant isolate in one of the studies (Chen et al., 2008). Acquisition of a plasmid-borne *bla*OXA-58 gene with an upstream IS1008 insertion is also shown to confer a high level of carbapenem resistance to *A. baumannii* (Chen et al., 2008). Therefore, as observed for the natural *bla*AmpC gene of *A. baumannii*, ISAba1 might provide promoter sequences that enhance expression of associated genes. These promoter sequences are probably extremely efficient in *A. baumannii*, so that insertion of ISAba1 upstream of *bla*OXA-51-like genes might represent a true mechanism of carbapenem resistance, or at least decreased susceptibility. Hence, it is sensible to believe that the association of *bla*OXA -51 like genes with IS elements may have a role in increasing carbapenem resistance. At least in one instance, it was conclusively shown that the reduced susceptibility to carbapenems was related to selection of the ISAba1-related overexpression of *bla*OXA-66 that belongs to *bla*OXA-51 subgroup (Figueiredo et al., 2009).

2.2 Modifications in target proteins

2.2.1 Penicillin binding protein

Carbapenem resistance in *A. baumannii* may be because of penicillin binding proteins (PBP) or porin modifications. The penicillin-binding domains of PBPs are transpeptidases or carboxypeptidases involved in peptidoglycan metabolism. Reduced expression level of PBP was observed in multidrug resistant strains in order to resist the activity of antibiotics. Some of the strategies adopted by *A. baumannii*, which have been uncovered, are the acquisition of an additional low-affinity PBP, overexpression of an endogenous low-affinity PBP and alterations in endogenous PBPs by point mutations or homologous recombination.

One recent study strongly indicated an association between down-regulation of PBPs and/or alteration in PBPs for β-lactam resistance in *A. baumannii* (Vashist et al., 2011). In this study, it was shown that one of the PBP designated PBP-7/8 is critical for the survival of *A. baumannii* strain AB307–0294 in the rat soft tissue infection and pneumonia models. Furthermore, it was shown PBP-7/8 either directly or indirectly contributes to the resistance of this strain to complement-mediated bactericidal activity (Russo, 2009).

2.2.2 *gyr*A and *par*C

Quinolone resistance is often caused by modifications in the structure of DNA gyrase secondary to mutations in the quinolone resistance determining regions (QRDR) of the *gyr*A and *par*C genes. DNA gyrase and DNA topoisomerase IV encoded by *gyr*A and *par*C genes respectively, are among the housekeeping genes involved in DNA replication and processing are the targets for ciprofloxacin and other fluoroquinones. A point mutation on the *gyr*A gene (Ser-83 to leu) was observed in MDR strains of *A. baumannii* which is consistent with fluoroquinolone resistant phenotype. Sequencing of the *par*C gene also indicated mutations in the *par*C gene that caused an amino acid change at either Ser-80 or Glu-84 (Deccache et al., 2011)

2.3 Alternations in permeability

2.3.1 Changes in OMPs & porins

Reducing the transport of β-lactam into the periplasmic space via changes in porins or OMPs reduces the access to PBPs. The outer membrane in MDR *A. baumannii* is less permeable to antimicrobial agents than that in other susceptible ones. Alternations in permeability characteristics disturbs the β-lactam assimilation into the periplasmic space, resulting in the weak activity of antibiotics. Several porins, including the 33-kDa CarO protein, that constitute a pore channel for influx of carbapenems, might be involved in such resistance. Sometimes disruption of OMP genes by ISAba10 element may lead to the inactivation of the OMPs like CarO thereby reducing the extent of which the antibiotic enters the cell. When the chromosomal locus containing the *car*O gene was cloned from clinical isolates and characterised, it was shown that only a single copy of *car*O, present in a single transcriptional unit, was present in the *A. baumannii* genome. The *car*O gene encodes a polypeptide of 247 aminoacid residues, with a typical N-terminal signal sequence and a predicted trans-membrane β-barrel topology (Siroy et al., 2006). Remarkably, many recent studies have revealed that disruption of the *car*O gene by the IS elements such as ISAba1, ISAba125, or ISAba825 results in loss of activity of CarO OMP leading to carbapenem resistance in *A. baumannii* (Mussi et al., 2005; Poirel et al., 2006). Many recent reports of outbreaks caused by carbapenem resistant phenotypes and their characterization having revealed the loss or reduction of porins such as OMPs of 22-29 kDa, 47, 44, and 37kDa and one of 31 to 36 kDa substantiates the findings of many previous investigations on OMPs. Additional gene expression studies, along with phenotypic characterization, of these membrane proteins will conclusively clarify the role of membrane permeability in β-lactam resistance.

2.4 Efflux pumps

Efflux pumps are the ones among the well studied mechanisms of resistance in *A. baumannii*, by which the bacterial cells overcome the action of antibiotics by expelling them out. For example the 3.9-Mb genome of *A. baumannii* AYE is reported to harbour 46 open reading frames (ORFs) encoding putative efflux pumps of different families (Fournier et al., 2006). The over expression of efflux pump genes have been reported in the antibiotic resistant strains which provides the evidence for the role of efflux pumps in making the bacteria multi-drug resistant. To date, five classes of efflux pumps have been reported to be present in *A. baumannii* such as ATP binding cassette (ABC), major facilitator superfamily (MFS), multidrug and toxic compound extrusion (MATE), resistance–nodulation–cell division (RND) and small multidrug resistance (SMR).

The efflux systems in *A. baumannii* that are completely characterized functionally so far include AdeABC, AdeFGH and AdeIJK (RND type), AbeM (MATE type), and CraA (MFS type) (Peleg, 2008; Roca, 2009; Damier-Piolle, 2009). We have only partial knowledge on the functionality of ABC and SMR efflux pumps (Iacono et al., 2008; Srinivasan et al., 2009)

2.4.1 RND type efflux pump

The RND class efflux pumps that are commonly found in Gram-negative bacteria are usually tripartite in nature, i. e. they comprise of three protein components such as cytoplasmic, inter-membrane or membrane fusion protein (MFP) and peripalsmic or outer membrane protein which are encoded by three different genes present in a single operon. The cytoplasmic protein is otherwise termed as transporter protein which is involved in the export of substrates such as drugs or antibiotics from the cell, MFP and OMP help in export mechanisms. Different classes of RND family efflux pumps have been reported till date in *Acinetobacter* sp. Among these *ade*ABC, *ade*FGH and *ade*IJK functions and specificities have been studied extensively and overexpression of all these efflux pumps is controlled by two-component regulatory systems such as sensor and regulator kinase cascade.

In *A. baumannii*, AdeABC is one of the common types of efflux pumps which are involved in posing resistance to antibiotics such as aminoglycosides, β-lactams, chloramphenicol, tetracyclin, trimethoprim, erythromycin and drugs such as ethidium bromide (Magnet et al., 2001; Peleg et al., 2008). However, many studies seemed to indicate that the presence of *ade*ABC and *ade*DE is species specific, wherein *ade*ABC is being restricted to *A. baumannii* and adeDE to *Acinetobacter* genomespecies 3 (Chau et al., 2004). Contrastingly, one recent study for the first time showed the involvement of AdeABC pump in a non-*A. baumannii* strain and this study also described it in detail and characterized this pump. This investigation had also revealed that all three types of RND pumps coexist in non-*A. baumannii* strains (Roca et al., 2011). In AdeABC pump, AdeB is the multidrug transporter protein, AdeA is the membrane fusion protein and AdeC is the OMP. The efflux transporter AdeB captures the substrates either from within the phospholipid bilayer or the cytoplasm and then transports them out via OMP (AdeC). The periplasmic protein AdeA acts as an intermediate component which acts as an overpass between AdeB and AdeC components. AdeR-S two-component system is likely to control the expression of AdeABC type pumps. Further, point mutations in components of AdeABC and its regulatory proteins have been associated with overexpression of AdeABC leading to multidrug resistance (Marchand et al., 2004).

One study supports the hypothesis that the increased expression of *ade*B is associated with increased MICs of tigecycline. However, in the absence of an *ade*B gene knockout experiments, it is difficult to ascertain the overall contribution of the AdeABC efflux pump to tigecycline nonsusceptibility (Peleg et al., 2007; Hornsey et al., 2010). But, one recent study demonstrated that overexpression of the *ade*ABC efflux pump resulted in tigecycline nonsusceptibility by quantizing transcripts of the *ade*B gene and demonstrating conversion of the tigecycline resistance pattern in the presence of an efflux pump inhibitor without any previously known mutation (Sun et al., 2010). When the isolates were analysed separately, there was an association between a higher MIC and elevated adeABC expression, although more isolates would need to be investigated to confirm this observation.

AdeIJK is the second RND type efflux pump reported in A. baumannii, in which adeI, adeJ, and adeK genes encode the MFP, transporter and outer membrane components of the pump, respectively. This type of pumps are found to be involved in exporting β-lactams, chloramphenicol, tetracycline, erythromycin, lincosamides, fluoroquinolones, fusidic acid, novobiocin, rifampin, trimethoprim, acridine, safranin, pyronine and sodium dodecyl sulphate (Piolle et al., 2008).

The third RND type efflux pump is AdeFGH, which was found to be functional in the mutant in which AdeABC and AdeIJK were non-functional. In one clinically relevant study, it was shown that the increased expression of AdeFGH in A. baumannii is an additional mechanism for high-level resistance to fluoroquinolones and decreased susceptibility to tigecycline. The efficiency of AdeFGH pump is less when compared to the other type of efflux pumps because its overexpression was not reported during antibiotic stress and is found be constitutively expressed in the cells. AdeL, a LysR type regulator controls the expression of AdeFGH operon. The presence of the adeFGH operon in 90% of the strains was shown in one study (Coyne et al., 2010). This work also revealed that overexpression of adeFGH is likely due to point mutation in adeL, suggesting that this event may possibly occur in all clinical strains under selection pressure. More molecular and biochemical studies on the transcriptional regulator AdeL should allow better understanding of the mechanism of AdeFGH expression in A. baumannii (Coyne et al., 2010)

2.4.2 MFS type efflux pump

Major facilitator superfamily (MFS) acts as efflux pumps to decrease the intracellular concentrations of multiple toxic substrates and confer multidrug resistance. TetA and TetB efflux pumps from the MFS, involved in the tetracycline and minocycline resistance in A. baumannii. Many believe that MFS efflux pump is also responsible for the intrinsic chloramphenicol resistance described in A. baumannii strains, and therefore it was suggested that it can be named CraA, for chloramphenicol resistance Acinetobacter (Magnet et al., 2001; Peleg et al., 2008). Recently, a novel efflux pump AmvA (Methyl Viologen resistance) that mediates antimicrobial and disinfectant resistance in A. baumannii has been characterized (Rajamohan et al., 2010). AmvA is known to be responsible for the transport of toxic substances such as acridine orange, acriflavine, benzalkonium chloride, DAPI, deoxycholate, ethidium bromide, methyl viologen, SDS and tetraphenylphosphonium chloride(TPPCl). In yet another study, two different MFS type efflux pumps such as CmlA and CraA that are specific for chloramphenicol resistance have been reported (Roca et al., 2009).

2.4.3 MATE type efflux pump

The MATE (Multidrug and Toxic Compound Extrusion) family is the most recently categorized, one among the five multidrug efflux transporter families. There are almost twenty different types of MATE type transporters reported in bacteria. A proton driven

MATE family of efflux pump AbeM is reported in *Acinetobacter* which was characterized to be responsible for exerting resistance to kanamycin, erythromycin, chloramphenicol, tetraphenylphosphonium chloride (TPPCl), norfloxacin, ciprofloxacin and trimethoprim (Su et al., 2005)

2.4.4 SMR type efflux pump

One most recent study for the first time described the role of the SMR efflux pump in *Acinetobacter* spp (Srinivasan et al., 2009). The regulatory protein of this pump AbeS mediates resistance to various antibiotics, hydrophobic compounds, detergents, and disinfectants in *A. baumannii* strain AC0037 (Srinivasan et al., 2009). The SMR type pump is composed of four transmembrane α-helices of approximately 100–140 amino acids in length driven by H+ gradient. A related study concluded that the coupling ion in the AbeM pump is H+ and not Na+. It is worthwhile to note that some H^+ - norfloxacin antiport activity is seen earlier in vesicles of *E. coli* KAM32/pUC18 (Su et al., 2005).

2.4.5 ABC transporters

ATP Binding Cassette (ABC) transporters form a special family of membrane proteins, characterized by homologous ATP-binding and large, multispanning transmembrane domains. Several members of this family are primary active transporters. Whole cell proteome analysis of *Acinetobacter* has revealed the presence ABC transporters which are proposed to be responsible for the transport of ferric ion and drug resistance (Iacono et al., 2008).

2.5 Aminoglycoside-modifying enzymes (AMEs)

Resistance to aminoglycosides by AMEs is also a major threatening feature which leads to resistant phenotypes which shows resistance to aminoglycoside antibiotics such as gentamycin, kanamycin and streptomycin in *Acinetobacter* spp. All three classes of aminoglycoside-modifying enzymes reported have been found in *Acinetobacter*. These enzymes are the O-nucleotidyltransferases (ANT) and O-phosphotransferases (APH) that catalyse the nucleotidylation (adenylation) and phosphorylation of the hydroxyl groups and finally the N-acetyltransferases (AAC) that catalyse acetylation of amino groups thereby rendering the antibiotics inactive. Studies have shown that the genes encoding all these enzymes to be present on plasmids, transposons or within integron-type structures.

In summary, emergence of MDR *A. baumannii* isolates that are resistant to almost all available antibiotics are a serious problem in clinical settings. More ominously, pan drug-resistant (PDR) and extremely drug-resistant (XDR) *A. baumannii* isolates that have been recently emerged (Park et al., 2009). As a consequence, colistin is now considered as a therapy of last resort against MDR *Acinetobacter* infections (Nation & Li, 2009). Unfortunately, colistin resistance has also been reported now (Adams et al., 2009). The overexpression of components of PmrAB two-component system such as *pmr*B and/or *pmr*A appear to be only partially responsible for colistin resistance as shown by Park et al (Park et al., 2011). All kinds of mechanisms of antimicrobial resistance in *Acinetobacter* species have been clearly illustrated in Figure – 1.

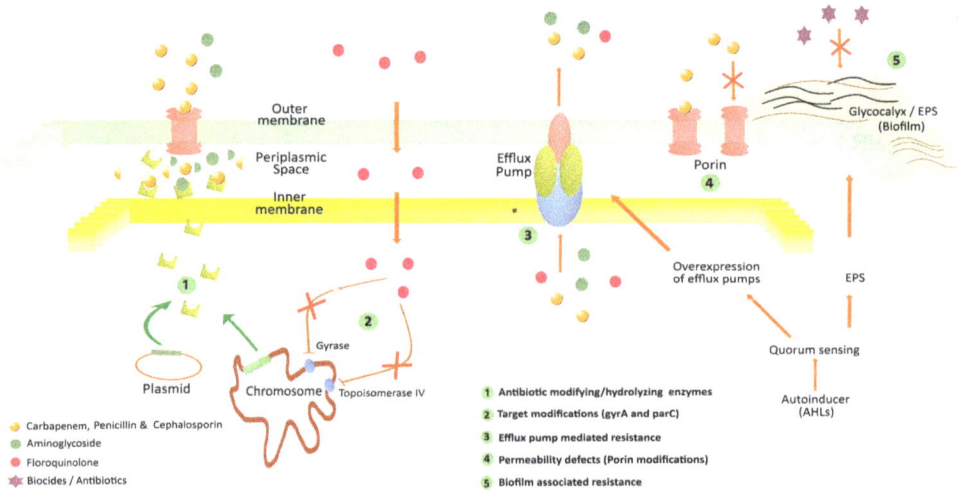

Fig. 1 Potential mechanisms of antimicrobial resistance in *Acinetobacter* species. General depiction of different kinds of antimicrobial resistance mechanisms operating in *Acinetobacter* spp. Five types resistance mechanisms are illustrated in the figure, which is of self explanatory

Finally, more experiments are in need that elucidates the performance of gene knockout studies particularly, knockout of the genes for β-lactamases and efflux systems and restoration of the genetic support for deficient mechanisms (e.g., porins) will further define their roles in *Acinetobacter* clinical isolates.

3. Biofilms and antibiotic resistance

The ability of *A. baumannii* to adhere to and form biofilms on biotic and abiotic surfaces (inanimate objects) may explain its success in the hospital environment. Biofilms might contribute to the environmental persistence of *Acinetobacter* leading to host infection and colonization

3.1 Bacterial biofilms

The bacterial biofilm have been in nature since very long but, it was not until 1970s that science could decipher and appreciate the biofilm lifestyle of bacteria. Biofilm is a complex aggregation of microorganisms, wherein the cells are embedded in a self-produced matrix of extracellular polymeric substance (EPS). The new definition of a biofilm is a microbially derived sessile community characterized by cells that are irreversibly attached to a substratum or interface or to each other, are embedded in a matrix of extracellular polymeric substances that they have produced, and exhibit an altered phenotype with respect to growth rate and gene transcription (Donlan & Costerton, 2002). It is now becoming clear that aggregation of bacterial cells are natural assemblages of bacteria within the biofilm matrix and it functions as a cooperative consortium, in a relatively complex and coordinated manner. Biofilm phenotype of a pathogen promotes increased colonization and persistence and therefore is the leading cause for device-related infections. The ability of these pathogens to adhere to human tissues and medical devices and produce biofilms is a major virulence factor that correlates with increase in antibiotic resistance, reduced phagocytosis, and overall persistence of the bacterial population. Moreover, these biofilms are notoriously difficult to eradicate and are a source of many recalcitrant infections. The medical importance of the scientific studies of biofilms and its architecture resides more in our ability to explain the characteristics of device-related infections and other chronic infections and to design strategies to counter their refractory nature.

3.1.1 Biofilms and resistance

The mechanisms by which biofilms contribute to reduced susceptibility still remain unclear, but a number of different explanations have been proposed. Biofilms are inherently resistant to the antimicrobial agents, reasons being failure of an agent to penetrate full depth to cells of biofilm or cells slow growing state due to the organism's slow metabolism. For chemically reactive disinfectants such as chlorine, iodine and peroxygens, and for highly charged antibiotics, such as the glycopeptides, the glycocalyx does indeed greatly affect the ability of the antimicrobial agent to reach those cells that are deep within the biofilm. On the other hand, for relatively unreactive, uncharged agents, such as the β-lactams, such reaction-diffusion limitation is unlikely to occur. The glycocalyx may however, contribute to reduced susceptibility to β-lactams, if the antibiotic is susceptible to inactivation by β–lactamases and if the β-lactamase is derepressed while the bacterium is in the biofilm mode of growth. In such cases, the enzyme is concentrated within the extracellular polymer matrix and hydrolyses the drug as it penetrates (Gilbert & Brown, 1998). Reduced susceptibility to β-lactams amongst biofilm bacteria is more likely to be a function of a diminished growth rate within the deeper recesses of the biofilm which causes the expression of penicillin-binding proteins that are unrepresentative of those normally targeted by these antibiotics (Gilbert & Brown, 1998). Retarded growth also affects the bactericidal action of the β-lactams because transpeptidase inhibition, which induces cellular injury, is directly related to growth rate. One investigation revealed that gene transfer in biofilms occurs far more frequently than previously noticed (Hausner & Wuertz, 1999) and horizontal gene transfer inside a biofilm matrix offers a great advantage in terms of both frequency and stability (Hausner & Wuertz, 1999). The knowledge that attached cells of the same species differ in their ability to maintain incoming plasmids hints at specific physiological conditions in biofilms which lead to individual cells experiencing different environmental pressures.

3.1.2 Biofilm cycle – a multistep process

Attachment to abiotic surface is mainly dependent on cell surface hydrophobicity, whereas surface proteins mediate adhesion to host matrix-covered implants. After adhesion to the surface, exopolysaccharide, specific proteins and accessory macromolecules aid in intercellular aggregation (Otto, 2009). At critical cell density, cells co-ordinate through a communication pathway involving signalling molecules, termed quorum sensing (QS), resulting in biofilm formation (Costerton et al., 1999). Further, at a later stage, due to physical forces or intercellular signalling, the cells detach and disperse to colonize new areas (Costerton et al., 1999).

3.1.3 Biofilm and disease

While many biofilm infections are "stealthy," in that they develop slowly and initially produce few symptoms, they may be very damaging because they promote immune complex sequelae and act as reservoirs for acute exacerbations in hosts. Many a times host immune response products of oxidative bursts rarely penetrate the biofilm matrix accounting for the inability of phagocytes to destroy the pathogen (Costerton et al., 1999). The exact processes by which biofilm associated organisms elicit disease in the human host are poorly understood. However, suggested mechanisms include: (i) detachment of cells or cell aggregates from indwelling medical device biofilms, resulting in bloodstream or urinary tract infections, (ii) production of endotoxins and (iii) resistance to the host immune system (Peleg et al., 2008). One should begin to examine any infection that is refractory to antibiotic therapy and to host defences in terms of the genes that are expressed to produce the refractory bacterial phenotype. Furthermore, one must begin to use the biofilm phenotype of each chronic pathogen in the development of new vaccines and antibiotics aimed at biofilm-specific targets that can be the means of controlling burgeoning group of diseases caused by biofilm phenotype.

3.2 Biofilm development mechanisms in *A. baumannii*

There are three important factors which contribute to the persistence of *A. baumannii* in the hospital environment, namely: resistance to major antimicrobial drugs, resistance to desiccation and resistance to disinfectants. This survival property is most likely to play a significant role in the outbreaks caused by this pathogen (Tomaras et al., 2003). The potential ability of *Acinetobacter* to form biofilms may explain its outstanding antibiotic resistance against a wide range of antibiotics (Rao et al., 2008; Dijkshoorn et al., 2007; Donlan & Costerton, 2002). *A. baumannii* has the ability to colonize both abiotic and medical devices (Tomaras et al., 2003) and form biofilms that display decreased susceptibility to multiple antibiotics (Uma Karthika et al., 2008). Adherence of *A. baumannii* to human bronchial epithelial cells and erythrocytes has already been demonstrated, with pilus like structures appear to be important for adherence (Gospodarek et al., 1998, Lee et al., 2006). This process is considered to be a first step in the colonization process of *A. baumannii*. Survival and growth on host skin and mucosal surfaces requires the clones that can resist inhibitory agents and the conditions that are exerted by these surfaces. Outgrowth on mucosal surfaces and medical devices, such as intravascular catheters and endotracheal tubes can result in *A. baumannii* biofilm formation, which enhances the risk of infection of the bloodstream and airways (Tomaras et al., 2003). One of the studies had showed that the common source of *Acinetobacter* bacteremia is intravascular catheters and the colonization of respiratory tract (Cisneros et al., 2002). Interestingly, it has also been demonstrated that biofilm formation in *Acinetobacter* is phenotypically associated with exopolysaccharide (EPS) production and pilus formation (Tomaras et al., 2004). The protein equivalent to CsuE of *Vibrio parahaemolyticus*, a chaperone has been identified as a key factor in pilus and biofilm formation in a pioneer study (Tomaras et al., 2004). Surprisingly, considerable variation in quantitative adherence was observed among different strains of *A. baumannii* isolated from the same geographical region (Lee et al., 2006). This observation of varying degree of adherence among the strains is in concordance with our studies (unpublished data). Our earlier investigation also demonstrated a high propensity among the clinical isolates of *A.*

baumannii to form biofilm and a significant association of biofilms with multiple drug resistance (Rao et al., 2008). Thus, biofilm production by *A. baumannii* promotes increased colonization and persistence leading to higher rates of device related infections. Identification of new genes involved in biofilm formation is required for better understanding of molecular basis of strain variation and various pathogenic mechanisms implicated in chronic *Acinetobacter* infections.

3.2.1 Factors associated with *A. baumannii* biofilm formation

3.2.2 Poly-β-(1, 6)-N-acetlyglucosamine (PNAG)

One of the important polysaccharides is poly-β-(1, 6)-N-acetlyglucosamine (PNAG), which has been now portrayed as a major component of biofilms of bacteria was first described in the genus *Staphylococci* (Maira-Litran et al., 2002). PNAG seems to be having profound effects on host-microbe interactions. PNAG affects colonization, virulence, and immune evasion in infections caused by both Gram-positive and Gram-negative species (Itoh et al., 2008). Apart from its role in surface and cell-to-cell adherence (Cramton et al., 1999), PNAG is described as an important virulence factor (Kropec et al., 2005) and provides protection against the antibiotics and shown to protect *Staphylococci* against innate host defences (Lewis 2001 and Voung et al., 2004). Pga locus encodes for the proteins involved in the synthesis and translocation of PNAG on to the bacterial surface (Kropec et al., 2005; Shiro et al., 1995; Vuong et al., 2004). In *S. aureus*, PNAG confers resistance to killing mediated by innate host immune mediators. Overall, PNAG production by *S. aureus* appears to be a critical virulence factor as assessed in murine models of systemic infection (Kropec et al., 2005). PgaB and IcaB (from *Staphylococci*) contain polysaccharide N-deacetylase domains belonging to carbohydrate esterase family 4. PNAG is also shown to be essential for the formation of the nonrandom or periodic cellular architecture in *E. coli* biofilm microstructure and for conversion from temporary polar cell surface attachment to permanent lateral attachment during the initial stages of biofilm development (Itoh et al., 2008). PgaB of *pga*ABCD peron of *E. coli* is predicted to be an outer membrane lipoprotein. The *hms* locus in *Yersinia pestis*, which is equivalent to PNAG operon apparently promotes the transmission of the plague bacillus *Y. pestis* from the flea vector to the mammalian host (Jarrett et al., 2004). PgaB ortholog in *Y. pestis* designated as HmsF, co-purifies with the outer membrane fraction in this bacterium.

PNAG, the most important EPS secreted by the bacterial population also forms the major component of the biofilms in *Acinetobacter* spp. (Choi et al., 2009). Recent study on *pga*ABCD of Gram-negative bacteria with the typical reference strain of *A. baumannii* showed that the four gene loci share a high degree of similarity with *E. coli* and *Y. pestis* (Choi et al., 2009). *A. baumannii pga*A encodes for a predicted 812-amino-acid OMP and it contains a porin domain suggesting that it facilitates PNAG translocation across the outer membrane and a superhelical periplasmic domain that is thought to play a role in protein-protein interaction (Itoh et al., 2008). PgaB is made up of 510 amino acids with a putative polysaccharide deacetylase domain. PgaB is an outer membrane lipoprotein that along with PgaA, is necessary for PNAG export (Itoh et al., 2008). *pga*C encodes for a 392-amino-acid N-glycosyltransferase that belongs to the glycosyltransferase 2 family. Gene *pga*D encodes for a 150 amino acid protein which localizes in the cytoplasm and assists PgaC in the synthesis of PNAG (Itoh et al., 2008). One recent investigation speculated that in a more dynamic environment with higher shear forces, PNAG is more essential for maintaining the integrity of *A. baumannii* biofilms (Choi et al., 2009).

3.2.3 Biofilm-associated protein (Bap)

Biofilm-associated proteins (Bap) were first characterized in *S. aureus* (Cucarella et al 2001) and recent research findings indicated that *Acinetobacter* has a homologue of Bap protein of *Staphylococcus*. Bap family members are high-molecular weight proteins present on the bacterial surface, contain a core domain of tandem repeats, and play a critical role in cell-cell interactions and biofilm maturation (Loehfelm et al., 2008; Lasa & Penades, 2006). Bap is made up of 8620 amino acids, arranged in tandemly repeated modules A-E (Rahbar et al 2010). It has a higher proportion of negatively charged amino acids in the tandem repeats compared to non-tandem repeat parts (Loehfelm et al., 2008). As it has no transmembrane anchoring domain, its interaction with the cell wall is unclear and yet to be investigated.

The mechanism by which the Bap contributes to biofilm development is unknown, though their large size and the presence of a high number of repeats suggest that these proteins could mediate homophilic or heterophilic intercellular interactions (Lasa & Penades, 2006). Structural studies suggest that the main target for Bap is carbohydrates, for maintenance of biofilm complex (Rahbar et al., 2010). Time course confocal laser scanning microscopy and three-dimensional image analysis of actively growing biofilms demonstrate that Bap mutant is unable to sustain biofilm thickness and volume, suggesting a role for Bap in supporting the development of the mature biofilm structure. In *A. baumannii*, Bap is identified as a specific cell surface protein and is involved in intercellular adhesion within the mature biofilm. Future studies in *A. baumannii* must explore Bap-mediated interactions like direct mediation of intercellular adhesion from one bacterium to a surface receptor on a neighboring bacterium, autoadhesion between Bap molecules on adjacent bacteria and/or whether cells may be linked indirectly via shared interactions with some extracellular biofilm matrix component. However, one can hope that Bap can be a potential target to develop a novel vaccine that can abolish biofilm development (Rahbar et al., 2010).

3.2.4 Chaperone-usher secretion system

A. baumannii require chaperone-usher pili assembly for the production of biofilm on inanimate surfaces as revealed from the study of Tomaras et al (2003). This secretion system encodes for a putative pili-like structure/adhesion protein essential for the initiation of biofilm formation. The *csu* operon expressing chaperone-usher pili assembly comprised of a gene cluster that encompasses six ORFs: *csu*AB-A-B-C-D-E and is polycistronic in nature (Tomaras et al., 2003). The translational products of the *csu*D and *csu*E are highly related to chaperone and usher bacterial proteins, respectively, the four remaining ORFs encode hypothetical proteins potentially involved in pili assembly (Tomaras et al., 2003). The *csu* operon is regulated by a two-component system, *bfm*RS. BfmS is a sensor kinase, which senses environmental conditions and activates a response regulator encoded by *bfm*R. Over-expression of the *csu*AB operon is caused by higher BfmR intracellular concentration (Tomaras et al., 2003). Current models on biofilm formation clearly implicate the participation of bacterial surface related flagella and pili (O' Toole & Kolter, 1998) and cellular appendages (Tolker-Nielson et al., 2000). Bacterial cells in the biofilm community are linked to each other through extracellular appendages that resemble pili structures (Tomaras et al., 2003).

All the above data suggest that there may be an overlap in factors required for the initiation and maturation of biofilms on abiotic and biotic surfaces, bacterial attachment and pathogenesis *in vivo*. Though one can articulate that quorum sensing may be a central mechanism for autoinduction of multiple virulence factors such as genes those involved in the cell envelope, EPS production, pilus biogenesis, iron uptake and metabolism (Smith, 2007) and type IV virulence/secretion systems.

4. Quorum sensing in bacteria

Many bacteria use cell to cell communication to monitor their population density, synchronize their behavior and socially interact. Such communication used by the bacteria is chemical in nature and generally designated as quorum sensing (QS) which is nothing but a coordinated gene regulation and is generally termed as QS. Small diffusible molecules produced by bacteria are 'signals' which can reach other cells and elicit 'answers'. This phenomenon relies mainly on cell density and with the increase in cell density, a critical concentration of signaling molecule will be reached that allows sensing of the signalling molecule and enables the other bacteria to respond. QS is a type of community behaviour prevalent among a diverse group of bacteria to switch between planktonic phenotype to high cell density biofilm phenotype. Irrespective of either Gram-negative or Gram-positive bacteria, the process of QS is analogous in both the groups. The stepwise process involving intracellular synthesis of low molecular weight molecules and secrete them to the extracellular milieu. When the number of cells in a population increases, the concentration of QS molecules also increases and once the minimal threshold level crosses, the molecules are recognised by the receptors that trigger signal transduction cascades that result in a population wide change in gene expression. Such molecular cascades enable the population to function in harmony to survive and proliferate. Depending upon the bacterial species, the physiological processes regulated by QS are extremely diverse, ranging from maintaining the biofilms to regulating the antibiotic resistance. A flurry of research over the past decade has led to significant understanding of many aspects of QS molecules including their synthesis, the receptors that recognize the signal and transduce this information to the level of gene expression and the interaction of these receptors with the transcriptional machinery. Recent studies have begun to integrate QS into global regulatory networks and establish its role in developing and maintaining the structure of bacterial communities.

QS network in Gram-negative bacteria regulate the expression of specific sets of genes in a cell density-dependent fashion (Ng & Bassler, 2009). Pathogenic bacteria typically use QS in the regulation of genes encoding extracellular virulence factors. Gram-positive bacteria like *S. aureus* secrete small peptides for cell to cell communication. On the other hand Gram-negatives like *A. baumannii* predominantly produce small molecules like acylated homoserine lactones (Acyl-HSL) as QS entities. Sometimes other signalling molecules such as 2-heptyl-3-hydroxy-4-quinolone and diketopiperazines are also produced by Gram-negative bacteria (Holden et al., 2000)

4.1 Quorum sensing molecules

Acyl homoserine lactones (AHLs) are a major class of autoinducer signals used by Gram-negative proteobacteria for intraspecies communication that are best characterised till date. AHLs of QS signalling system seem to control diverse physiological functions such as biofilm formation, Ti plasmid conjugation, production of antibiotics, and competence in certain bacteria (Fuqua et al., 2001; Antunes et al., 2010). AHLs are composed of HSL rings carrying acyl chains of C4 to C18 in length. These side chains harbour occasional modification, notably at the C3 position or unsaturated double bonds. The first AHL autoinducer and its cognate regulatory circuit has been first discovered in the bioluminescent marine bacterium *Vibrio fischeri*. Two proteins, LuxI and LuxR, are essential for QS control of bioluminescence in *V. fischeri*. The LuxI/LuxR regulatory system of *V. fischeri* is considered the paradigm for the control of gene expression by QS in Gram-negative bacteria. Homologs of *luxI* and *luxR* have been identified in a large number of bacterial genomes and these other LuxIR-type QS systems control global cell density dependent gene expression. In *V. fischeri*, LuxI is the synthase of the QS autoinducer N-3-(oxo-hexanoyl)-homoserine lactone (3OC6HSL). LuxI catalyzes acylation and lactonization reactions between the substrates S-adenosylmethionine (SAM) and hexanoyl-ACP. Following synthesis, 3OC6HSL diffuses freely in and out of the cell and its concentration increases as the cell density of the population increases (Stevens et al., 1994). LuxR is the cytoplasmic receptor for 3OC6HSL as well as the transcriptional activator of the luciferase operon. Without the 3OC6HSL ligand, the LuxR protein is unstable and is rapidly degraded. When 3OC6HSL accumulates, it is bound by LuxR and the LuxR-AHL complex recognizes a consensus binding sequence (*lux* box) upstream of the luciferase operon and activates its expression. Because expression of luxI is also activated by 3OC6HSL-bound LuxR, when the QS circuit engages, autoinducer production is induced, and the surrounding environment is flooded with the signal molecule. This autoinduction positive feedback loop is presumed to enforce synchrony as the population of cells switches from low cell density mode to high cell density QS mode (Stevens et al., 1994; Schaefer et al., 1996).

The QS networks are increasingly gaining importance in clinical isolates as they function as global regulators. One of the well studied organisms in clinical context is *P. aeruginosa*, which uses AHL as a QS signaling molecule. In *P. aeruginosa*, the QS network is found to play a major role in maintaining biofilm, this biofilm matrix in turn helps the bacteria to survive hostile conditions by becoming resistance to bactericidal agents, resisting nutrition depleted conditions and thereby helps them to remain persistent in hospital environment that makes complete eradication of this organism a challenging quest.

4.2 Quorum sensing in *A. baumannii*

Quorum sensing (QS) in *A. baumannii* appears to have a regulatory role in biofilm formation (Smith et al., 2007). Environmental survival and growth require attributes such as resistance to desiccation and antibiotics, versatility in growth requirements, biofilm forming capacity and possibly, QS activity (Dijkshoorn et al., 2007; Smith, 2007). QS has been shown to regulate a wide array of virulence mechanisms in many Gram-negative organisms (Antunes et al., 2010) and *Acinetobacter* is no different. The presence of QS has been inferred from the detection of a gene that is involved in autoinducer production (Gaddy et al., 2009) that could control the various metabolic processes, production of virulence factors, including biofilm formation. QS network in *Acinetobacter* is mediated by acyl homoserine lactones (AHL). Up to five different QS signal molecules that are more detectable (produced abundantly) during the stationary phase have been identified in *Acinetobacter*, indicating that this may be a central mechanism for autoinduction of multiple virulence factors (Gonzalez et al., 2001;Joly-Guillou et al., 2005; Niu et al., 2008; Gonzalez et al., 2009). In one most recent study, different species of *Acinetobacter* were analyzed for the production of AHL and it was shown that QS sensors were not homogenously distributed among species, though one particular AHL was specifically present in most of the strains belonging to *A. calcoaceticus-A. baumannii* complex (Gonzalez et al., 2009). Furthermore, it was revealed that no distinction could be made between the QS signals secreted by typical opportunistic strains of the *A. calcoaceticus-A. baumannii* complex isolated from patients and strains belonging to other species of the genus (Gonzalez et al., 2009). In our investigation, we have also identified more than six different QS signal molecules in majority of the *A. baumannii* clinical isolates wherein chromatographic separation (Thin Layer Chromatography) of ethyl acetate extracts followed by β-galactosidase assay for determining QS activity using *A. tumefaciens* reporter strain NT1, containing plasmid pZLR4 carrying traR and a traG::lacZ reporter fusion was used. However, among these only one kind of QS molecule was produced abundantly (Figure – 2).

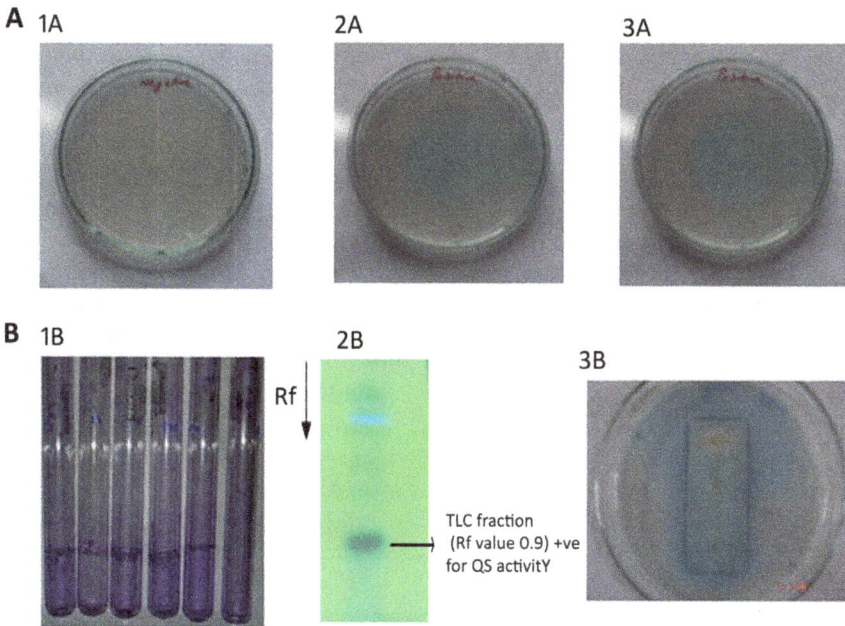

A:- Biosensor overlay test using reporter strain (*Agrobacterium tumefaciens* pZLR4) for detection of quorum sensing (QS) molecules; 1A – Negative control; 2A *A. tumefaciens* Positive control NTL4(pTiC58ΔaccR); 3A - QS activity positive reaction produced ethyl acetate extract of *A. baumannii* clinical isolate confirming the production Acyl Homoserine lactone
B:- 1B- Biofilm production in *A. baumannii* isolates detected through Tube method using 1% crystal violet stain. Thick violet ring was witnessed between liquid air interfaces; 2B - Thin layer chromatography (TLC) of crude ethyl acetate extract of *A. baumannii* culture supernatant; 3B - Ethyl acetate extracts obtained from *A. baumannii* culture supernatants were separated by TLC and over laid with *A. tumefaciens* (pZLR4).

Fig. 2. Quorum sensing activity in *A. baumannii*

Another recent investigation on *A. baumannii* M2 strain characterized an AHL and one AHL synthase gene was identified, which was held responsible for predominant of kind QS molecule produced (Niu et al., 2008). Although additional AHLs were detected in this study, they were not able detect any other gene related to them. Hence, it appears that the auto inducer synthase that was discovered has low specificity and may be capable of synthesizing other QS signals as well. Some interesting questions arising out of above study are: do the diversity of QS signals observed respond only to particular synthase? or is there any existence of more than one AHL synthase?

However, since AHL signals produced by acyltransferases do not have similarity to LuxI or LuxM/AinS, it cannot be ruled out that additional AHL signals are present in *A. baumannii* M2. The AbaI protein was similar to members of the LuxI family of autoinducer synthases and was predicted to be the only autoinducer synthase encoded by *A. baumannii*. The expression of *aba*I at the transcriptional level was activated by ethyl acetate extracts of *A. baumannii* culture supernatants or by synthetic 3-hydroxy-C12-HSL. Further an *aba*I mutant failed to produce any detectable AHL signals and was impaired in biofilm development indicting that there is direct role QS molecules in biofilm development (Niu et al., 2008). QS machinery in *A. baumannii* appear to be mediated by a two component system AbaIR (Niu et al., 2008). This two-component system is homologous to a typical LuxIR family of proteins found in Gram- negative bacteria. This system includes a sensor protein AbaI that functions as an enzyme synthesizing AHLs and AbaR that functions as receptor by recognizing the AHL and induces a cascade of signaling pathway(s). QS was found to play a major role in biofilm maintenance and maturation in *Acinetobacter*. Niu et al (2008) have revealed that in abaI null mutants, there is about 40% reduction of biofilm and this was restored when AHL supplied externally. Consistent with this study, scanning electron microscopy (SEM) analysis data from our laboratory has shown biofilm formation in biofilm-negative clinical isolates when AHL was provided exogenously, as well there was enhanced biofilm formation in weakly adherent clinical isolates after such supplementation (Figure– 3). *A. baumannii* was found to produce more than 5 types of AHLs with varying fatty acid chains (Gonzalez et al., 2001 & 2009; Niu et al., 2008). The *aba*I autoinducer synthase was found to produce N-(3-hydroxydodecanoyl)-L-HSL (3-hydroxy-C12-HSL) when cloned and expressed in *E. coli*. Genomic sequence analysis of *A. baumannii* ATCC 17978 has revealed that *aba*I and acyltransferase may be the core mediator for synthesis of AHLs with varying chemical nature. Such observations as whole underpin a positive correlation between QS and biofilm formation

A comparative study using *in silico* tools have shown that the autoinducer synthase gene *aba*I is more than 45% identical to autoinducer synthase gene from environmental non-pathogenic organisms like *Halothiobacillus neapolitanus*, *Acidithiobacillus ferrooxidans* ATCC23270 and less identical to RhlI and LasI system of pathogenic *P. aeruginosa* but about 47.3% identical to autoinducer synthase genes of an environmental strain *Pseudomonas* sp RW10S (Bhargava et al., 2010). These similarities and dissimilarities between environmental and clinical isolates clearly demonstrates how *Acinetobacter* as evolved from an environmental form to a pathogenic individual. Further, in-depth analysis has revealed that *A. baumannii* has more similarity with *Burkholderia ambifaria* at organism level and in stark contrast, its *aba*I gene shares similarity with *H. neapolitanus*. Similarly, *aba*R was found to share more similarity to *H. neapolitanus* but it is unrelated to *B. ambifaria*. This can raise another question that *aba*I and *aba*R are two different genes yet they share similarity with homologs of another organism and it is because *aba*R is present just 63 base pairs upstream of *aba*I and it can be easily transferred as a single unit from one organism to the other.

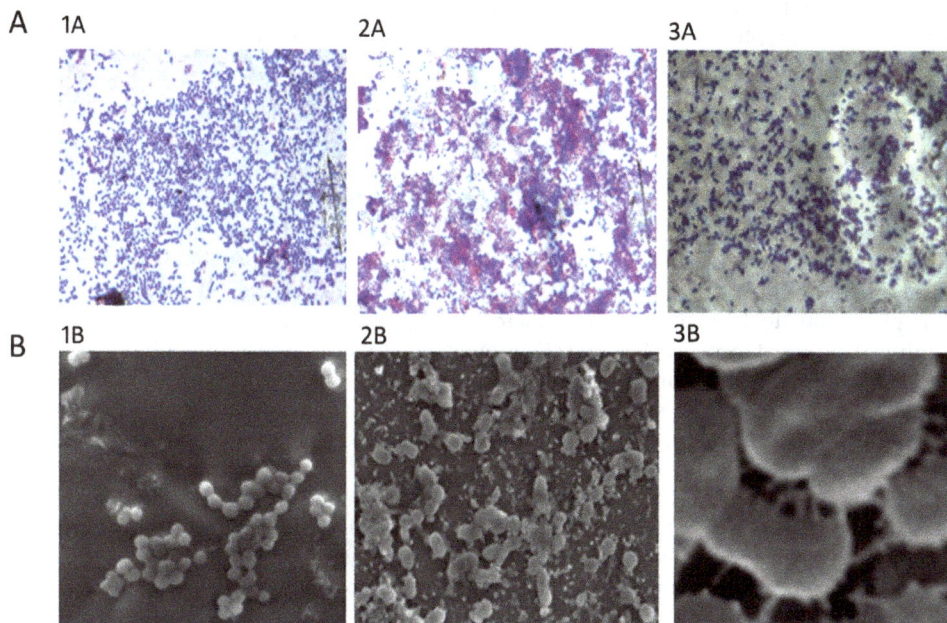

1A- Growth of *A. baumannii* (biofilm-negative) on glass cover slip stained with 0.1% of crystal violet; 2A- Effect of N-AHL (200µM) extracted from *A. baumannii* biofilm phenotype on growth of biofilm non-producer; biofilm development can be observed. 3A - Effect of garlic extract on growth and biofilm formation; inhibition of biofilm was observed.
1B & 2B - SEM images of preparations similar to 1A & 2A respectively (X 5000 magnification); 3B magnified images showing cell to cell adherence through pili-like appendages (X 15000 magnifiction).

Fig. 3. A & B – Microscopic and scanning electron microscopic (SEM) analysis of effect of N-Acyl homoserine lactone (AHL) and garlic extract (Quorum quenching agent) on biofilm-negative strains of *A. baumannii* of clinical origin.

The likely lateral gene transfer between two distinct bacteria can be attributed to the natural competence of *A. baumannii* that has made them to acquire genetic information from other organisms. Interestingly, QS sensing is well known to increase competence in bacteria which further illuminates the importance of these chemical mediators.

A. baumannii being found to be a major threat in many hospitals, recent studies have clearly demonstrated the alarming need for an intense research on QS in *A. baumannii*. Pandrug resistance of *A. baumannii* is attributed to a number of antibiotic resistance mechanisms and biofilm formation. This biofilm formation is in turn regulated by QS networks, which make them to be considered as an important drug target to combat these multidrug resistant superbugs.

4.3 Quorum sensing and Antibiotic resistance

Multiple drug resistance can be attributed to a number of mechanisms, which includes synthesis of enzymes that degrade the drugs, modified targets that does not respond to the drug and presence of efflux pumps that pumps out the bactericidal drugs from the bacterial system to the extracellular milieu. QS was found to be regulating multidrug resistance in two ways, one involves up regulation of biofilm associated EPS matrix and other by up regulation of efflux pump genes.

The production of an EPS matrix is one of the distinguishing characteristics of biofilm and it has been suggested that EPS prevents the access of antibiotics into the bacterial community. Our investigations reveal that there is a strong association between multidrug resistance and biofilms wherein majority of our clinical isolates, which were strong biofilm producers were also exhibiting multidrug resistance (Rao et al., 2008). Compared to non-biofilm producers, biofilm producers showed a significantly higher resistance to cephotaxime, amikacin, ciprofloxacin and aztreonam. Thus, it is clear that clinical isolates of *A. baumannii* have a high propensity to form biofilm and there is a significant association of biofilms with multiple drug resistance. Further investigation showed that presence of antibiotic resistant determinant *bla*PER-1 is more critical for cell adherence, which is the first step in biofilm formation cycle. One of the success stories of *Acinetobacter* is its ability to withstand stress conditions like exposure to high dose of antibiotics. Previous studies on *Pseudomonas* have shown that exposure to the macrolide antibiotics found to enhance biofilm formation. Such responses suggest biofilm as a potential defence mechanism against antibiotics. Similar mechanism is seen in *A. baumannii* in which strong biofilm producers are commonly multidrug resistant. The role of QS molecule as a key player in antibiotic resistance can be understood from their mechanism of enhancing replication and transfer of plasmids, which are the major carriers of antibiotic resistant genes. Thus in a biofilm microstructure there is an increased possibility of gene transfer including genes for antibiotic resistance. Consequently, the biofilm forming capacity of *A. baumannii* combined with its multidrug resistance contributes to the organism's survival and further dissemination in the hospital settings.

Evidences for the role of QS in upregulating efflux pumps arise from studies in *E. coli* in which over expression of *E. coli* luxR homologue SdiA lead to the overexpression of AcrAB efflux pumps and its knockout lead to decrease in AcrAB efflux gene expression. This study clearly demonstrates how QS directly play an indispensable role in regulating efflux pump gene expression. SdiA as well regulates cell division in a cell density-dependent manner. It was also shown that SdiA controls multidrug resistance by positively regulating the MDR pump AcrAB and overproduction of SdiA confers multidrug resistance and increased levels of AcrAB. Conversely, *sdi*A null mutants are hypersensitive to drugs and have decreased levels of AcrB protein. These observations provide a direct link between QS and MDR achieved through efflux pump. Combined with earlier reports, this data support a model in which a role of drug efflux pumps is to mediate cell–cell communication in response to cell density (Rahmati et al., 2002). Now, it is clear that *sdi*A positively regulates the AcrAB efflux pump to mediate multiple drug resistance in *E. coli*.

In *P. aeruginosa*, when the cells are in the logarithmic growth phase, the MexR repressor negatively regulates *mex*AB-*opr*M efflux pump expression by binding at the MexR-MexAB-OprM operator-promoter region. As the cells enter the stationary growth phase, they sense a high population density and turn on a QS switch producing an autoinducer, C4-HSL, which independently induces the expression of *mex*AB-*oprM* operon directly or it inactivates the MexR repressor, as a consequence it enhances the transcription of MexAB–OprM efflux pump (Maseda et al., 2004). This study also revealed that MexAB mutants accumulate 3O-C12-HSL intracellularly, which shows how QS signals form a part of efflux pump networks. In *A. baumannii*, antibiotic resistance is also brought about by a number efflux pump genes and the RND efflux genes which are found to share about 47% similarity with MexAB pumps are the major efflux pumps in *A. baumannii*. *A. baumannii* also produces C12-HSL compounds as QS molecules, which shows that there may be an interconnecting role between efflux pumps and QS that imparts multiple drug resistance.

To overcome stress, cells express various factors and one of them is RpoS which is regulated by the global regulator Hfq. In one of the studies conducted in *P. aeruginosa*, *las*R knockout mutants showed decreased resistance to ofloxacin, whereas the resistance was restored when RpoS was over expressed in *las*R knockouts. This finding suggests the strong role of stress regulators in multiple-drug resistance. As Hfq was found to regulate RpoS which in turn involved in orchestrating QS controlling antibiotic resistance, one can understand the pivotal role of stress regulators in QS and multidrug resistance. *Acinetobacter* genome analyses provide evidences for the presence of both Hfq and RpoS in *A. baumannii* though their interconnecting role is not yet elucidated.

4.4 Biofilm associated gene expression and virulence factors

Many recent investigations have revealed differential gene expression of genes during biofilm formation. Since biofilm helps in persistence of the organism in various stressful environments including survival in human hosts, many stress tolerating factors (can also termed as virulence factors) are produced to overcome a range of stress conditions. In this regard, our investigations have shown a positive correlation between biofilm and virulence factors. Our study which included majority of clinical isolates of *A. baumannii* that are biofilm producers were also found to be positive for production of virulence factors like protease, gelatinase, phospholipase, serum resistance and haemolysis (unpublished data). These factors are highly helpful for the pathogens survival in human hosts. Thus our observation sturdily supports a positive correlation between biofilm and virulence factors. Some cells in biofilm have slow growth rate, which is related to general stress response rather than nutrient limitations. To overcome stress, cells express various factors and one of them is RpoS which is regulated by the global regulator Hfq. As Hfq was found to regulate RpoS which in turn leads to QS controlled expression of virulence factors, one can understand the pivotal role of Hfq during harsh conditions. A general model of QS network with overall role of AHL in signal transduction regulated by AbaR, possible role of AbaI, Hfq, RpoS in *Acinetobacter* spp. is depicted in Figure – 4.

In conclusion, QS sensing works as a global regulator in regulating a diversified network of signalling cascades which helps the organism to resist infinite hostile conditions that are yet to be unveiled. Bacterial virulence being shown as one of the functions regulated by QS may therefore be a right target for designing newer therapeutics. Consequently, interference with QS-based inter-cellular communication might become the basis of new therapeutic schemes. Moreover, understanding QS cascades apart from revealing the communal relationships between the cells may help in designing potential drugs which can tackle multidrug resistant superbug *A. baumannii*.

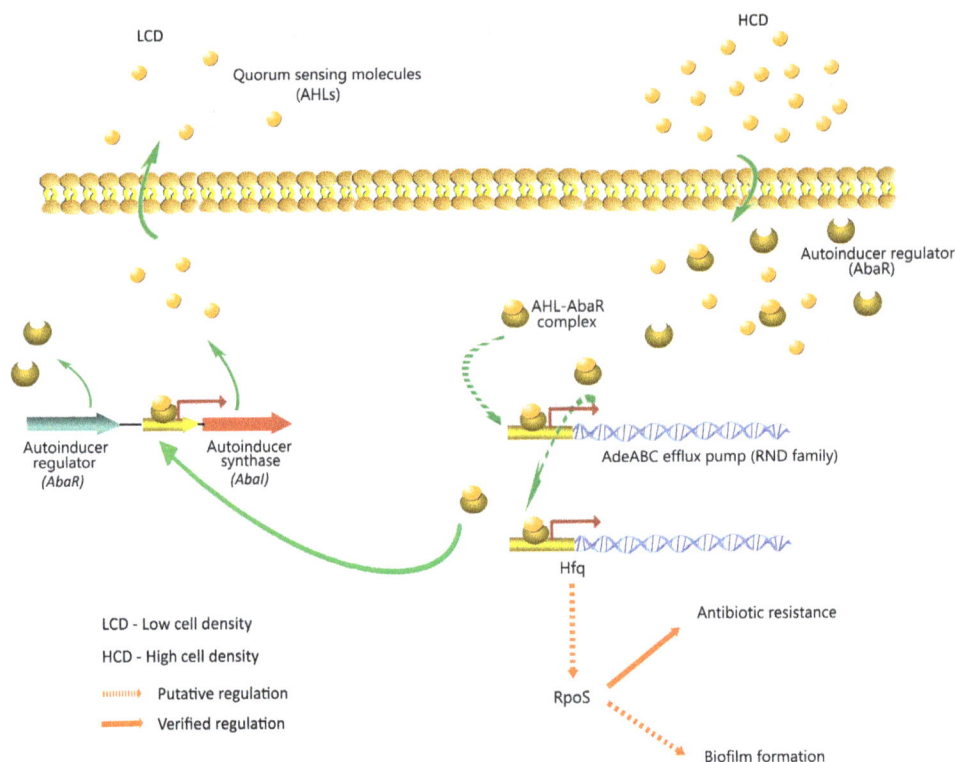

Fig. 4. A General model of acyl-homoserine lactone (AHL) signal transduction in *Acinetobacter* spp. by quorum sensing is shown. Tentative model for AHL synthesis (*left side*) and AHL interaction with AbaR-type regulatory proteins (*right side*) are depicted. Green solid arrows on the outer membrane indicate the potential two-way traffic of AHLs into and out of the cell. Putative regulatory role of AbaR and its interaction with AbaI or AbaI-type protein is shown at left side. Putative activation and overexpression of AdeABC efflux pump by AHL- AbaR complex is depicted by green dotted arrows at the right side. The presumed role of AHL- AbaR complex in up regulation of Hfq expression and putative regulation of RpoS by Hfq are shown. Finally, role of RpoS in antibiotic resistance and its probable role in biofilm development are illustrated.

5. Future prospective

Ironically, many have started believing that we are nearing the post antibiotic era as no new groups of antibiotics have been discovered after 1980s. As such, we are in a desperate need for searching new therapeutic solutions for infections caused pan-drug resistant bacteria. We might achieve this with respect to nosocomial pathogen *A. baumannii* after some careful studies of the genomics and proteome of *Acinetobacter* species looking for possible promising targets. In the following paragraphs, we describe one of the potential targets as an example, where we have tried to relate iron metabolism to biofilm production, which is based entirely on indirect evidences but strong correlation of *A. baumannii* with its other close relatives in a genomic perspective.

The remarkable similarities between the prokaryote and eukaryote iron transport systems underscore the importance of our analysis with respect to the host-bacteria interactions leading to disease. An increased knowledge of the molecular mechanisms of microbial pathogenicity mediated by iron and host resistance will undoubtedly help in finding potential drug targets. The iron-scarce environment of a vertebrate host generates a non-specific defence mechanism as most iron is bound with host proteins such as haemoglobin, or complexed with high affinity ligands such as transferrin and lactoferrin (Neilands et al., 1995). To overcome this, *A. baumannii* and other Gram-negatives secrete high affinity iron chelators, called siderophores that gather this micro- but essential nutrient (Neilands et al., 1995; Crosa, 1989). Siderophores (from the Greek: "iron carriers") are defined as relatively low molecular weight, ferric ion specific chelating agents elaborated by bacteria and fungi growing under low iron stress environment. The role of these compounds is to scavenge iron from the environment and to make the mineral and make it available to the cell. The ability to extract iron from these iron-scarce environments of the host often contributes to the virulence of a successful pathogen.

5.1 Iron metabolism in *Y. pestis* and *A. baumannii*

Indeed, there have been reports that iron deficient media suppress biofilm formation and hence decrease virulence (Weinberg, 2004; Yang et al., 2007). But, this would do nothing to hinder the growth of the pathogen as the siderophores perform superbly, the task of iron acquisition with their extremely high affinity for ferric ion (Neilands et al., 1995; Braun and Hantke, 2011). We certainly have a choice of targeting the iron acquisition system so as to abolish the virulence. Recent studies on human Gram-negative pathogen *Y. pestis* suggest that the HmsHFRS and HmsT operons regulating hemin-binding and storing system are also involved in biofilm formation (Perry et al., 1990; Kirillina et al., 2004). In fact, *Y. pestis* Hms+ phenotype, described by enormous adsorption of hemin or congo red to become red coloured, is a manifestation of biofilm formation during growth at 26–34 °C (Perry et al., 2004). *A. baumannii* has genes homologous to HmsH, HmsF and HmsR that occur end-to-end and (may) constitute an operon having a pair of hypothetical genes and spanning about a 4.7 kb region along the complementary strand of the genome (Figure-5).

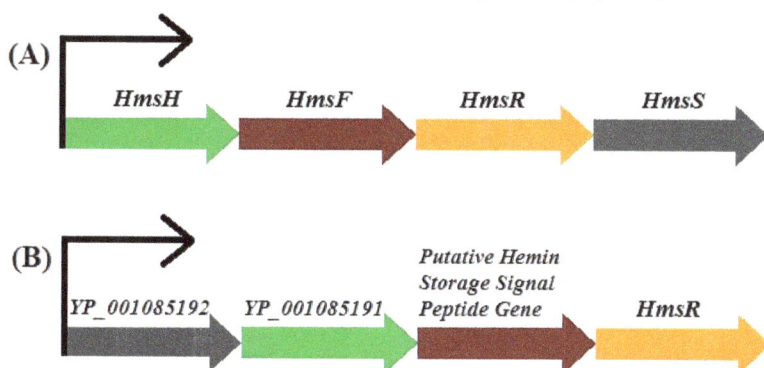

Fig. 5. A comparison between (A) *Y. pestis* Hms operon and (B) a 4.7 kb region of *A. baumannii* genome (see text) having four genes. Matching colours except dark grey colour showing homologues. Dark grey segments do not match. Promotor and intergenic sequences are ignored for the sake of simplicity.

Y. pestis HmsH is an outer membrane protein with a predicted β-barrel domain (Wortham et al., 2010) and has a weak homology to *A. baumannii* poly-beta-1, 6-N-acetyl-D-glucosamine (PGA) synthesis protein. HmsF is also an outer membrane protein with a predicted deacetylase domain. HmsR and HmsS are inner membrane proteins (Wortham et al., 2010). HmsR has a putative glycosyl-transferase domain where as HmsS homologue Ica is linked to the *Y. pestis* biofilm PGA synthesis protein PgaD. *Y. pestis* HmsH, HmsF, HmsR and HmsS have 58.2%, 60.8%, 83% and 50% sequence similarities to *E. coli* PgaA, PgaB, PgaC, PgaD respectively (Forman et al., 2006). But, they have very weak similarities with their (predicted) *A. baumannii* counterparts. Yet, from some recent investigations, it is now becoming obvious that genes from Hms operon have corresponding counterparts in *A. baumannii* (Zhou and Yang, 2001).

The above mentioned 4.7 kb region in genome of *A. baumannii* contains 4 genes in tandem, which consists of a pair of hypothetical proteins, bearing IDs YP_001085192 and YP_001085192 followed by a putative hemin storage signal peptide protein and hemin storage system protein HmsR. Neither the sequence nor the structural topology of YP_001085192 fits into any of the genes of *Y. pestis* HmsHFRS operon. Rather, according to UniProtKB annotations, it is a putative phosphotransferase, containing a nucleotide (possibly ATP) binding motif. There have been some evidences of phosphoenolpyruvate phosphotransferase (PTS) systems being involved in biofilm formation in *Vibrio cholerae*, *E. coli* and *Streptococcus gordonii* (Houot and Watnick, 2008; Lazazzera, 2010; Houot et al., 2010). YP_001085191, when searched against RefSeq (Pruitt et al., 2000) database, comes to be *A. baumannii* poly-beta-1, 6 N-acetyl-D-glucosamine export porin PgaA, which could be involved in the export of PGA to the cell exterior. The putative hemin storage signal peptide gene, as the name suggests, is involved in hemin storage. Searching results in the Conserved Domain Database (CDD) (Marchler- Bauer et al., 2011) suggested further that it has one each of polysaccharide deacetylase and poly-beta-1,6-N-acetyl-D-glucosamine N-deacetylase PgaB domains. The polysaccharide deacetylase domain is found in polysaccharide deacetylase. This family of polysaccharide deacetylases includes NodB (nodulation protein B from *Rhizobium*), which is a chito-oligosaccharide deacetylase. It also includes chitin deacetylase from yeast and endoxylanases which hydrolyses glucosidic bonds in xylan (Fukushima et al., 2004). Poly-beta-1, 6-N-acetyl-D-glucosamine N-deacetylase PgaB produces polysaccharides based on N-acetyl-D-glucosamine in straight chains with beta-1, 6 linkages. Deacetylation by this protein appears necessary to allow export through the porin PgaA (Itoh et al., 2008). The last one in the order, HmsR, as resulted in the CDD search, belongs to the cellulose synthase superfamily (Roberts and Bushoven, 2007) and also contains a DXD motif which binds to a metal ion that is used to coordinate the phosphates a nucleotide-sugar at the active site. These features suggest that *A. baumannii*, like its near relatives, depends on hemin-adsorption and storage for biofilm formation.

Neither the hemin acquisition (Zimbler et al., 2009) nor the biofilm function has remained uncharacterized in *A. baumannii*. But the above discussion correlates these two and suggests that they are not independent of each other. Even *A. baumannii* is able to survive without the help of iron chelators, if its Hms system is functional (Zimbler et al., 2009). On the contrary, an Hms negative almost does not develop biofilms (Figure-6) (Jarrett et al., 2004). One previous work (James et al., 2006) had revealed that genes coding for hemin and iron acquisition systems in *Porphyromonas gingivalis* are regulated by QS protein LuxS. Again QS is well known for inducing biofilm formation.

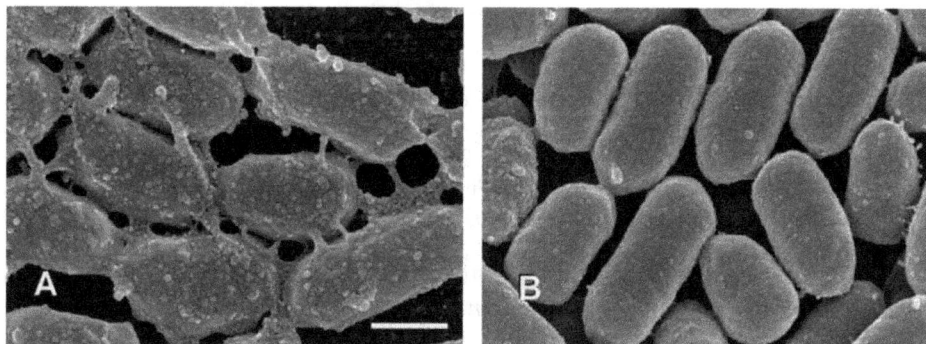

Fig. 6. Scanning electron microscopy of Hms-positive (A) and Hms-negative (B) *Yersinia pestis* grown on agar plates at 21°C. Bar, 0.5 μm. Reproduced with the permission from Jarret et al., 2004.

6. Conclusion

This review attempted to give a glimpses of multiple mechanisms of antimicrobial resistance adopted by various species of *Acinetobacter*, described the current understanding of biofilm development and various factors regulating the biofilm formation in *Acinetobacter*. This write up also explained about the biofilm development and different virulence factors elaborated by *Acinetobacter* and its correlation with antibiotic resistance. Finally, quorum sensing has been elucidated in detail, which works as a global regulator in controlling and regulating diverse physiological functions such as biofilm formation, pilus biogenesis, production of multiple virulence factors, development of antibiotic resistance and increasing the competence of cells that helps in gene transfer. All the information discussed here will definitely help the future research in this area.

In conclusion, all the available evidence implies that *A. baumannii* is very important human pathogen that is gradually gaining more attention as a major global public health problem. It is responsible for a significant proportion of nosocomial infections among patients who are critically-ill receiving intensive care in the ICUs. With this situation together with the fact that certain biofilm phenotypes of *A. baumannii* being highly refractile and recalcitrant that are highly resistant to multiple drugs due to intrinsic resistance properties and those that can acquire resistant determinants with increasing propensity, makes this pathogen one of the most difficult challenges of the present days.

7. Acknowledgment

We are very grateful to **Dr. Stephen K. Farrand**, Departments of Crop Sciences and of Microbiology, University of Illinois at Urbana-Champaign, USA for generously providing *Agrobacterium tumefaciens* NTL4 (pZLR4) indicator strain, *A. tumefaciens* Positive control NTL4(pTiC58ΔaccR) and *A. tumefaciens* NTL4 negative control strains and for helpful discussions.

Authors would also like to thank Indian Council of Medical Research (ICMR), Government of India for funding the Project No.5/3/3/14/2007-ECD and University Grant Commission (UGC), Government of India for funding under Special Assistance Programme (UGC-SAP)

8. References

Adams, M.D. Nickel, G.C. Bajaksouzian, S. Lavender, H. Murthy, A.R. Jacobs, M.R. & Bonomo, R.A. (2009). Resistance to colistin in *Acinetobacter baumannii* associated with mutations in the PmrAB two-component system, *Antimicrob. Agents and Chemother*, Vol. 53, No. 9, (September 2009), pp. 3628-3634, ISSN 0066-4804

Antunes, L.C. Ferreira, R.B. Buckner, M.M. Finlay B.B (2010). Quorum sensing in bacterial virulence. *Microbiology*, Vol. 156, No. 8, (August 2010), pp. 2271-2282, ISSN 1350-0872

Bhargava, N. Sharma,P. Capalash,N. (2010). Quarum sensing in *Acinetobacter*: an emergingPathogen. *Critical Reviews in Microbiology*, Vol.36, No.4, (November 2010), pp.349-360, ISSN 1040-841X

Braun, V. & Hantke, K. (2011). Recent insights into iron import by bacteria. *Current Opinion in Chemical Biology*, Vol.15, No.2, (April 2011), pp. 328–334, ISSN 1367-5931

Chau, S.L. Chu, Y.W. Houang, E.T. (2004). Novel resistance-nodulation-cell division efflux system AdeDE in *Acinetobacter* genomic DNA group 3. *Antimicrob Agents and Chemotherapy* Vol. 48, No. 10, (October 2004) pp. 4054-4055, ISSN 0066-4804

Chen, T. Wu, R. Shaio, M. Fung, C. & Cho, W. (2008). Acquisition of a plasmid-borne blaOXA-58 gene with an upstream IS1008 insertion conferring a high level of carbapenem resistance to *Acinetobacter baumannii*. *Antimicrobial Agents and Chemotherapy* Vol.52, (July 2008) pp.2573–2580, ISSN 0066-4804

Chen, Y. Zhou, Z. Jiang, Y. & Yu, Y. (2011). Emergence of NDM-1-producing *Acinetobacter baumannii* in China. *Journal of Antimicrobial Chemotherapy* Vol. 66, No. 6 (June 2011) pp. 1255-9, ISSN 0305-7453

Choi, AHK; Slamti, L; Avci, FY; Pier, GB; & Maira-Litra´n, T. (2009) The *pga*ABCD locus of *Acinetobacter baumannii* encodes the production of Poly--1-6-N-acetylglucosamine, which is critical for Biofilm formation. *Journal of Bacteriology*. Vol. 191, No. 19, pp. 5953–5963, ISSN 1098-5530

Cisneros, J.M. & Rodríguez-Baño, J. (2002). Nosocomial bacteremia due to *Acinetobacter baumannii*: epidemiology, clinical features and treatment. *Clinical Microbiology Infection*, Vol. 8, No. , pp. 687-693, ISSN 1469-0691

Coelho, J. Woodford, N. Afzal-Shah, M. & Livermore, D. (2006). Occurrence of OXA-58-like carbapenemases in *Acinetobacter* spp. collected over 10 years in three continents. *Antimicrobial Agents and Chemotherapy* Vol. 50, No. 2, (February 2006) pp. 756–758, ISSN 0066-4804

Coelho, J.M. Turton, J.F. Kaufmann, M.E. Glover, J. Woodford, N. Warner, M. Palepou, M.F. Pike, R. Pitt, T.L. Patel, B.C. & Livermore, D.M. (2006). Occurrence of carbapenem-resistant *Acinetobacter baumannii* clones at multiple hospitals in London and Southeast England, *Journal of Clinical Microbiology* Vol.44, No.10 (October 2006) pp.3623–3627, ISSN 0095-1137

Costerton, J.W. Stewart, P. S. & Greenberg, E.P. (1999). Bacterial biofilms: a common cause of persistent infections. *Science* Vol. 284, No. 5418, (May 1999) pp. 1318-1322, ISSN 0036-8075

Coyne, S. Rosenfeld, N. Lambert, T. Courvalin, P. & Perichon, B. (2010). Overexpression of Resistance-Nodulation-Cell Division Pump AdeFGH Confers Multidrug Resistance in *Acinetobacter baumannii*, *Antimicrobial Agents and Chemotherapy* Vol.54, No.10, (October 2010) pp. 4389-4393, ISSN 0066-4804

Crosa J. H. (1989). Genetics and molecular biology of siderophore-mediated iron transport in bacteria. *Microbiological Reviews*, Vol.53, No.4, (December 1989), pp. 517-530, ISSN 1098-5557.

Cucarella, C; Solano, C; Valle, J; Amorena, B; Lasa, I & Penades, JR (2001). Bap, a *Staphylococcus aureus* surface protein involved in biofilm formation. *Journal of Bacteriology* Vol. 183, pp. 2888–2896, ISSN 1098-5530

Deccache, Y. Irenge, L.M. Savov, E. Ariciuc, M. Macovei, A. Trifonova, A. Gergova, I. Ambroise, J. Vanhoof, R. & Gala, J.L. (2011). Development of a pyrosequencing assay for rapid assessment of quinolone resistance in *Acinetobacter baumannii* isolates. *Journal of Microbiol Methods* Vol.86, No. 1, (July 2011), pp. 115-118, ISSN 0167-7012

Donlan, RM & Costerton, JW. (2002) Biofilms: Survival mechanisms of clinically relevant microorganisms. *Clinical Microbiology Reviews*. Vol. 15, No. 2, pp. 167-193, ISSN: 0983-8512.

Dijkshoorn, L. Nemec, A. & Seifert, H. (2007). An increasing threat in hospitals: multidrug resistant *Acinetobacter baumannii*. *Nature Reviews Microbiology*. Vol. 5, No. pp. 939-950, ISSN 1740-1526

Endimiani, A. Luzzaro, F. Migliavacca, R. Mantengoli, E. Hujer, A.M. Hujer, K.M. Pagani, L. Bonomo, R. A. Rossolini, G. M. & Toniolo, A. (2007). Spread in an Italian Hospital of a Clonal *Acinetobacter baumannii* Strain Producing the TEM-92 Extended-Spectrum β-Lactamase. *Antimicrobial agents and chemotherapy* Vol. 51, No. 6 (June 2007) pp. 2211–2214, ISSN 0066-4804

Figueiredo, S. Poirel, L. Croize, J. Recule, C. & Nordmann, P. (2009). In Vivo Selection of Reduced Susceptibility to Carbapenems in *Acinetobacter baumannii* Related to ISAba1-Mediated Overexpression of the Natural blaOXA-66 Oxacillinase Gene, *Antimicrob. Agents and Chemother*, Vol.53, No.6, (June 2009) pp. 2657-2659, ISSN 0066-4804

Forman, S., Bobrov, A. G., Kirillina, O., Craig, S. K., Abney, J., Fetherston, J. D. & Perry, R. D. (2006). Identification of critical amino acid residues in the plague biofilm Hms proteins. *Microbiology*, Vol.152, No.11, (November 2006), pp. 3399–3410, ISSN 1465-2080.

Forster, D.H. & Daschner, F.D. (1998). *Acinetobacter* Species as Nosocomial Pathogens. *European Journal of Clinical Microbiology Infectious* Disease Vol. 17, No. 2, (February 1998), pp.73–77, ISSN 0934-9723

Fournier, P.E. Vallenet, D. Barbe, V. Audic, S. Ogata, H. Poirel, L. Richet, H. Robert, C. Magnet, S. Abergel, C. Nordmann, P. Weissenbach, J. Raoult, D. & Claverie, J.M. (2006), *PLoS genetics*, Comparative Genomics of Multidrug Resistance in *Acinetobacter baumannii*, Vol.2, No.1 (January 2006) pp. 62-72, ISSN 1553-7390

Fukushima, T., Tanabe, T., Yamamoto, H., Hosoya, S., Sato, T., Yoshikawa, H. & Sekiguchi, J. (2004). Characterization of a polysaccharide deacetylase gene homologue (pdaB) on sporulation of *Bacillus subtilis*. *Journal of Biochemistry*, Vol.136, No.3, (September 2004), pp. 283-291, ISSN 1098-5530.

Fuqua, C. Parsek, M.R. Greenberg, E.P. (2001). Regulation of gene expression by cell-to-cell communication: acyl-homoserine lactone quorum sensing. *Annual Reviews Genetics*, Vol. 35, (December 2009), pp.439–68, ISSN 0066-4197.

Gaddy, J.A. & Actis, L.A. (2009). Regulation of *Acinetobacter baumannii* biofilm formation. *Future Microbiol* Vol. 4, No.3, (Aril 2009), pp.273-278, ISSN 1746-0913

Gilbert, P. & Brown, M. R. W. (1998). Biofilms and β-lactam activity. *Journal of Antimicrobial Chemotherapy* Vol. 41, No. 5 (May 1998), pp 571-572, ISSN 0305-7453

Gonzalez, R.H, Nusblat A. & Nudel B. C. (2001). Detection and characterization of quorum sensing signal molecules in *Acinetobacter* strains. *Microbiology Research* Vol. 155, No. 4, (March 2001), pp. 271–277.

González, R.H. Dijkshoorn, L. Van den Barselaar, M. Nudel, C. (2009). Quorum sensing signal profile of *Acinetobacter* strains from nosocomial and environmental sources. *Revista Argentina de Microbiología*, Vol.41, (March 2009), pp. 73-78, ISSN 0325-757413

Gospodarek E, Grzanka A, Dudziak Z et al. (1998). Electron-microscopic observation of adherence of *Acinetobacter baumannii* to red blood cells. *Acta Microbiol Pol* Vol. 47, No. 2, (February 1998), pp.213–217.

Hausner, M & Wuertz, S. (1999) High rates of conjugation in bacterial biofilms as determined by quantitative in situ analysis. *Applied Environmental Microbiology*. Vol 65, pp. 3710–3713, ISSN 0099-2240

Henwood C. J, Gatward T. & Warner M et al. (2002). Antibiotic resistance among clinical isolates of *Acinetobacter* in the UK and in-vitro evaluation of tigecycline (GAR-936). *Journal of Antimicrobial Chemotherapy* Vol. 49, No. 3, (March 2002), pp. 479–487, ISSN 0305-7453

Higgins, P.G. Poirel, L. Lehmann, M. Nordmann, P. Seifert, H. (2009). OXA-143 a novel carbapenem hydrolyzing class D β-lactamase in *Acinetobacter baumannii*. *Antimicrobial Agents and Chemotherapy* Vol. 53, No. 12, (December 2009), pp.5035–5038, ISSN 0066-4804

Holden I, Swift I, Williams I. (2000). New signal molecules on the quorum-sensing block. *Trends Microbiology* Vol. 8, No. 3, (March 2000), pp. 101-104. ISSN 0966-842X

Hornsey, M. Ellington, M.J. Doumith, M. Thomas, C.P. Gordon, N.C. Wareham, D.W. Quinn, J. Lolans, K. Livermore, D.M. & Woodford, N. (2010). AdeABC-mediated efflux and tigecycline MICs for epidemic clones of *Acinetobacter baumannii*, *J Antimicrob Chemother*, Vol. 65, (June 2010), pp. 1589-1593, ISSN 0305-7453

Houot, L. & Watnick, P. I. (2008). A novel role for enzyme I of the *Vibrio cholerae* phosphoenolpyruvate phosphotransferase system in regulation of growth in a biofilm. *Journal of Bacteriology*, Vol.190, No.1, (January 2008), pp. 311–320, ISSN 1098-5530.

Houot, L., Chang, H., Pickering, B. S., Absalon, C. & Watnick, P. I. (2010). The phosphoenolpyruvate phosphotransferase system regulates *Vibrio cholerae* biofilm formation through multiple independent pathways. *Journal of Bacteriology*, Vol.192, No.12, (June 2010), pp. 3055-3067, ISSN 1098-5530.

Itoh, Y., Rice, J. D., Goller, C., Pannuri, A., Taylor, J., Meisner, J., Beveridge, T. J., Preston, J. F. 3rd & Romeo, T. (2008). Roles of *pgaABCD* genes in synthesis, modification, and export of the *Escherichia coli* biofilm adhesin poly-beta-1, 6-N-acetyl-D-glucosamine. *Journal of Bacteriology*, Vol.190, No.10, (May 2008), pp. 3670-3680, ISSN 1098-5530.

James, C. E., Hasegawa, Y., Park, Y., Yeung, V., Tribble, G. D., Kuboniwa, M., Demuth, D. R. & Lamont, R. J. (2006). LuxS involvement in the regulation of genes coding for hemin and iron acquisition systems in *porphyromonas gingivalis*. *Infection & Immunity*, Vol.74, No.7, (July 2006), pp. 3834–3844, ISSN 1098-5522.

Jarrett, C. O., Deak, E., Isherwood, K. E., Oyston, P. C., Fischer, E. R., Whitney, A. R., Kobayashi, S. D., DeLeo, F. R. & Hinnebusch, B. J. (2004). Transmission of Yersinia pestis from an Infectious Biofilm in the Flea Vector. *The Journal of Infectious Diseases*, Vol.190, No.4, (August 2004), pp. 783–92, ISSN 1537-6613

Joly-Guillou M. L. (2005). Clinical impact & pathogenicity of *Acinetobacter*. *Clinical Microbiology and Infection* Vol. 11, No. 11, (November 2005), pp.868–873. ISSN 1469-0691

Karthikeyan, K., Thirunarayan, M.A. & Krishnan, P (2010). Coexistence of blaOXA-23 with blaNDM-1 and armA in clinical isolates of *Acinetobacter baumannii* from India, *J Antimicrob Chemother*, Vol.65, (July 2010) pp. 2253-2270, ISSN 0305-7453

Kirillina, O., Fetherston, J. D., Bobrov, A.G., Abney, J. & Perry, R. D. (2004). HmsP, a putative phosphodiesterase, and HmsT, a putative diguanylate cyclase, control Hms dependent biofilm formation in *Yersinia pestis*. *Molecular Microbiology*, Vol.54, No.1, (October 2004), pp. 75–88, ISSN 1365-2958.

Kropec, A; Maira-Litran, T; Jefferson, KK; Grout, M; Cramton, SE; Gotz, F; Goldmann, DA & Pier, GB. (2005) Poly-N-acetylglucosamine production in *Staphylococcus aureus* is essential for virulence in murine models of systemic infection. *Infection and. Immunity*. Vol 73, pp. 6868–6876, ISSN: 0019-9567.

Lasa, I & Penades, JR. (2006) Bap: A family of surface proteins involved in biofilm formation. *Research in Microbiology* Vol. 157, pp. 99–107. ISSN: 0923-2508.

Lazazzera, B. A. (2010). The phosphoenolpyruvate phosphotransferase system: as important for biofilm formation by *Vibrio cholerae* as it is for metabolism in *Escherichia coli*. *Journal of Bacteriology*, Vol.192, No.16, (August 2010), pp. 4083-4085, ISSN 1098-5530.

Lee, K. Lee, W. G. Uh, Y. et al. (2003). VIM- and IMP-type metallo-blactamase-producing *Pseudomonas* spp. and *Acinetobacter* spp. in Korean hospitals. *Emerging Infectious Disease* Vol. 9, No. 7, (July 2003) pp. 868–871, ISSN1080-6059

Lee, K. Yum, J.H. Yong, D. Lee, H.M. Kim, H.D. Docquier, J.D. Rossolini, G.M. & Chong, Y. (2005). Novel Acquired Metallo- β -Lactamase Gene, blaSIM-1, in a Class 1 Integron from *Acinetobacter baumannii* Clinical Isolates from Korea, *Antimicrobial Agents and Chemotherapy* Vol. 49, No. 11, (November 2005) pp. 4485-4491, ISSN 0066-4804

Lee JC, Koerten H, van den Broek P, et al. (2006). Adherence of *Acinetobacter baumannii* strains to human bronchial epithelial cells. *Research Microbiology* Vol. 157, No. 4, (May 2006), pp. 360–366. ISSN - 0923-2508

Lewis, K. (2001). Riddle of biofilm resistance. *Antimicrobial Agents and Chemotherapy*. Vol. 45, No. 4, (April 2001), pp. 999-1007, ISSN: 0066-4804.

Loehfelm, T.W. Luke, N. R. & Campagnari, A. A.. (2008). Identification and characterization of an *Acinetobacter baumannii* biofilm-associated protein. *Journal of Bacteriology*. Vol. 190, No. 3, (February 2006), pp. 1036-1044, ISSN: 1098-5530.

Livermore, D.M. & Woodford, N. (2006). The beta-lactamase threat in *Enterobacteriaceae, Pseudomonas* and *Acinetobacter*. *Trends in Microbiology* Vol. 14, No. 9 (September 2006), pp. 413-420. ISSN 0966-842X

Livermore, D. (2007). The zeitgeist of resistance. *Journal of Antimicrobial Chemotherapy* Vol. 60, No. suppl 1, (August 2007) pp. i59-61. ISSN 0305-7453

Lu, P.L. Doumith, M. Livermore, D.M. Chen, T.P. & Woodford, N. (2009). Diversity of carbapenem resistance mechanisms in *Acinetobacter baumannii* from a Taiwan hospital: spread of plasmid-borne OXA-72 carbapenemase. *Journal of Antimicrobial Chemotherapy* Vol.63 (April 2009), pp.641–647, ISSN 0305-7453

Maglott, D.R., Katz, K. S., Sicotte, H. & Pruitt, K. D. (2000) NCBI's LocusLink and RefSeq. Nucleic Acids Research Vol. 28, No. 1, (January 2000), pp. 126-128, ISSN 0305-1048

Magnet, S. Courvalin, P. & Lambert, T. (2001). Resistance-Nodulation-Cell Division-Type Efflux Pump Involved in Aminoglycoside Resistance in *Acinetobacter baumannii*

Strain BM4454, *Antimicrob. Agents and Chemother,* Vol.45, No.12, (December 2011) pp. 3375-3380, ISSN 0066-4804

Maira-Litrán, T. Kropec, A. Abeygunawardana, C. Joyce, J. Mark, G. Goldmann, D. A. & Pier, G. B. Immunochemical properties of the staphylococcal poly-N-acetylglucosamine surface polysaccharide. (2002). *Infection Immunity* Vol. 70, No. 8 (August 2002) pp. 4433-4440, ISSN 0019-9567

Marchler-Bauer, A., Lu, S., Anderson, J. B., Chitsaz, F., Derbyshire, M. K., Deweese-Scott, C., Fong, J. H., Geer, L. Y., Geer, R. C., Gonzales, N. R., Gwadz, M., Hurwitz, D. I., Jackson, J. D., Ke, Z., Lanczycki, C. J., Lu, F., Marchler, G. H., Mullokandov, M., Omelchenko, M. V., Robertson, C. L., Song, J. S., Thanki, N., Yamashita, R. A., Zhang, D., Zhang, N., Zheng, C. & Bryant, S. H. (2011). CDD: a Conserved Domain Database for the functional annotation of proteins. *Nucleic Acids Research*, Vol.39, Database issue (January 2011), pp. D225-D229, ISSN 1362-4962

Marchand, I. Piolle, L.D. & Courvalin, P. (2004). Expression of the RND-type efflux pump AdeABC in Acinetobacter baumannii is regulated by the AdeRS two-component system. *Antimicrob Agents Chemother*, Vol.48 (September 2004) pp. 3298– 30, ISSN 0066-4804

Maseda, H. Sawada, I. Saito, K. Uchiyama, H. Nakae, T. Nomura, N. (2004). Enhancement of the *mexAB-oprM* efflux pump expression by a quorum-sensing autoinducer and its cancellation by a regulator, MexT, of the*mexEF-oprN* efflux pump operon in *Pseudomonas aeruginosa. Antimicrobial Agents Chemother*apy, Vol.48, No.4, (Apirl 2004), pp. 1320-1328, ISSN 0066-4804

Mussi, M.A. Limansky, A.S. & Viale, A.M. (2005). Acquisition of resistance to carbapenems in multidrug-resistant clinical strains of *Acinetobacter baumannii*: natural insertional inactivation of a gene encoding a member of a novel family of b-barrel outer membrane proteins. *Antimicrob Agents Chemother*, Vol.49 (April 2005), pp.1432–1440, ISSN 0066-4804

Naas, T. Namdari, F. Poupet, H.R. Poyart, C & Nordmann, P. (2007). Panresistant extended-spectrum β-lactamase SHV-5-producing *Acinetobacter baumannii* from New York City. *Journal of Antimicrobial Chemotherapy* Vol. 60, No. 5, (November 2007) pp. 1174–1176, ISSN 0305-7453

Naiemi, N.A. Duim, B. Savelkoul, P.H.M. Spanjaard, L. Jonge, E.D. Bart, A. Grauls, C.M.V. & Jong, M.D. (2005). Widespread Transfer of Resistance Genes between Bacterial Species in an Intensive Care Unit: Implications for Hospital Epidemiology, *J. Clin. Microbiol.* Vol.43, No.9 (September 2005), pp. 4862-4864, ISSN 0095-1137

Nation, R. L. & Li, J. (2009). Colistin in the 21st century. *Current Opinion in Infectious Disease* Vol. 22, No. 6 (December 2009) pp. 535-543. ISSN 0951-7375

Navon-Venezia, S. Ben-Ami, R. Carmeli, Y. (2005). Update on *Pseudomonas aeruginosa* and *Acinetobacter baumannii* infections in the healthcare setting. *Current Opinion in Infectious Disease* Vol. 18, No. 4, (August 2005) pp. 306–313, ISSN 0951-7375

Neilands, J. B. (1995). Siderophores: structure and function of microbial iron transport compounds. *Journal of Biological Chemistry*, Vol.270, No.45, (November 1995), pp. 26723-26726, ISSN 1083-351X.

Ng, W.L., & Bassler, B.L. (2009). Bacterial quorum-sensing network architectures. *Annual Reviews Genetics*, Vol. 43, (August 2009), pp.197–222, ISSN 0066-4197

Niu, C. Clemmer, K.M. Bonomo, R.A. Rather, P.N. (2008). Isolation and characterization of an autoinducer synthase from *Acinetobacter baumannii*. *Journal of Bacteriology*, Vol.190, No.9, (February 2008), pp.3386-3392, ISSN 0021-9193

Otto, M. (2009) *Staphylococcus epidermidis* – the 'accidental' pathogen. *Nature Reviews Microbiology*. Vol. 7, No. 8, (August 2009), pp. 555-567, ISSN: 1740-1526.

O'Toole, GA & Kolter, R. (1998). Flagellar and twitching motility are necessary for *Pseudomonas aeruginosa* biofilm development. *Molecular Microbiology*. Vol. 30, No. 2, (October 1998), pp. 295–304, ISSN: 1365-2958.

Park, Y.K. Jung, S.I. Park, K.W. Cheong, H.S. Peck, K.R. Song, J.H. Ko, K.S. (2009). Independent emergence of colistin-resistant *Acinetobacter spp*. Isolates from Korea, *Diagnostic Microbiology and Infectious Disease*, Vol.64, (January 2009), pp.43-51, ISSN 0732 8893

Park, Y.K. Choi, J.Y. Shin, D. & Ko, K.S. (2011), Correlation between overexpression and amino acid substitution of the PmrAB locus and colistin resistance in *Acinetobacter baumannii*, *International Journal of Antimicrobial Agents*, Vol. 37, (February 2011) pp. 525-530, ISSN 0924-8579

Peleg, A.Y. Franklin, C. Walters, L. J. Bell, J.M. & Spelman, D.W. (2006). OXA-58 and IMP-4 carbapenem-hydrolyzing b-lactamases in an *Acinetobacter junii* blood culture from Australia. *Antimicrobial Agents and Chemotherapy* Vol. 50, No. 1, (January 2006) pp. 399–400, ISSN 0066-4804.

Peleg, A.Y. Adams, J. & Paterson, D.L. (2007). Tigecycline Efflux as a Mechanism for Nonsusceptibility in *Acinetobacter baumannii*, *Antimicrobial Agents and Chemotherapy* Vol. 51, No. 6, (June 2007) pp. 2065-2069, ISSN 0066-4804

Peleg, A.Y. Seifert, H. & Paterson, D.L. (2008). *Acinetobacter baumannii*: Emergence of a Successful Pathogen, *Clin. Microbiol. Rev.* Vol.21, No.3, (July 2008), pp. 538–582, ISSN 0893-8512

Perry, R. D., Pendrak, M. L. & Schuetze, P. (1990). Identification and cloning of a hemin storage locus involved in the pigmentation phenotype of *Yersinia pestis*. *Journal of Bacteriology*, Vol.172, No.10, (October 1990), pp. 5929–5937, ISSN 1098-5530.

Perry, R. D., Bobrov, A. G., Kirillina, O., Jones, H. A., Pedersen, L., Abney, J. & Fetherston, J. D. (2004). Temperature regulation of the hemin storage (*Hms+*) phenotype of *Yersinia pestis* is posttranscriptional. *Journal of Bacteriology*, Vol.186, No.6, (March 2004), pp. 1638–1647, ISSN 1098-5530.

Piolle, L.D. Magnet, S. Bremont, S. Lambert, T. & Courvalin, P. (2008). AdeIJK, a Resistance-Nodulation-Cell Division Pump Effluxing Multiple Antibiotics in *Acinetobacter baumannii*, *Antimicrob. Agents and Chemother*, Vol.52, No.2, (February 2008) pp. 557-562, ISSN 0066-4804

Rahbar, MR; Rasooli, I; Gargavi, SLM; Amani, J & Fattahian, Y. (2010) In silico analysis of antibody triggering biofilm associated protein in *Acinetobacter baumannii*. *Journal of Theoretical Biology*. Vol. 266, pp. 275-290, ISSN: 0022-5193.

Poirel, L. Lebessi, E. Heritier, C. Patsoura, A. Foustoukou, M & Nordmann, P (2006). Nosocomial spread of OXA-58-positive carbapenem-resistant *Acinetobacter baumannii* isolates in a paediatric hospital in Greece, *Clinical Microbiology and Infection*, Vol.12 No.11, (November 2006) pp.1138-1141, ISSN 1198-743X

Poirel, L. & Nordmann, P. (2006). Genetic structures at the origin of acquisition and expression of the carbapenem-hydrolyzing oxacillinase gene blaOXA-58 in *Acinetobacter baumannii*. *Antimicrobial Agents and Chemotherapy* Vol. 50, No. 4, (April 2006) pp. 1442–1448. ISSN 0066-4804.

Poirel, L. Mansour, W. Bouallegue, O & Nordmann, P (2008). Carbapenem-Resistant *Acinetobacter baumannii* isolates from Tunisia Producing the OXA-58-Like Carbapenem-Hydrolyzing Oxacillinase OXA-97, *Antimicrob. Agents and Chemother,* Vol.52, No.5, (May 2008) pp. 1613-1617, ISSN 0066-4804

Pournaras, S. Maniati, M. Petinaki, E. Tzouvelekis, L. S. Tsakris, A. Legakis, N. J. & Maniatis, A.N. (2003). Hospital outbreak of multiple clones of *Pseudomonas aeruginosa* carrying the unrelated metallo-beta-lactamase gene variants blaVIM-2 and blaVIM-4. *Journal of Antimicrobial Chemotherapy* Vol. 51, No. 6 (June 2003) pp. 1409-1414, ISSN 0305-7453

Pruitt, K., Brown, G., Tatusova, T., & Maglott, D., (2002). Chapter 18, The Reference Sequence (RefSeq) Project, *The NCBI Handbook,* http://www.ncbi.nlm.nih.gov/books/NBK21091/

Rahbar, M. R. Rasooli, I. Mousavi Gargari, S. L. Amani, J. & Fattahian, Y. (2010). In silico analysis of antibody triggering biofilm associated protein in *Acinetobacter baumannii. Journal of Theoretical Biology* Vol. 266, No. 2 (September 2010) pp. 275-90, ISSN 0022-5193

Rahmati, S. Yang, S. Davidson, A.L. Zechiedrich, E.L. (2002). Control of the AcrAB multidrug efflux pump by quorum-sensing regulator SdiA. *Molecular Microbiology,* Vol. 43, No.3, (February 2002), pp.677–685, ISSN 0950-382X

Rajamohan, G. Srinivasan, V.B, & Gebreyes, W.A. (2010). Molecular and functional characterization of a novel efflux pump, AmvA, mediating antimicrobial and disinfectant resistance in *Acinetobacter baumannii, J Antimicrob Chemother,* Vol.65, (June 2010), pp.1919-1925, ISSN 0305-7453

Rao, RS; Karthika, RU; Singh, SP; Shashikala, P; Kanungo, R; Jayachandran, S & Prashanth, K. (2008) Correlation between biofilm production and multiple drug resistance in imipenem resistant clinical isolates of *Acinetobacter baumannii. Indian Journal of Medical Microbiology.* Vol. 26, No. 4, pp. 333-337, ISSN: 02550857

Roberts, A. W. & Bushoven, J. T. (2007). The cellulose synthase (CESA) gene superfamily of the moss *Physcomitrella patens. Plant Molecular Biology,* Vol.63, No.2, (January 2007), pp. 207-219, ISSN 1573-5028.

Roca, I. Marti, S. Espinal, P. Martínez, P. Gibert, I. & Vila, J. (2009). CraA, a major facilitator superfamily efflux pump associated with chloramphenicol resistance in *Acinetobacter baumannii. Antimicrobial Agents and Chemotherapy* Vol. 53, No. 9 (September 2009) pp. 4013-4014. ISSN 0066-4804.

Roca, I., Espinal, P. Marti, S. & Vila, J. (2011). First Identification and Characterization of an AdeABC-Like Efflux Pump in *Acinetobacter* Genomospecies 13TU, *Antimicrob. Agents and Chemother,* Vol.55, No.3, (March 2011) pp. 1285-1286, ISSN 0066-4804

Rosenbusch, J. P. (1974). Characterization of the major envelope protein from *Escherichia coli. Journal of Biological Chemistry* Vol. 249, No. 24, (December 1974) pp. 8019-8029, ISSN 0021-9258

Russo, T.A. Donald, U.M. Beanan, J.M. Olson, R., MacDonald, I.J. Sauberan, S.L. Luke, N.R. Schultz, L.W. & Umland, T.C. (2009). Penicillin-Binding Protein 7/8 Contributes to the Survival of *Acinetobacter baumannii* In Vitro and In Vivo, *The Journal of Infectious Diseases,* Vol. 199, (February 2009) pp. 513-21, ISSN 0022-1899

Sato, K. & Nakae T. (1991). Outer membrane permeability of *Acinetobacter calcoaceticus* and its implication in antibiotic resistance. *Journal of Antimicrobial Chemotherapy* Vol. 28, No. 1, (July 1991) pp. 35-45, ISSN 0305-7453

Schaefer, A.L. Hanzelka, B.L. Eberhard, A. Greenberg, E.P. (1996). Quorum sensing in *Vibrio fischeri*: probing autoinducer–LuxR interactions with autoinducer analogs. *J ournal of Bacteriology*, Vol.178, No.10, (May 1996), pp. 2897–2901, ISSN 0021-9193

Shiro, H. Meluleni, G. Groll, A. Muller, E. Tosteson T. D, Goldmann, D.A. Pier, G. B. (1995). The pathogenic role of *Staphylococcus epidermidis* capsular polysaccharide/adhesin in a low-inoculum rabbit model of prosthetic valve endocarditis. *Circulation* Vol. 92, No. 9 (November 1995) pp. 2715-2722, ISSN 0009-7322

Siroy, A. Molle, V. Guillier, C.L. Vallenet, D. Caron, M.P. Cozzone, A.J. Jouenne, T. & De, E. (2006). Channel Formation by CarO, the Carbapenem Resistance-Associated Outer Membrane Protein of *Acinetobacter baumannii*, *Antimicrobial Agents and Chemotherapy* Vol.49, No.12, (December 2005) pp. 4876-4883, ISSN 0066-4804

Smith MG, Gianoulis TA, Pukatzki S et al. (2007). New insights into *Acinetobacter baumannii* pathogenesis revealed by high-density pyrosequencing and transposon mutagenesis. Genes and Development Vol. 21, No. 5, (March 2007), pp.601–614. ISSN - 0890 9369

Srinivasan, V.B. Rajamohan, G. & Gebreyes, W.A. (2009). Role of AbeS, a Novel Efflux Pump of the SMR Family of Transporters in Resistance to Antimicrobial Agents in *Acinetobacter baumannii*. *Antimicrobial Agents and Chemotherapy* Vol. 53, No. 12, (December 2009) pp. 5312-5316, ISSN 0066-4804

Stevens, A.M. Dolan, K.M. Greenberg E.P. (1994). Synergistic binding of the *Vibrio fischeri* LuxR transcriptional activator domain and RNA polymerase to the *lux* promoter region. *Proceedings of National Academy of Sciences*, Vol. 91, (December 1994), pp.12619–12623, ISSN 0027-8424

Su, X.Z. Chen, J. Mizushima, T. Kuroda, T. & Tsuchiya.T. (2005). AbeM an H⁺ Coupled *Acinetobacter baumannii* Multidrug Efflux Pump Belonging to the MATE Family of Transporters, *Antimicrobial Agents and Chemotherapy* Vol. 49, No. 10, (October 2005) pp. 4362-4364, ISSN 0066-4804

Sun, J.R. Chan, M.C. Chang, T.Y. Wang, W.Y. Chiueh, T. S. (2010). Overexpression of the adeB gene in clinical isolates of tigecycline-nonsusceptible *Acinetobacter baumannii* without insertion mutations in adeRS. *Antimicrobial Agents and Chemotherapy* Vol. 54, No. 11, (November 2010) pp. 4934-4938, ISSN 0066-4804.

Toleman, M.A. Biedenbach, D. Bennett, D.M. Jones, R. N. & Walsh, T.R. (2005). Italian metallo-beta-lactamases: a national problem? Report from the SENTRY Antimicrobial Surveillance Programme. *Journal of Antimicrobial Chemotherapy* Vol. 55, No. 1, (January 2005) pp. 61-70, ISSN 0305-7453

Tolker-Nielsen, T; Brinch, UC; Ragas, PC; Andersen, JB; Jacobsen, CS & Molin, S. (2000). Development and dynamics of Pseudomonas sp. biofilms. *Journal of Bacteriology*. Vol. 182, pp. 6482–6489, ISSN: 1098-5530.

Tomaras, AP; Dorsey, CW; Edelmann, RE & Actis, LA. (2003) Attachment to and biofilm formation on abiotic surfaces by *Acinetobacter baumannii*: involvement of a novel chaperone-usher pili assembly system. *Microbiology*. Vol. 149, pp. 3473–3484, ISSN: 0099-2240.

Tsakris, A. Ikonomidis, A. Pournaras, S. Tzouvelekis, L.S. Sofianou, D. Legakis, N.J. & Maniatis, A.N. (2006). VIM-1 Metallo-β-lactamase in *Acinetobacter baumannii*, *Emerg Infect Dis*. Vol.12, No. 6, (June 2006) pp. 981-983, ISSN 1080-6059

Tsakris, A. Ikonomidis, A. Spanakis, N. Pournaras, S. & Bethimouti, K. (2007). Identification of a novel blaOXA-51 variant, blaOXA-92, from a clinical isolate of *Acinetobacter baumannii*, *Clinical Microbiology and Infection*, Vol.13, No.3 (March 2007) pp.347-349, ISSN 1198-743X

Tsakris, A. Ikonomidis, A. Poulou, A. Spanakis, N. Vrizas, D. Diomidous, M. Pournaras, S. & Markou, F. (2008). Clusters of imipenem-resistant *Acinetobacter baumannii* clones producing different carbapenemases in an intensive care unit. *Clinical Microbiology and Infection* Vol. 14, No. 6, (June 2008) pp. 588-594, ISSN 1198-743X

Turton, J.F. Ward, M.E. Woodford, N. Kaufmann, M.E. Pike, R. Livermore, D.M. & Pitt, T.L. (2006). The role of ISAba1in expression of OXA carbapenemase genes in *Acinetobacter baumannii*, *FEMS Microbiol Lett*, Vol.258 (March 2006) pp.72–77, ISSN 0378-1097

Uma Karthika, R. Srinivasa Rao, R. Sahoo, S. Shashikala, P., Kanungo, R. Jayachandran, S. & Prashanth, K. (2009). Phenotypic and Genotypic assays for detecting the prevalence of Metallo-β- lactamases in clinical isolates of *Acinetobacter baumannii* from a South Indian tertiary care hospital. *Journal of Medical Microbiology*, Vol. 58, No. 4, (April 2009) pp 430-435, ISSN 0022-2615

Vashist, J. Tiwari, V. Das, R. Kapil, A. & Rajeswari, M.R. (2011). Analysis of penicillin-binding proteins (PBPs) in carbapenem resistant *Acinetobacter baumannii*, *Indian J Med Res*, Vol.133, (March 2011) pp. 332-338, ISSN 0971-5916

Vila, J. Marti, S. & Cespedes, J.S. (2007). Porins, efflux pumps and multidrug resistance in *Acinetobacter baumannii*, *J Antimicrob Chemother*, Vol.59, (February 2007) pp. 1210-1215, ISSN 0305-7453.

Vuong, C; Voyich, JM; Fischer, ER; Braughton, KR; Whitney, AR; DeLeo, FR & Otto, M. (2004) Polysaccharide intercellular adhesin (PIA) protects *Staphylococcus epidermidis* against major components of the human innate immune system. *Cellular Microbiology*. Vol 6, pp. 269–275, ISSN: 1462-5822.

Weinberg, E. D. (2004). Suppression of bacterial biofilm formation by iron limitation. *Medical Hypotheses*, Vol.63, No.5, (August 2004), pp. 863–865, ISSN 0306-9877.

Wieczorek P, Sacha P, Hauschild T et al. (2008). Multidrug resistant *Acinetobacter baumannii* – the role of AdeABC (RND family) efflux pump in resistance to antibiotics. Folia *Histochemica Et Cytobiologica* Vol. 46, No. 3, (March 2008), pp.257-267, 0239-8508

Wortham, B. W., Oliveira, M, A., Fetherston, J. & Perry, R. D. (2010). Polyamines are required for the expression of key Hms proteins important for *Yersinia pestis* biofilm formation. *Environmental Microbiology*, Vol.12, No.7, (July 2010), pp. 2034–2047, ISSN 1462-2920.

Yang, L., Barken, K. B., Skindersoe, M. E., Christensen, A. B., Givskov, M. & Tolker-Nielsen, T. (2007). Effects of iron on DNA release and biofilm development by *Pseudomonas aeruginosa*. *Microbiology*, Vol.153, No.5, (May 2007), pp. 1318–1328, ISSN 1465-2080.

Zhou, D. & Yang, R. (2011). Formation and regulation of *Yersinia* biofilms. *Protein & Cell*, Vol.2, No.3, (March 2011), pp. 173-179, ISSN 1674-8018.

Zimbler, D. L., Penwell, W. F., Gaddy, J. A., Menke, S. M., Tomaras, A. P., Connerly, P. L. & Actis, L. A. (2009). Iron acquisition functions expressed by the human pathogen *Acinetobacter baumannii*. *Biometals*, Vol.22, No.1, (February 2009), pp. 23–32, ISSN 1572-8773.

9

Staphylococcal Infection, Antibiotic Resistance and Therapeutics

Ranginee Choudhury[1], Sasmita Panda[1],
Savitri Sharma[2,*] and Durg V. Singh[1,*]
[1]*Infectious Disease Biology, Institute of Life Sciences, Bhubaneswar*
[2]*Ocular Microbiology Service, LV Prasad Eye Institute, Bhubaneswar*
India

1. Introduction

Staphylococcus spp. are a challenge for the modern day medicine due to the complexity of disease process and presence and expression patterns of their respective virulence factors. The members of this genus possess many known toxins, multiple immunoavoidance mechanisms and adherence factors, most of which demonstrate transient, timed, and disease-specific expression. They cause different types of infections in a host that are either planktonic, biofilm mediated or both. Sepsis and pneumonia are mainly caused by planktonic forms whereas, a whole range of diseases, namely, endophthalmitis, osteomyelitis, endocarditis, chronic skin infections, indwelling medical device infections, chronic rhino-sinusitis, and dental implantits are caused by the biofilmic form of the bacteria. Abscess can be caused by both of the forms (Harro et al., 2010). Staphylococci are human pathogen, known for their ability to become resistant to antibiotics. They have been associated, besides causing ophthalmic infections, with skin infections and sepsis. Methicillin resistant *S. aureus* (MRSA), in addition to resistance to other drugs, have emerged as a widespread cause of community infection as well. In this chapter, we describe the epidemiology and antibiotic resistance among *S. aureus* and other species with special reference to ophthalmic infections and focus on newer approaches for treatment of staphylococcus infection like phage therapy and vaccines.

2. Staphylococcus in wound and eye infections

Staphylococcus aureus, a gram-positive bacterium, discovered in 1880's has been shown to be a potential pathogen causing infections such as minor skin infections and post-operative wound infection. Since the introduction of penicillin for the treatment, the mortality rate of individuals caused by *S. aureus* infection was about 80%. After emergence of penicillin resistance and introduction of methicillin in 1961, *S. aureus* developed resistance to methicillin due to acquisition of the *mecA* gene. During last 47 years, various hospital-associated methicillin-resistant *S. aureus* (HA-MRSA) and later virulent community-associated MRSA (CA-MRSA) clones characterised by the presence of toxin Panton-Valentine-leukocidin (PVL), were reported (Deurenberg and Stobberingh, 2008).

Staphylococci have a special relationship with the eye. On one hand, almost all species of staphylococci may be present in the lid margins or conjunctiva as normal commensals without causing disease and on the other hand, they may cause severe eye infections which may result in irreversible blindness. Colonization by resident bacteria on the ocular surface can provide a defense by inhibiting the growth of virulent bacterial strains (Iskeleli et al., 2005). However, in cases of trauma, or alteration of ocular tissue, indigenous flora may cause significant external and internal ocular infection (Speaker et al., 1991). In previous studies, native ocular flora has been shown to be predominantly *Staphylococcus* species (Iskeleli et al., 2005). While normal ocular flora has been well established in the developed world, there have been very few publications from rest of the world. In a study of the normal conjunctiva from Rajasthan, India, 86% of eyes were culture positive for bacteria and 12% positive for fungi. The most common bacterial isolates were *S. albus* (32%) followed by *S. aureus* (28%) (Tomar et al., 1971). In another study from Masungbo, Sierra Leone where analysis of conjunctival swabs obtained from healthy eyes of 276 residents showed presence of coagulase-negative staphylococci (28.6%), fungus (26.0%) and *S. aureus* (19.9%) (Capriotti et al., 2009). Many studies have not speciated the staphylococci from normal lids and conjunctiva, however, *S. epidermidis* is reported to be the most common species (McCulley et al., 1982).

Both coagulase negative and positive staphylococci are responsible for a variety of anterior and posterior segment of eye infections such as blepharitis, canaliculitis, dacryocystitis, conjunctivitis, keratitis, scleritis, endophthalmitis, preseptal and orbital cellulitis etc. Important attributes of organisms causing ocular infections include virulence, invasiveness, numbers of organism entering the host tissues and the site of entry. Coagulase, lipase and esterase are important bacterial enzymes produced by staphylococci associated with blepharitis. Several characteristics of the host also determine the effect of bacterial virulence and development of disease. Age, use of drugs and contact lens use, trauma, surgery etc. may also influence the effect of virulence factors besides presence of risk factors e.g., dry eye states, chronic nasolacrimal duct obstruction, previous ocular disease etc. Tissue injury can result from direct action of bacteria and their toxins, as well as from bacteria induced inflammation. Immunopathologic activities include recruitment of polymorphonuclear cells, macrophages and lymphocytes. Mediators of inflammation such as histamine, tumour necrosis factor, cytokines, leukotrienes, prostaglandins etc. play important role in interaction with the bacteria and their removal or proliferation.

Type of endophthalmitis	Geographic area	Duration of study	No. of patients	No, of isolates	% of CoNS	References
Posttraumatic	India	7 years	182	139	17.3	(Kunimoto et al., 1999b)
Postoperative	India	7 years	206	176	46.0	(Kunimoto et al., 1999a)
Postoperative	Singapore	5 years	34	21	57.0	(Wong and Chee, 2004)
Postoperative	India	--	80	37	62.6	(Srinivasan et al., 2002)
Postoperative	USA	5 years	278	313	49.9	(Benz et al., 2004)

Table 1. Prevalence of *Staphylococcus* species in endophthalmitis in various studies

Inflammation of the lid margin or blepharitis may be anterior or posterior, the former involving the lash line and the latter meibomian glands. Both the conditions may be associated with skin diseases such as dermatitis (seborrhoeic or atopic) and rosacea. The anterior blepharitis with lash collarettes, crusting, lid ulceration and folliculitis is usually associated with *S. aureus*. The most common form of bacterial conjunctivitis is the acute mucopurulent form of *S. aureus*. This may be associated with obstruction of the Naso-lacrimal duct. *S. aureus* conjunctivitis can become chronic due to its affinity for the eyelid margin and the resultant blepharitis. Coagulase negative staphylococci (CoNS), characteristically the endogenous flora of the ocular surface, are most of the common cause of postoperative endophthalmitis world over (Callegan et al., 2002; Kunimoto et al., 1999a, Benz et al., 2004, Wong and Chee, 2004). CoNS also rank first among bacteria causing posttraumatic endophthalmitis of which 45.3% isolates belong to gram positive cocci and 17.3% of these were belong to gram positive bacilli (Kunimoto et al., 1999b). Whereas CoNS do not commonly cause endogenous endophthalmitis, *S. aureus* have been reported from such infection (Callegan et al., 2002). **Table 1.** shows the prevalence of *Staphylococcus* species in patients with endophthalmitis.

Microbial keratitis is a serious infection of the cornea that may be caused by a variety of organisms including staphylococci. Most of the studies from developed countries such as the USA (Liesegang and Forster, 1980, Ormerod et al., 1987, Asbell and Stenson, 1982) (except southern USA) and Australia (McClellan et al., 1989) have listed *S. epidermidis* or coagulase negative staphylococci as the leading cause of bacterial keratitis. In India, the leading cause of bacterial keratitis varies; however, some investigators have listed staphylococci as the commonest bacteria (Gopinathan et al., 2009). It is possible that some investigators may have considered *S. epidermidis* or coagulase negative staphylococci as a normal commensal of the conjunctiva and underreported the isolation of these organisms from corneal samples. Few studies have recommended application of certain criteria to determine significance of a positive culture from corneal scrapings (Gopinathan et al., 2009). Since *S. epidermidis* form the commonest commensal of the extraocular surfaces, it is highly probable that these organisms invade corneal tissues compromised by antimicrobial and / or corticosteroid therapy or trauma.

For treatment of eye infections, antibiotics are usually administered topically as eye drops or intraocular injections, depending on the clinical condition. Other routes of administration such as subconjunctival injection are rarely used. Topically administered drugs have major advantage of localized drug effects, avoidance of hepatic first pass metabolism, and convenience. The disadvantage is low bioavailability to intraocular tissues, estimated to be only 1-10% (Davies, 2000). A large number of eye drops for topical therapy are available for extraocular eye infections, that include fluoroquinolones, macrolides, aminoglycosides, glycopeptides, tetracyclines, chloramphenicol, Neosporin (bacitracin, neomycin, polymyxin).

A broad range of three generations of fluoroquinolones are available such as ciprofloxacin (0.3%), ofloxacin (0.3%), levofloxacin (0.5% and 1.5%) , gatifloxacin (0.3%) and moxifloxacin (0.5%, preservative free) as eye drops also. Gatifloxacin and moxifloxacin, the newer fourth generation fluoroquinolones that target both DNA gyrase and topoisomerase IV are highly effective against gram positive bacteria including staphylococci in human and animal corneal ulcer model (Romanowski et al., 2005, Aliprandis et al., 2005). However, gatifloxacin was shown to be more effective than moxifloxacin against staphylococci (Reddy et al., 2010).

Fluoroquinolone eye drops are widely used for prophylaxis before eye surgery to prevent postoperative infection, most commonly caused by CoNS. Recently, intracameral injection of moxifloxacin has been found to be safe and effective in reducing the rate of postoperative endophthalmitis following cataract surgery (Lane et al., 2008).

Historically, the aminoglycosides have been the mainstay in the treatment of ocular infections. However, increasing resistance has limited their use in recent years in the treatment of staphylococcal infections. Glycopeptides such as vancomycin and teicoplanin the bactericidal antibiotics which inhibit peptidoglycan synthesis in the bacterial cell wall by complexing with cell wall precursors are highly effective against staphylococci including methicillin resistant staphylococci. However, eye drops are not yet available. Injectable vancomycin is routinely used for intravitreal injection (1mg/0.1ml) for the treatment of bacterial endophthalmitis. Emergence of vancomycin resistance has been reported in CoNS (Schwalbe et al., 1987). Topical ocular formulations of erythromycin are effective for conjunctivitis and blepharitis, however clarithromycin and azithromycin are derivatives that offer significant advantage over erythromycin owing to their expanded spectra (Barry et al., 1988).

Systemic infection with methicillin resistant *S. aureus* (MRSA) is known to cause morbidity and mortality. The prevalence of MRSA in ocular infections varies in different studies. While it is reported to be as low as 3% in England (Shanmuganathan et al., 2005), it is high (25-64%) in Japan (Fukuda et al., 2002). However, Indian workers have also reported increasing prevalence of MRSA over the years (Bagga et al., 2010). These authors showed decreased susceptibility to fluoroquinolones among MRSA from ocular infections. Shanmuganathan et al. (2005) found the MRSA susceptible to chloramphenicol and gentamicin and resistant to third generation fluoroquinolones (ciprofloxacin and ofloxacin) and cefazolin. Topical administration of fortified cefazolin (5%) was recommended for the treatment of staphylococcal keratitis based on in vitro susceptibility of *S. aureus* and CoNS (Sharma et al., 1999, Sharma et al., 2004). In an ongoing study, 4 of the 45 isolates (8.9%) of *S. aureus* from eye infections were MRSA (Kar et al., 2010). Using microbroth dilution and E test, a high level of resistance to fluoroquinolones but susceptibility to cefazolin, vancomycin and chloramphenicol was found among both MRSA and MSSA strains (Kar et al., 2010).

3. Antibiotic resistance

Antibiotics that are used against *Staphylococcus* spp. basically target cell wall synthesis, protein synthesis, nucleic acid synthesis and other metabolic pathways. The selection pressure applied by the antibiotics that are used in clinical and agricultural settings has promoted the evolution and spread of genes that confer resistance (Allen et al., 2010). Resistance to various antibiotics can be either internal or acquired by horizontal gene transfer via various mobile genetic elements like plasmids, transposons, integrons, etc. Internal mechanisms include mutational modification of gene targets, over expression of various efflux pumps; whereas acquired resistance involves enzymatic inactivation of the drug and bypassing of the target.

Exposure to antibiotics may lead to the formation of persister cells, small colony variants (SCVs), biofilms and over-expression of efflux pumps (Lewis, 2008, Singh et al., 2009, Proctor et al., 1998, Kwon et al., 2008, Martinez et al., 2009b) (Fig. 1). Persisters are dormant, multidrug tolerant variants of regular cells that are formed through a combination of stochastic and deterministic events in microbial populations (Lewis, 2010). Persisters over express genes such as chromosomal toxin-antitoxin modules that shut down their cellular functions, therefore, antibiotictarget inducing dormant cell to become tolerant to the lethal action of antibiotics (Keren et al., 2004, Singh et al., 2009). Another major problem posed by persister cells is they hide at various niches evading the host immune system, such as central nervous system (*Treponema pallidum*), macrophages or granulomas (*Mycobacterium tuberculosis*), stomach (*Helicobacter pylori*), gallbladder (*Salmonella typhi*) etc. (Jayaraman, 2008).

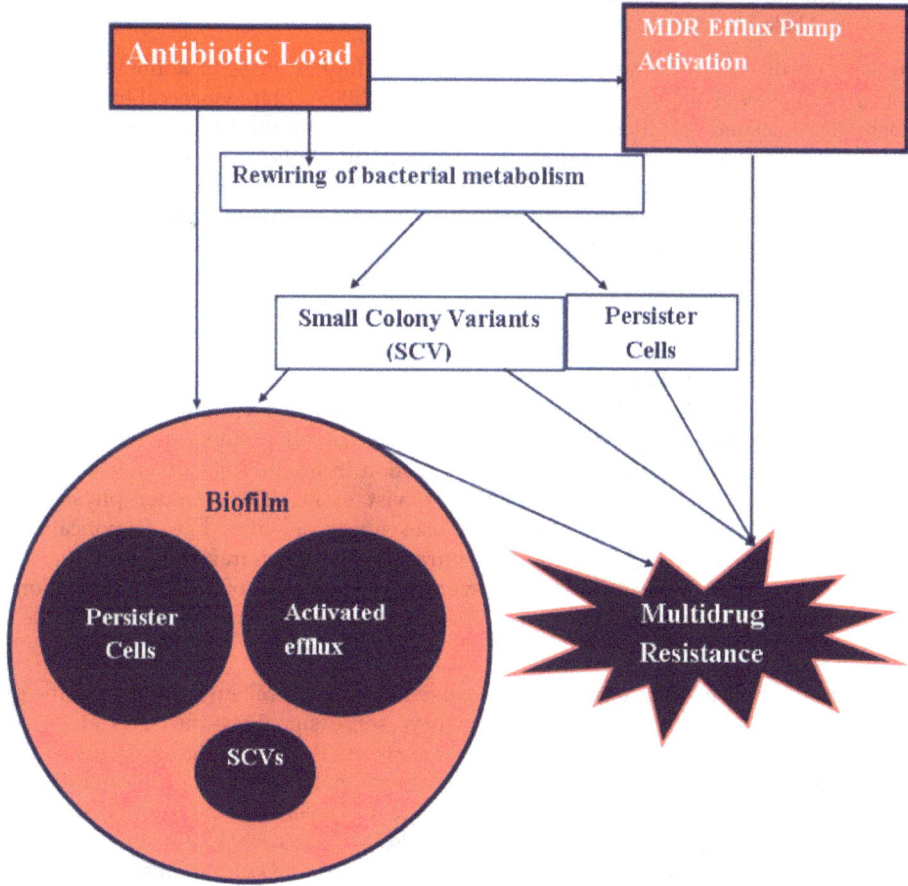

Fig. 1. Sub-inhibitory concentrations of antibiotics lead to formation of persister cells (Lewis, 2010), small colony variants (Proctor et al., 1998), biofilms (Kwon et al., 2008) and over-expression of efflux pumps (Martinez et al., 2009b). Biofilms are known to harbor cells with these kinds of modifications (Singh et al., 2010, Allegrucci and Sauer, 2007, Kvist et al., 2008). SCVs have enhanced biofilm forming capability (Singh et al., 2010). Each of these mechanisms may lead to multidrug resistance or it may be the combinatorial effect of all the above-mentioned processes.

SCVs constitute a slow-growing subpopulation of bacteria with distinctive phenotype and pathogenic traits (Proctor, 2006). They differ from the normal phenotype in their colony size, growth rate, pigmentation, haemolysis, expression of virulence factors, haemin and menadione auxotrophy, aminoglycosides and cell wall inhibitors action (Singh et al., 2009). Defective respiratory activity serves as the biochemical basis for the development of SCVs (Proctor et al., 1998). SCV of *S. epidermidis* may play a role in the pathogenesis of prosthetic valve endocarditis (Baddour and Christensen, 1987), and catheter-induced endocarditis (Baddour et al., 1988). Several findings mandate the investigation of small colony variants for persistent infections (Proctor et al., 1994, Proctor et al., 1998, Spearman et al., 1996, Kahl et al., 1998, Abele-Horn et al., 2000).

Bacteria in biofilms can tolerate ten to thousand fold higher levels of antibiotics than the genetically equivalent planktonic bacteria (Resch et al., 2005). Staphylococcal biofilms cause biomaterial-associated infections which do not respond to antimicrobial treatment often requiring removal of the same leading to substantial morbidity and mortality (Gotz and Peters, 2000). It has also been observed that biofilms harbour persister cells and small colony variants (Singh et al., 2010, Allegrucci and Sauer, 2007) (Fig. 1). Whereas planktonic persisters are eliminated by the immune system *in vivo*, persisters in biofilms serve as a shield evading the immune response (Lewis, 2010). According to Levin and Rozen (Levin and Rozen, 2006), a reservoir of such shielded persisters is a potential source for the emergence of heritable antibiotic resistance.

Kvist et al., (2008) reported the enhanced activity of efflux pumps in the bacteria residing in the biofilms (Fig. 1). The authors argued that the cramped environment in the biofilm demands better waste management leading to escalation of efflux pumps thereby increasing the antibiotic resistance of the biofilm cells. Reduction in biofilm formation was observed with the addition of efflux pump inhibitors (Kvist et al., 2008). Under physiological conditions, efflux pumps are involved in housekeeping activities like detoxification of intracellular metabolites, cell homeostasis, intracellular signal trafficking and bacterial virulence in animal and plant hosts. However, in the presence of high concentration of antibiotics and other environmental factors, they can shift their functional roles (Martinez et al., 2009a).

Antibiotics and their resistance genes were evolved in non-clinical environments in the pre-antibiotic usage era. Some antibiotics which may serve signalling purposes at the low concentration are probably found in natural ecosystems. Resistance determinants to these antibiotics were originally selected in their hosts for metabolic purposes or signal trafficking. Other antibiotic-resistance genes have been obtained by virulent bacteria through horizontal gene transfer (Martinez et al., 2009a). For example, *S. aureus mecA* gene is located on a mobile genetic element, the staphylococcal cassette chromosome *mec* (SCCmec) (Tsubakshita et al., 2010), horizontally acquired from other staphylococcal species *S. sciuri* (Couto et al., 1996) and *S. fleurettii* (Katayama et al., 2000). Also high level of vancomycin resistance is associated with carriage of *vanA* cluster encoded by Tn1546 transposon, first reported in *Enterococcus* species (Uttley et al., 1988). VRSA isolates from Michigan and Pennsylvania were found to harbor plasmids of 57.9Kb and 120Kb respectively carrying the transposon (Weigel et al., 2003, Tenover et al., 2004).

Resistance to fluoroquinolones offer a classic example of point mutations (e.g., *gyrA&B*, *grlA&B*) and efflux mediated resistance (Morar and Wright, 2010). Point mutations in particular regions of each enzyme subunit, known as Quinolone-Resistance-Determining-Region (QRDR) makes the enzyme less susceptible to inhibition by fluoroquinolones. The level of resistance increases in a stepwise manner each time with an additional mutation in target enzyme (Hooper, 2001). Selection pressure exerted by enhanced use of quinolones have led to the emergence of resistant strains carrying mutations within the endogenous transport system that improve affinity of the efflux system for quinolones (Ohshita et al., 1990, Chopra, 1992). The quinolone resistance in *S. aureus* also involves enhanced efflux by the Nor family of multidrug efflux pumps (McCallum et al., 2010). Several reports have linked increased expression of NorA to reduced susceptibility to chloramphenicol, beta-lactams, tetracycline, puromycin and some dyes, such as ethidium bromide (McCallum et al., 2010, Hooper, 2001, Ruiz, 2003). Point mutations in *norA* gene have been associated with reduced uptake of norfloxacin by the cell (Ohshita et al., 1990). NorB and NorC are the other members of Nor family encoding fluroquinolone resistance (Truong-Bolduc et al., 2006).

Although fluoroquinolones are considered first-line treatment of ocular infections, 85% of MRSA are resistant to ophthalmic fluoroquinolones (McDonald and Blondeau, 2010). This rise in resistance mandates the need for new agents. Basifloxacin, a novel fluoroquinolone was approved as a topical agent for treatment of bacterial conjunctivitis in May 2009 demonstrated rapid bactericidal activity against isolates that showed in vitro resistance to other fluoroquinolones, beta-lactams, macrolides and aminoglycosides (Haas et al., 2010). Moreover, basifloxacin lack systemic counterpart, thereby eliminating the contribution of systemic use of this drug to the emergence of resistance, although cross resistance from other systemic fluoroquinolones is possible (McDonald and Blondeau, 2010).

The direct relationship between the development of Linezolid (the last-line agent) resistance and prolonged exposure of the drug among cystic fibrosis patients was reported by Endimiani et al., (2011). Linezolid resistance in *S. aureus* is uncommon though there are reports of mutations in 23S rRNA and ribosomal protein L3 and L4 encoded by *rplD* gene and *rplC* genes (Locke et al., 2009). However, the most worrisome mechanism involving acquisition of the methytransferase *cfr* that methylates the 23S rRNA associated with mobile genetic elements had first been identified in 16.5 kb multi-drug resistance plasmid in *Staphylococcus sciuri* (Kehrenberg et al., 2005).

4. Therapeutics & therapy

With the ample evidence of strong association between antibiotic resistance and antibiotic consumption the scientific community should also come up with alternative means of antibacterial therapies, besides legitimately using available antibiotics, which can be used either alone or in conjunction with the antibiotics. Here we discuss some of the alternative strategies including vaccine development, phage therapy, use of lytic enzymes and plant-derived antibacterials. There are some reports on the use of nanoparticles as an efficient means of delivering antibacterials.

4.1 Staphylococcal vaccines

S. aureus has devised various mechanisms to evade the immune system. (i) two immunoglobulin binding proteins (protein A and Sbi), (ii) immune cell lysing toxins (Hlg, PVL), (iii) proteins interfering with complement activation (SCIN– staphylococcal complement inhibitor) and (iv) chemotaxis of neutrophils inhibiting peptides. Production of superantigens by *S. aureus* leads to allergy and immunosuppression. *S. epidermidis* relies primarily on cell-surface polymers and the ability to form a biofilm to survive in the host (Foster, 2005). However, protective role of antistaphylococcal antibodies from staphylococcal infection has been well documented in literature (Dryla et al., 2005). Holtfreter and Broker (2005) reported that carriers have high titers of neutralizing antibodies specific for those superantigens that are expressed by their colonizing strain. This carriage status confers strain specific humoral immunity, which may contribute to protection during *S. aureus* septicemia. Substantial controversy exists as to whether staphylococcal infections may be prevented by vaccination and, if so, which antigens should be selected and patients targeted for vaccination. In a comprehensive review on immune-therapeutics for staphylococcal infections by Ohlsen and Lorenz (2010) described the necessity for the development of both passive and active immunotherapies against *Staphylococcus*. The underlying criteria for the selection of targets e.g. gene products or toxins, should be conservability and expression in most of the clinical isolates.

4.1.1 MSCRAMM (Microbial Surface Component Recognizing Adhesive Matrix Molecules)

Some of the surface proteins of *S. aureus* have been exploited for immunotherapy. MSCRAMM protein family represents prototype of targets because of their exposed location and virulence involvement (Ohlsen and Lorenz, 2010, Flock, 1999). The best characterized MSCRAMM proteins include (i) clumping factor B (clfB), (ii) collagen-binding protein (Cna), and (ii) fibronectin-binding protein (FnBPA) (Ohlsen and Lorenz, 2010, Garcia-Lara et al., 2005). Veronate (Inhibitex) was developed by including anti-clfA and SdrG (*S. epidermidis* protein) from selected human donors (Patti, 2005), but failed to reach its target endpoints for the protection because of low birth weight babies at clinical trial III (Ohlsen and Lorenz, 2010).

Aurexis® is a humanized monoclonal antibody that recognizes clumping factor A (ClfA), a cell surface protein expressed by virtually all strains of *S. aureus*. Aurexis® binds with high affinity and specificity and interferes with *S. aureus* ability to colonize and spread to fibrinogen containing substrates such as wound sites, biomaterial coated implants, and damaged endovascular tissues. Inhibitex is actively seeking a corporate partner(s) for the continued clinical development of Aurexis® (http://www.inhibitex.com/Pipeline/Partnerships.html). Antibodies against clumping factor B (clfB) (Schaffer et al., 2006), Cna (Mamo et al., 2000), FnBPA (Zhou et al., 2006) have shown promising results. However, antibodies against against these targets have not yet been included in clinical trials (Ohlsen and Lorenz, 2010). Stranger-Jones et al., (2006) reported that the combination of four surface proteins IsdA, IsdB, SdrB, and SdrE afforded high level of protection against invasive disease or lethal challenge with human clinical *S. aureus* isolates.

4.1.2 Capsule

Capsular polysaccharides (CPs) represent the best established targets for vaccine-induced immunity to bacterial cells. About 70%–80% of *S. aureus* strains produce one of two CP antigens e.g. CP5 or CP8 (Skurnik et al., 2010). Nabi pharmaceuticals developed a vaccine StaphVax™ conjugating CP5 and CP8 to detoxified *Pseudomonas aeruginosa* exoprotein A, that failed to protect haemodialysis patients against *S. aureus* infections (Ohlsen and Lorenz, 2010,

Shinefield et al., 2002). To enhance the efficacy of StaphVax™, Pentastaph™ -pentavalent *S. aureus* vaccine was developed that included surface polysaccharide component 336, PVL and alpha-toxin to eliminate *S. aureus* by phagocytosis and neutralizing bacterial toxins. This vaccine has been evaluated in Phase II for safety and immunogenicity (Ohlsen and Lorenz, 2010).

4.1.3 Biofilm as the vaccine target

Although the significance of biofilm in infections has been recognized, there has not been much effort to develop vaccine targeting biofilms. The possible target sites for vaccine development may be the bacterial cells within the biofilm and/or biofilm matrix (Harro et al., 2010). Cerca et al., (2007) reported that an antibody developed against *Staphylococcus* Poly-N-acetyl glucosamine (PNAG) was found effective against different strains of *E. coli*. In another report, effectiveness of PNAG as vaccine candidate in *S. aureus* mediated skin abcesses and lethal *E. coli* peritonitis was demonstrated (Gening et al., 2010). However, PNAG may not be an ideal vaccine candidate against those strains possessing *icaADBC* locus because it is not produced in all biofilm-producing staphylococcal strains (Harro et al., 2010, Rohde et al., 2001). Therefore, it was suggested that vaccine studies should be focussed on the cell embedded in the matrix rather than the matrix. A proteomic approach of looking into the comparative proteomes of the planktonic and biofilm cells may be an interesting area to start with (Harro et al., 2010).

4.1.4 Whole cell vaccine

Vaccine Research International (http://www.vri.org.uk/) is developing a vaccine (SA75) using chloroform killed whole cells of *S. aureus*. Phase I clinical trials have been successfully completed. The whole cell preparation could provide a broad spectrum of *S. aureus* antigens in a single vaccine some of which had immune-stimulatory affect and act as an adjuvant generating higher antibody response against protective antigens. However, the mechanism of action is unknown and down-regulation of immune pathways by components of the vaccine cannot be ruled out (Ohlsen and Lorenz, 2010).

4.1.5 Staphylococcal enterotoxin as a vaccine candidate

Virulence factor-specific antibodies derived from vaccination or employed as therapeutics represent a potential defense against bacterial diseases (Larkin et al., 2010). Staphylococcal enterotoxins are considered potential biowarfare agents that can be spread through ingestion or inhalation (Drozdowski et al., 2010). Staphylococcal enterotoxins (SEs) and related toxic shock syndrome toxin-1 (TSST-1) act as superantigens. These protein toxins can cause acute gastroenteritis and toxic shock syndrome. There are more than twenty different SEs described to date with varying amino acid sequences, common conformations, and similar biological effects. Picomolar concentrations of these superantigenic toxins activate specific T-cell subsets after binding to major histocompatibility complex class II. Activated T-cells vigorously proliferate and release proinflammatory cytokines plus chemokines that can elicit fever, hypotension, and other ailments which include a potentially lethal shock (Larkin et al., 2009, Varshney et al., 2010).

Studies on the protective effect of non-toxic mutant GST–mTSST-1 fusion protein against staphylococcal infection, was purified and tested. Mice were immunized with the GST–mTSST-1 plus alum adjuvant and challenged with viable *S. aureus*. The results indicate the efficacy of this protein in the elimination of bacterial load from the organs as well as in the inhibition of production of pro-inflammatory cytokines due to TSST-1 in the splenic cells. Furthermore immunization with GST–mTSST-1 strongly induced the production of TSST-1 specific antibodies, especially immunoglobulin G1 and immunoglobulin G2b (Cui et al., 2005).

Varshney et al., 2010 showed that four murine monoclonal antibodies bind to conformational epitopes that are destroyed by deletion of the distal C-terminal 11 Amino acids (Varshney et al., 2010). This study, for the first time, showed that MRSA derived SEB (staphylococcal enterotoxin B) contains a deletion in the C-terminal, which affects binding of certain protective Abs. This study also demonstrated enhanced protection against SEBILS (SEB induced Lethal Shock) when two non-protective mAbs were combinedly administered *in vivo*.

Drozdowski et al., (2010) generated high-affinity SEB-specific antibodies capable of neutralizing SEB *in* vitro as well as *in vivo* in a mouse model. They described for the first time recombinantly-derived human monoclonal antibodies against SEB that possess high affinity, target specificity, and therapeutic potential for superantigen-induced toxic shock. These antibodies prevent intoxication by interfering with toxin binding to MHC II and/or TCR. In addition to potential applications for treating toxic shock syndrome, human monoclonal antibodies recognizing SEB or other bacterial superantigens may be useful if employed as an adjunct therapy with antibiotics in treating *S. aureus* infections.

STEBvax is a new vaccine developed against toxic shock syndrome. It is currently under clinical trial phase I. The vaccine is being tested for prophylactic and therapeutic use (http://clinicaltrials.gov/ct2/show/NCT00974935) .

Larkin et al., (2010) selected human monoclonal antibodies from a phage display library, using a recombinant SEB vaccine (STEBVax) incorporating site-specific mutations that prevent MHC II interactions. This group discovered that some antibody clones cross-react with SEC1, SEC2, and streptococcal pyrogenic exotoxin C (SpeC), while others were highly specific for SEB. Many of the antibodies effectively inhibited T-cell activation by SEB in vitro, bound to toxin with nanomolar affinity, and prevented SEB-induced toxic shock in vivo. This recombinantly-derived, human monoclonal antibodies against SEB had high affinity, target specificity, and therapeutic potential for superantigen-induced toxic shock. These antibodies prevented intoxication by interfering with toxin binding to MHC II and/or T-cell antigen receptors. The author suggested the potential applications for treating toxic shock syndrome, human monoclonal antibodies recognizing SEB or other bacterial superantigens may be useful if employed as an adjunct therapy along with antibiotics in treating difficult *S. aureus* infections (Larkin et al., 2010).

4.1.6 Future perspectives in vaccine development

As discussed earlier, comparative proteomic analysis of planktonic and biofilm cells is an interesting area to look for vaccines against biofilm. Another important strategy is to look for immunodominant antigens. This strategy has led to the identification of a wide range of surface and extracellular target antigens such as IsdB, GrfA, IsaA, IsaB, Atl, IsdA, IsdH,

FmtB, SspA, SspB and Lip (Lorenz et al., 2000, Etz et al., 2002, Clarke and Foster, 2006). The rationale behind such a strategy is that the patients may develop antibodies against specific staphylococcal antigens during infection that may be critical for combating the infections (Ohlsen and Lorenz, 2010).

Another promising strategy is the reduction of nasal colonization by *S. aureus* as several studies have shown that nasal carriers have increased risk of developing infections by endogenous strains (von Eiff et al., 2001, Wertheim et al., 2004). Vaccination with clumping factor B, iron-responsive surface determinants (Isd) A and H, teichoic acid and capsular polysaccharides have been reported to reduce the nasal colonization with *S. aureus* (Dryla et al., 2005, Clarke and Foster, 2006).

4.2 Phage therapy

The rise of multidrug resistant bacteria has enforced the resurgence of phage therapy in the West, though this mode of therapy is being practiced for several years in Eastern Europe. Some of the success stories on phage therapy are described here. The Eliava Institute in Tbilisi, Republic of Georgia, has developed a highly virulent, monoclonal staphylococcal bacteriophage active against 80-95% of *S. aureus* strains including MRSA. This product was used for local and generalized infections, including neonatal sepsis, osteomyelitis, wound infections, pneumonia etc. (Hanlon, 2007). There are some polyvalent obligate lytic *S. aureus* phages e.g. phage phi812, phageK and phage44AHJD which have been successfully tested for their efficacy in killing *S. aureus* including MRSA strains (Mann, 2008). Evaluation of phageK showed marked reduction of pathogenic and antibiotic resistant coagulase positive and negative staphylococci associated with bovine and human infections that included *S. aureus*, *S. epidermidis*, *S. saprophyticus*, *S. chromogenes*, *S. capitis*, *S. hominis*, *S. haemolyticus*, *S. caprae*, and *S. hyicus*. The modified phage generated by passing through less susceptible target strain can be used in combination with phageK to increase the host range. This study had also shown the potential of delivering the phage in the form of handwash or antistaphylococcal cream (O'Flaherty et al., 2005b). Merabishvili and colleagues (2009), demonstrated laboratory-based production and quality control of a cocktail, currently under evaluation, consisting of exclusively lytic bacteriophages for the treatment of *Pseudomonas aeruginosa* and *S. aureus* infections of burn wound.

Curtin and Donlan (2006), reported use of phage *e.g.* phage456, in reducing the biofilm formation and adherence of *S. epidermidis* biofilms on both hydrogel-coated and serum/hydrogel coated silicone catheters. The presence of divalent cations in the growth medium (Mg^{++}, Ca^{++}) further increased the efficacy of phage456 in reducing biofilm formation. Polyvalent *Staphylococcus* phage combined with highly efficient *Pseudomonas* T7-like phage (phage phiIBB-PF7A) effectively showed reduction in dual species biofilms, killing and finally removal of bacteria from the host substratum (Sillankorva et al., 2010).

There were efforts to engineer bacteriophage by over-expressing proteins to target gene networks, particularly non-essential genes, to enhance bacterial killing by antibiotics. Using this approach, Lu and Collins (2007), engineered a T7 phage which significantly reduced *Escherichia coli* biofilm. They claim that this combinatorial approach may reduce the incidence of antibiotic resistance and enhance bacterial killing.

There are many advantages of using phage in therapeutics. (i) Dysbiosis can be avoided due to their specificity, (ii) Multiple administrations are not required because phage replicates at the site of infection, (iii) Phage could select resistant mutants of the selected bacteria, and (iv) Selection of new phages is rapid compared to the development of new antibiotic which may take several years. However, the disadvantage is that the causal organism needs to be identified before administering the phage (Sulakvelidze et al., 2001). Moreover, prior to the extensive therapeutic use of phages it is prudent to ensure the safety of therapeutic phages. The phages should not carry out generalized transduction and possess gene sequences having significant homology with known antibiotic resistances, phage-encoded toxins and other bacterial virulence factors (Sulakvelidze et al., 2001).

4.3 Antistaphylococcal lytic enzymes

Antistaphylococcal lytic enzymes can be broadly divided into two groups: (i) Staphylococcal phage lysins (endolysins) and (ii) Bacteriocins (e.g. Lysostaphin) (Borysowski and Gorski, 2009a).

4.3.1 Lysins

Lysins are enzymes, consist of N-terminal catalytic domain and C-terminal bacterial cell-wall binding domain, and are produced by bacteriophage that digests the bacterial cell wall (Fischetti, 2010, Borysowski and Gorski, 2009a). LysK, highly specific for the genus *Staphylococcus*, was obtained from phageK, has been effectively used in the treatment of staphylococcal infections (O'Flaherty et al., 2005a). Interestingly MV-L derived from bacteriophage phiMRII was found specific to *S. aureus* and *S. simulans* infection (Rashel et al., 2007). This phage also acted synergistically with glycopeptide antibiotics against VISA and MRSA. Moreover, MV-L induced antibodies could not abolish the bacteriolytic activity. Endolysin from another phi11 showed elimination of *S. aureus* NCTC8325 biofilm but not of *S. epidermidis* O-47 biofilm (Sass and Bierbaum, 2007). Purified endolysin (MW 53.3kDa) from virulent *S. aureus* bacteriophage Twort, *plyTW*, demonstrated cleavage of staphylococcal peptidoglycan. Upstream of *plyTW* there is Twort holin gene, *holTW*, which produces unspecific holes in the bacterial cytoplasmic membrane, degrade staphylococcal peptidoglycan through hydrolysis of alanine amino bonds (Loessner et al., 1998). CHAP (cysteine-histidine dependent amidohydrolase/ peptidase) exhibits lytic activity against staphylococcal isolates including MRSA, was identified by deletion analysis of LysK domain. CHAP can be used as single domain for therapeutic purposes over the whole enzyme as this may lower the risk of immunogenic response (Horgan et al., 2009).

4.3.2 Synergistic effect of lysins

Manoharadas et al., (2009) constructed a chimeric endolysin (P16-17) consisting of N-terminal D-alanyl-glycyl endopeptidase domain and C-terminal P16 endolysin domain and P17 minor coat protein, targeting cell wall of *S. aureus* phage. This domain swapping approach and subsequent purification resulted in finding soluble P16-17 protein, which exhibited antimicrobial activity against *S. aureus*. This protein further augmented the antimicrobial efficacy of gentamicin suggesting synergistic effect in reducing effective dose of aminoglycosides. Synergistic effect of nisin and LysH5, the endolysin encoded by phi-SauS-IPLA88 was demonstrated (Garcia et al., 2010). It was suggested that better lytic enzymes can be constructed by using methods like protein engineering, domain swapping and gene shuffling. Owing to the non-existence of bacterial resistance to lysins someday phage lytic enzymes could be an essential strategy to combat pathogenic bacteria (Fischetti et al., 2010).

4.3.3 Lysostaphin as a therapeutic agent

Lysostaphin, a 25kDa protein possessing two functional domains: N-terminal catalytic domain and C-terminal cell wall binding domain B, is a plasmid-encoded extracellular enzyme produced by *S. simulans* biovar *staphylolyticus* (Borysowski and Gorski, 2009b). It is a Zn-containing endopeptidase that specifically cleaves the bonds between the glycine residues in the interpeptide cross-bridges of the staphylococcal peptidoglycan resulting in the hypotonic lysis of the bacterial cell (Kumar, 2008). There are several reports of lysostaphin mediated lysis of clinically relevant antibiotic resistant staphylococcal strains. Lysostaphin which is readily absorbed onto catheter surfaces without losing lytic property shows promise in the prevention of catheter-related bloodstream infections caused by CoNS and *S. aureus* (Shah et al., 2004, Borysowski and Gorski, 2009a). Lysostaphin has successfully eradicated nasal colonization of MSSA, MRSA and mupirocin-resistant *S. aureus* in experimental cotton rats (Kokai-Kun et al., 2003). In combination with lysostaphin, oxacillin or vancomycin, showed increased efficacy against MRSA (Kokai-Kun et al., 2007, Patron et al., 1999). Several workers demonstrated the effectiveness of lysostaphin in the treatment of biofilms formed by *S. aureus* and *S. epidermidis* and disruption of biofilms on glass and plastic surfaces (King et al., 1980, Walencka et al., 2005, Wu et al., 2003). Evaluation of PEGylation potential in improving lysostaphin pharmacokinetics showed substantial increase in serum drug half-life and reduced binding to anti-lysostaphin antibodies while maintaining the enzyme's lytic activity (Walsh et al., 2003).

4.3.4 Lysostaphin therapy in ocular infections

Lysostaphin was also tested as a potential means of treating some ocular infections, especially endophthalmitis and keratitis. Dajcs et al., (2001) demonstrated the effect of lysostaphin on MRSA endophthalmitis in the rabbit model. Lysostaphin when administered twice after 8h and 24h post-infection showed 88% and 50% sterilization compared to 0% sterilization in untreated controls. However, the severity of ocular inflammation could be controlled only on 8h post-infection treatment models. Lysostaphin as a probable immunizing agent was also investigated. In this study, rabbits were immunized with lysostaphin by subcutaneous, intranasal or intraocular route that showed successful retention of bactericidal activity in vivo, in spite of the high titre of anti-lysostaphin antibodies (Dajcs et al., 2002, Balzli et al., 2010).

4.3.5 Synergistic effects

Synergistic inhibition by ranalexin (a cationic peptide) in combination with lysostaphin resulted in an enhanced bactericidal effect. This finding, therefore, suggested that dressings could be impregnated with ranalexin and lysostaphin to treat wound infections caused by MRSA (Graham and Coote, 2007, Desbois et al., 2010). Furthermore lysozyme has been reported enhancing lysostaphin activity (Cisani et al., 1982). Combinatorial action of various beta-lactam antibiotics or mupirocin or gentamicin enhancing lysostaphin activity was reported by various groups (Polak et al., 1993, Climo et al., 2001, Kiri et al., 2002, LaPlante, 2007). Thus, it is concluded that lysostaphin is an effective agent as pre- and post-treatment option for staphylococcal infections though CoNS showed generally weaker effect than *S. aureus* (Borysowski and Gorski, 2009a). This was because of presence of higher amount of serine than glycine in peptidoglycan of coagulase-negative staphylococci (Kumar, 2008).

4.4 Plant-derived antibacterials

Plant-derived antibacterials are of three types: (i) traditional antibiotics, (ii) antibacterials that target bacterial virulence, and (iii) inhibitors of MDR pump. The first two categories have not been explored in detail (Lewis and Ausubel, 2006). The details of third category of compounds obtained from plant sources, their properties as MDR/ EPI inhibitors and its use as antibacterial against staphylococcal infection are summarized in Table 2.

Identification of EPIs from natural sources is still in infancy. However, the chemical diversity of plants and microorganisms and their requirement for nutrients to synthesize such compounds should make the search for EPIs from such sources an attractive option (Stavri et al., 2007).

4.5 Nature's backyard

Resistance of microbial pathogens to antibiotics is a serious threat to the well-being of mankind. Recently, two small molecules, platensimycin, identified from strain of *Streptomyces platensis* isolated from soil sample in South Africa, by using antisense differential sensitivity whole-cell screening program, targeting the fatty acid biosynthesis pathway of gram-positive bacteria. The platensimycin ($C_{24}H_{27}NO_7$, MW 441.47) comprises of two distinct structural element connected by an amide bond, is active against MRSA, VISA, Vancomycin-resistant enterococci and linezolid and macrolide resistant pathogens (Wang et al., 2006) (Fig. 2A).

Continued screening led to the discovery of platencin ($C_{24}H_{27}NO_6$, MW 425.2), a novel product that is chemically and biologically related to platensimycin which exhibits broad-spectrum antibacterial activity against gram positive bacteria which inhibit fatty acid biosynthesis (Fig. 2B). These molecule targets two essential proteins, beta-ketoacyl synthase II (FabF) and III (FabH) (Wang et al., 2007). These studies reflect upon the fact that nature holds the treasure trove of antibiotics which are yet to be explored.

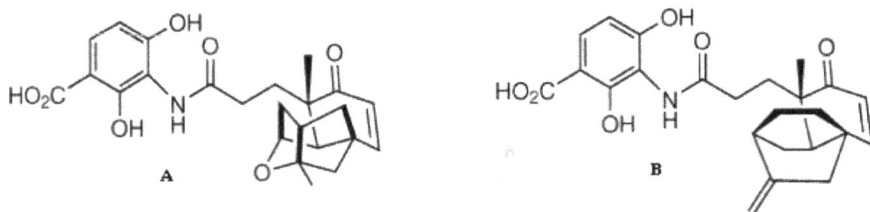

Fig. 2. Chemical structure of Platensimycin (A) and Platencin (B).

	Common name & plant species name	Compound	Properties	Total effect	Synergistic effect	References
1	Barberry & *Berberis* species	Berberine & 5'-methoxyhydnocarpin	Hydrophobic cation increases membrane permeability and intercalate DNA	Inhibit MDR	Antibacterial	(Stermitz et al., 2000)
2	Golden seal & *Hydrastis canadensis*	Berberine & 5'-methoxyhydnocarpin	5'-methoxyhydnocarpin-linking of berberine to INF_{55}	Inhibit MDR	Antibacterial	(Ball et al., 2006)
3	Silvery lupine & *Lupinus argenteus*	Isoflavones	Enhances activity of berberine and norfloxacin	Inhibit MDR	Antibacterial	(Morel et al., 2003)
4	Fabaceae & *Dalea versicolor*	Phenolic metabolites	Enhances activity of berberine, erythromycin and tetracycline	Inhibit MDR	Antibacterial	(Belofsky et al., 2004)]
5	Smoke tree & *Dalea spinosa*	2-arylbenzofuran aldehyde & Phenolic compounds; SpinosanA, Pterocarpan & Isoflavone	Enhances activity of berberine	Inhibit MDR	Antibacterial	(Belofsky et al., 2006)
6	Tea	Epicatechin gallate & Epigallocatechin gallate	Enhances activity of norfloxacin and tetracycline	Inhibit MDR	Antibacterial	(Gibbons et al., 2004, Sudano Roccaro et al., 2004)
7	Rosemery & *Rosmarinus officinalis*	Diterpines, Carnosic acid & Carnesol	Potentiate activity of tetracycline and erythromycin	Inhibit MDR	Antibacterial	(Oluwatuyi et al., 2004)
8	Gipsywort & *Lycopus europaeus*	Lipophilic extract	Potentiate activity of tetracycline and erythromycin	Inhibit MDR	Antibacterial	(Gibbons et al., 2003)
9	Grapefruit oil & *Citrus paradisi*	Coumarin derivative: Bergamottin epoxide & Coumarin epoxide	Enhances activity of ethidium bromide and norfloxacin	Inhibit MDR	Antibacterial	(Abulrob et al., 2004)
10	Piperine & *Piper nigrum* & *Piper longum*	Piperine	Potentiating action of piperine in combination with ciprofloxacin	Inhibit MDR	Antibacterial	(Khan et al., 2006)

Table 2. Properties of MDR/ EPI inhibitors isolated from medicinal plants and its use as antibacterial agent against Staphylococcal infection.

5. Conclusions

Extensive applied and basic research is needed to come up with strategies combating the major challenges of staphylococcal infections. Recently, folic acid tagged chitosan nanoparticles were effectively used to deliver vancomycin. It proved to be an efficient method to increase the bioavailability of the same (Chakraborty et al., 2010). Researchers have developed Nitric oxide releasing nanoparticles as treatment for skin and soft tissue infections successfully tested in murine models (Han et al., 2009, Englander and Friedman, 2010).

Use of vaccines and phages for the treatment and control staphylococcal infections might be a sustainable alternative to antibiotics. The advent of high throughput sequencing has led to the analysis of phage genomes and better understanding of phage evolution, phage-host interaction, bacterial pathogenicity, phage ecology and origin of phages (O'Flaherty et al., 2009). With the background knowledge of phage genomics, it will be possible to approach phage therapeutics cautiously and effectively. Future research should focus on multidisciplinary approach on the development of alternative/conjunctive strategies for treatment and prevention of staphylococcal infections.

6. Acknowledgement

This study, in part, was supported by Department of Science and Technology, New Delhi, grant no: SR/SO/HS-117/2007 to SS and DVS, DST-WOS-A grant no: SR/WOS-A/208/2009 to RC, and fund contributed by Department of Biotechnology, New Delhi to Institute of Life Sciences, Bhubaneswar. Junior Research Fellowship awarded by Department of Science and Technology, New Delhi to SP is gratefully acknowledged.

7. References

Abele-horn, M.; Schupfner, B.; Emmerling, P.; Waldner, H. & Goring, H. (2000). Persistent wound infection after herniotomy associated with small-colony variants of *Staphylococcus aureus*. *Infection*, Vol.28, pp. 53-54, ISSN: 0300-8126

Abulrob, AN.; Suller, MT.; Gumbleton, M.; Simons, C. & Russell, AD. (2004). Identification and biological evaluation of grapefruit oil components as potential novel efflux pump modulators in methicillin-resistant *Staphylococcus aureus* bacterial strains. *Phytochemistry*, Vol.65, pp. 3021-3027, ISSN: 0031-9422

Aliprandis, E.; Ciralsky, J.; Lai, H.; Herling, I. & Katz, HR. (2005). Comparative efficacy of topical moxifloxacin versus ciprofloxacin and vancomycin in the treatment of *P. aeruginosa* and ciprofloxacin-resistant MRSA keratitis in rabbits. *Cornea*, Vol.24, pp. 201-205, ISSN: 0277-3740

Allegrucci, M. & Sauer, K. (2007). Characterization of colony morphology variants isolated from *Streptococcus pneumoniae* biofilms. *J Bacteriol*, Vol.189, pp. 2030-2038, ISSN: 0021-9193

Allen, HK.; Donato, J.; Wang, HH.; Cloud-hansen, KA.; Davies, J. & Handelsman, J. (2010). Call of the wild: antibiotic resistance genes in natural environments. *Nat Rev Microbiol*, Vol.8, pp. 251-259, ISSN: 1740-1526

Asbell, P. & Stenson, S. (1982). Ulcerative keratitis. Survey of 30 years' laboratory experience. *Arch Ophthalmol*, Vol.100, pp. 77-80, ISSN: 0003-9950

Baddour, LM. & Christensen, GD. (1987). Prosthetic valve endocarditis due to small-colony staphylococcal variants. *Rev Infect Dis*, Vol.9, pp. 1168-74, ISSN: 0162-0886

Baddour, LM.; Simpson, WA.; Weems, JJ Jr.; Hill, MM. & Christensen, GD. (1988). Phenotypic selection of small-colony variant forms of *Staphylococcus epidermidis* in the rat model of endocarditis. *J Infect Dis*, Vol.157, pp. 757-763, ISSN: 0022-1899

Bagga, B.; Reddy, AK. & Garg, P. (2010). Decreased susceptibility to quinolones in methicillin-resistant *Staphylococcus aureus* isolated from ocular infections at a tertiary eye care centre. *Br J Ophthalmol*, Vol.94, pp. 1407-1408, ISSN: 0007-1161

Ball, AR.; Casadei, G.; Samosorn, S.; Bremner, JB.; Ausubel, FM.; Moy, TI. & Lewis, K. (2006). Conjugating berberine to a multidrug efflux pump inhibitor creates an effective antimicrobial. *ACS Chem Biol*, Vol.1, pp. 594-600, ISSN: 1554-8929

Balzli, CL.; McCormick, CC.; Caballero, AR. & O' Callaghan, RJ. (2010). Sustained anti-staphylococcal effect of lysostaphin in the rabbit aqueous humor. *Curr Eye Res*, Vol.35, pp. 480-486, ISSN: 0271-3683

Barry, AL.; Jones, RN. & Thornsberry, C. (1988). In vitro activities of azithromycin (CP 62.;993).; clarithromycin; erythromycin.; roxithromycin.; and clindamycin. *Antimicrob Agents Chemother*, Vol.32, pp. 752-754, ISSN: 1502-2307

Belofsky, G.; Carreno, R.; Lewis, K.; Ball, A.; Casadei, G. & Tegos, GP. (2006). Metabolites of the "smoke tree".; *Dalea spinosa*.; potentiate antibiotic activity against multidrug-resistant *Staphylococcus aureus*. *J Nat Prod*, Vol.69, pp. 261-264, ISSN: 0163-3864

Belofsky, G.; Percivill, D.; Lewis, K.; Tegos, GP. & Ekart, J. (2004). Phenolic metabolites of *Dalea versicolor* that enhance antibiotic activity against model pathogenic bacteria. *J Nat Prod*, Vol.67, pp. 481-484, ISSN: 0163-3864

Benz, MS.; Scott, IU.; Flynn, HW Jr.; Unonius, N. & Miller D. (2004). Endophthalmitis isolates and antibiotic sensitivities: a 6-year review of culture-proven cases. *Am J Ophthalmol*, Vol.137, pp. 38-42, ISSN: 0002-9394

Borysowski, A. & Gorski, A. (2009a). Enzybiotics and their potential applications in medicine, In: *Enzybiotics: Antibiotic Enzymes as Drugs and Therapeutics*, Villa, TG. & Patricia Veiga Crespo, PV. (Ed.)., pp. 1-26 ISBN: 978-0-470-37655-3, John Wiley and Sons, Inc., Hoboken, NJ, USA

Borysowski, A. & Gorski, A. (2009b). Anti-staphylococcal lytic enzymes, In: *Enzybiotics: Antibiotic Enzymes as Drugs and Therapeutics*, Villa, TG. & Crespo, PV. (Ed.)., pp. 149-172 ISBN: 978-0-470-37655-3, John Wiley and Sons, Inc., Hoboken, NJ, USA

Callegan, MC.; Engelbert, M.; Parke, DW 2nd.; Jett, BD. & Gilmore, MS. (2002). Bacterial endophthalmitis: epidemiology.; therapeutics.; and bacterium-host interactions. *Clin Microbiol Rev*, Vol.15, pp. 111-124, ISSN: 0893-8512

Capriotti, JA.; Pelletier, JS.; Shah, M.; Caivano, DM. & Ritterband, DC. (2009). Normal ocular flora in healthy eyes from a rural population in Sierra Leone. *Int Ophthalmol*, Vol.29, pp. 81-84, ISSN: 0165-5701

Cerca, N.; Maira-litran, T.; Jefferson, KK.; Grout, M.; Goldmann, DA. & Pier GB. (2007). Protection against *Escherichia coli* infection by antibody to the *Staphylococcus aureus* poly-N-acetylglucosamine surface polysaccharide. *Proc Natl Acad Sci U S A*, Vol.104, pp. 7528-7533, ISSN: 1091-6490

Chakraborty, SP.; Sahu, SK.; Mahapatra, SK.; Santra, S.; Bal, M.; Roy, S. & Pramanik P. (2010). Nanoconjugated vancomycin: new opportunities for the development of anti-VRSA agents. *Nanotechnology*, Vol.21, pp. 1-9, ISSN: 0957-4484

Chopra, I. (1992). Efflux-based antibiotic resistance mechanisms: the evidence for increasing prevalence. *J Chemother*, Vol.30, pp. 737-739, ISSN: 1502-2307

Cisani, G.; Varaldo, PE.; Grazi, G. & Soro, O. (1982). High-level potentiation of lysostaphin anti-staphylococcal activity by lysozyme. *Antimicrob Agents Chemother*, Vol.21, pp. 531-535, ISSN: 1502-2307

Clarke, SR. & Foster, SJ. (2006). Surface adhesins of *Staphylococcus aureus*. *Adv Microb Physiol*, Vol.51, pp. 187-224, ISSN: 0065-2911

Climo, MW.; Ehlert, K. & Archer GL. (2001). Mechanism and suppression of lysostaphin resistance in oxacillin-resistant *Staphylococcus aureus*. *Antimicrob Agents Chemother*, Vol.45, pp. 1431-1437, ISSN: 1502-2307

Couto, I.; de Lencastre, H.; Severina, E.; Kloos, W.; Webster, JA.; Hubner, RJ.; Sanches, IS. & Tomasz, A. (1996). Ubiquitous presence of a *mecA* homologue in natural isolates of *Staphylococcus sciuri*. *Microb Drug Resist*, Vol.2, pp. 377-391, ISSN: 1076-6294

Cui , JC.; Hu, DL.; Lin, YC.; Qian, AD. & Nakane, A. (2005). Immunization with glutathione S-transferase and mutant toxic shock syndrome toxin 1 fusion protein protects against *Staphylococcus aureus* infection. *FEMS Immunol Med Microbiol*, Vol.45, pp. 45-51, ISSN: 0928-8244

Curtin, JJ. & Donlan, RM. (2006). Using bacteriophages to reduce formation of catheter-associated biofilms by *Staphylococcus epidermidis*. *Antimicrob Agents Chemother*, Vol.50, pp. 1268-1275, ISSN: 1502-2307

Dajcs, JJ.; Thibodeaux, BA.; Girgis, DO.; Shaffer, MD.; Delvisco, SM. & O'Callaghan, RJ. (2002). Immunity to lysostaphin and its therapeutic value for ocular MRSA infections in the rabbit. *Invest Ophthalmol Vis Sci*, Vol.43, pp. 3712-3716, ISSN: 0146-0404

Dajcs, JJ.; Thibodeaux, BA.; Hume, EB.; Zheng , X.; Sloop, GD. & O'Callaghan RJ. (2001). Lysostaphin is effective in treating methicillin-resistant *Staphylococcus aureus* endophthalmitis in the rabbit. *Curr Eye Res*, Vol.22, pp. 451-457, ISSN: 0271-3683

Davies, NM. (2000). Biopharmaceutical considerations in topical ocular drug delivery. *Clin Exp Pharmacol Physiol*, Vol.27, pp. 558-562, ISSN: 0305-1870

Desbois , AP.; Gemmell, CG. & Coote, PJ. (2010). In vivo efficacy of the antimicrobial peptide ranalexin in combination with the endopeptidase lysostaphin against wound and systemic meticillin-resistant *Staphylococcus aureus* (MRSA) infections. *Int J Antimicrob Agents*, Vol.35, pp. 559-565, ISSN: 0924-8579

Deurenberg, RH. & Stobberingh, EE. (2008). The evolution of *Staphylococcus aureus*. *Infect Genet Evol*, Vol.8, pp. 747-763, ISSN: 1567-1348

Drozdowski, B.; Zhou, Y.; Kline, B.; Spidel, J.; Chan, YY.; Albone, E.; Turchin, H.; Chao, Q.; Henry, M.; Balogach, J.; Routhier, E.; Bavari, S.; Nicolaides, NC.; Sass, PM. & Grasso, L. (2010). Generation and characterization of high affinity human monoclonal antibodies that neutralize staphylococcal enterotoxin B. *J Immune Based Ther Vaccines*, Vol.8, pp. 1-9, ISSN: 1476-8518

Dryla, A.; Prustomersky, S.; Gelbmann, D.; Hanner, M.; Bettinger, E.; Kocsis, B.; Kustos, T.; Henics, T.; Meinke, A. & Nagy, E. (2005). Comparison of antibody repertoires against *Staphylococcus aureus* in healthy individuals and in acutely infected patients. *Clin Diagn Lab Immunol*, Vol.12, pp. 387-398, ISSN: 1071-412X

Endimiani, A.; Blackford, M.; Dasenbrook, EC.; Reed, MD.; Bajaksouszian, S.; Hujer, AM.; Rudin, SD.; Hujer, KM.; Perreten, V.; Rice, LB.; Jacobs, MR.; Konstan, MW. & Bonomo, RA. (2011). Emergence of linezolid-resistant *Staphylococcus aureus* after prolonged treatment of cystic fibrosis patients in Cleveland. *Antimicrob Agents Chemother*, epub. 24 January 2011, ISSN: 1502-2307

Englander, L. & Friedman, A. (2010). Nitric oxide nanoparticle technology: a novel antimicrobial agent in the context of current treatment of skin and soft tissue infection. *J Clin Aesthet Dermatol*, Vol.3, pp. 45-50, ISSN: 1941-2789

Etz, H.; Minh, DB.; Henics, T.; Dryla, A.; Winkler, B.; Triska, C.; Boyd, AP.; Sollner, J.; Schmidt, W.; Von Ahsen, U.; Buschle, M.; Gill, SR.; Kolonay, J.; Khalak, H.; Fraser, CM.; von Gabain, A.; Nagy, E. & Meinke, A. (2002). Identification of in vivo expressed vaccine candidate antigens from *Staphylococcus aureus*. *Proc Natl Acad Sci U S A*, Vol.99, pp. 6573-6578, ISSN: 1091-6490

Fischetti, VA. (2010). Bacteriophage endolysins: a novel anti-infective to control Gram-positive pathogens. *Int J Med Microbiol*, Vol.300, pp. 357-362, ISSN: 0022-2615

Flock, JI. (1999). Extracellular-matrix-binding proteins as targets for the prevention of *Staphylococcus aureus* infections. *Mol Med Today*,Vol.5 pp. 532-537, ISSN: 1357-4310

Foster, TJ. (2005). Immune evasion by staphylococci. *Nat Rev Microbiol*, Vol.3, pp. 948-958, ISSN: 1740-1526

Fukuda, M.; Ohashi, H.; Matsumoto, C.; Mishima, S. & Shimomura, Y. (2002). Methicillin-resistant *Staphylococcus aureus* and methicillin-resistant coagulase-negative *Staphylococcus* ocular surface infection efficacy of chloramphenicol eye drops. *Cornea*, Vol.21, pp. S86-89, ISSN: 0277-3740

Garcia-Lara, J.; Masalha, M. & Foster, SJ. (2005). *Staphylococcus aureus*: the search for novel targets. *Drug Discov Today*, Vol.10, pp. 643-651, ISSN: 1359-6446

Garcia, P.; Martinez, B.; Rodriguez, L. & Rodriguez, A. (2010). Synergy between the phage endolysin LysH5 and nisin to kill *Staphylococcus aureus* in pasteurized milk. *Int J Food Microbiol*, Vol.141, pp. 151-155, ISSN: 0168-1605

Gening, ML.; Maira-Litran, T.; Kropec, A.; Skurnik, D.; Grout, M.; Tsvetkov, YE.; Nifantiev, NE. & Pier, GB. (2010). Synthetic {beta}-(1->6).-linked N-acetylated and nonacetylated oligoglucosamines used to produce conjugate vaccines for bacterial pathogens. *Infect Immun*, Vol.78, pp. 764-772, ISSN: 0019-9567

Gibbons, S.; Moser, E. & Kaatz, GW. (2004). Catechin gallates inhibit multidrug resistance (MDR). in *Staphylococcus aureus*. *Planta Med*, Vol.70, pp. 1240-1242, ISSN: 0032-0943

Gibbons, S.; Oluwatuyi, M. & Kaatz, GW. (2003). A novel inhibitor of multidrug efflux pumps in *Staphylococcus aureus*. *J Antimicrob Chemother*, Vol.51, pp. 13-17, ISSN: 0305-7453

Gopinathan, U.; Sharma, S.; Garg, P. & Rao, GN. (2009). Review of epidemiological features.; microbiological diagnosis and treatment outcome of microbial keratitis: experience of over a decade. *Indian J Ophthalmol*, Vol.57, pp. 273-279, ISSN: 0301-4738

Götz, F., and Peters, G. (2000). Colonization of medical devices by coagulase-negative staphylococci, In: *Infections Associated with Indwelling Medical Devices*, Waldvogel, FA. & Bisno, AL. (Ed.)., pp. 55 - 88, ASM Press, ISBN: 978-1555811778, Washington DC, USA

Graham, S. & Coote, PJ. (2007). Potent.; synergistic inhibition of *Staphylococcus aureus* upon exposure to a combination of the endopeptidase lysostaphin and the cationic peptide ranalexin. *J Antimicrob Chemother*, Vol.59, pp. 759-762, ISSN: 0305-7453

Haas, W.; Pillar, CM.; Hesje, CK.; Sanfilippo, CM. & Morris, TW. (2010). Bactericidal activity of besifloxacin against staphylococci.; *Streptococcus pneumoniae* and *Haemophilus influenzae*. *J Antimicrob Chemother*, Vol.65, pp. 1441-1447, ISSN: 0305-7453.

Han, G.; Martinez, LR.; Mihu, MR.; Friedman, AJ.; Friedman, JM. & Nosanchuk, JD. (2009). Nitric oxide releasing nanoparticles are therapeutic for *Staphylococcus aureus* abscesses in a murine model of infection. *PLoS One*, Vol.4, e7804, ISSN: 1932-6203

Hanlon, GW. (2007). Bacteriophages: an appraisal of their role in the treatment of bacterial infections. *Int J Antimicrob Agents*, Vol.30, pp. 118-128, ISSN: 0924-8579

Harro, JM.; Peters, BM.; O'May, GA.; Archer, N.; Kerns, P.; Prabhakara, R. & Shirtliff, ME. (2010). Vaccine development in *Staphylococcus aureus*: taking the biofilm phenotype into consideration. *FEMS Immunol Med Microbiol*, Vol.59, pp. 306-323, ISSN: 0928-8244

Holtfreter, S. & Broker, BM. (2005). Staphylococcal superantigens: do they play a role in sepsis? *Arch Immunol Ther Exp (Warsz)*, Vol.53, pp. 13-27, ISSN: 0004-069X

Hooper, DC. (2001). Emerging mechanisms of fluoroquinolone resistance. *Emerg Infect Dis*, Vol.7, pp. 337-341, ISSN: 1080-6059

Horgan, M.; O'Flynn, G.; Garry, J.; Cooney, J.; Coffey, A.; Fitzgerald, GF.; Ross, RP. & Mcauliffe, O. (2009). Phage lysin LysK can be truncated to its CHAP domain and retain lytic activity against live antibiotic-resistant staphylococci. *Appl Environ Microbiol*, Vol .5, pp. 872-874, ISSN: 0099-2240

Iskeleli, G.; Bahar, H.; Eroglu, E.; Torun, MM. & Ozkan, S. (2005). Microbial changes in conjunctival flora with 30-day continuous-wear silicone hydrogel contact lenses. *Eye Contact Lens*, Vol.31, pp. 124-126, ISSN: 1542-2321

Jayaraman, R. (2008). Bacterial persistence: some new insights into an old phenomenon. *J Biosci*, Vol.33, pp. 795-805, ISSN 0250-5991

Kahl, B.; Herrmann, M.; Everding, AS.; Koch, HG.; Becker, K.; Harms, E.; Proctor RA. & Peters, G. (1998). Persistent infection with small colony variant strains of *Staphylococcus aureus* in patients with cystic fibrosis. *J Infect Dis*, Vol.177, pp. 1023-1029, ISSN: 0022-1899

Kar, S.; Panda, S.; Sharma, S.; Singh, DV.; Das, S. & Sahu, SK. (2010). Antibiogram of methicillin resistant and sensitive *Staphylococcus aureus* isolates from ocular infections. *Proceedings of MICROCON 2010 34th Annual conference of Indian Association of Medical Microbiologists*, Kolkata, India, November 26-28, 2010

Katayama, Y.; Ito, T. & Hiramatsu, K. (2000). A new class of genetic element.; staphylococcus cassette chromosome mec.; encodes methicillin resistance in *Staphylococcus aureus*. *Antimicrob Agents Chemother*, Vol.44, pp. 1549-1555, ISSN: 1502-2307

Kehrenberg, C.; Schwarz, S.; Jacobsen, L.; Hansen, LH. & Vester, B. (2005). A new mechanism for chloramphenicol, florfenicol and clindamycin resistance: methylation of 23S ribosomal RNA at A2503. *Mol Microbiol*, Vol.57, pp. 1064-1073, ISSN: 0950-382X

Keren, I.; Kaldalu, N.; Spoering, A.; Wang, Y. & Lewis, K. (2004). Persister cells and tolerance to antimicrobials. *FEMS Microbiol Lett*, Vol.230, pp. 13-18, ISSN: 0378-1097

Khan, IA.; Mirza, ZM.; Kumar, A.; Verma, V. & Qazi, GN. (2006). Piperine.; a phytochemical potentiator of ciprofloxacin against *Staphylococcus aureus*. *Antimicrob Agents Chemother*, Vol.50, pp. 810-812, ISSN: 1502-2307

King, BF.; Biel, ML. & Wilkinson, BJ. (1980). Facile penetration of the *Staphylococcus aureus* capsule by lysostaphin. *Infect Immun*, Vol.29, pp. 892-896, ISSN: 0019-9567

Kiri, N.; Archer, G. & Climo, MW. (2002). Combinations of lysostaphin with beta-lactams are synergistic against oxacillin-resistant *Staphylococcus epidermidis*. *Antimicrob Agents Chemother*, Vol.46, pp. 2017-2020, ISSN: 1502-2307

Kokai-Kun, JF.; Chanturiya, T. & Mond, JJ. (2007). Lysostaphin as a treatment for systemic *Staphylococcus aureus* infection in a mouse model. *J Antimicrob Chemother*, Vol.60, pp. 1051-1059, ISSN: 0305-7453

Kokai-Kun, JF.; Walsh, SM.; Chanturiya, T. & Mond, JJ. (2003). Lysostaphin cream eradicates *Staphylococcus aureus* nasal colonization in a cotton rat model. *Antimicrob Agents Chemother*, Vol.47, pp. 1589-1597, ISSN: 1502-2307

Kumar, JK. (2008). Lysostaphin: an antistaphylococcal agent. *Appl Microbiol Biotechnol*, Vol.80, pp. 555-561, ISSN: 0175-7598

Kunimoto, DY.; Das, T.; Sharma, S.; Jalali, S.; Majji, AB.; Gopinathan, U.; Athmanathan, S.; Rao, TN. (1999a). Microbiologic spectrum and susceptibility of isolates: part I. Postoperative endophthalmitis. Endophthalmitis Research Group. *Am J Ophthalmol*, Vol.128, pp. 240-242, ISSN: 0002-9394

Kunimoto, DY.; Das, T.; Sharma, S.; Jalali, S.; Majji, AB.; Gopinathan, U.; Athmanathan, S.; Rao, TN. (1999b). Microbiologic spectrum and susceptibility of isolates: part II. Posttraumatic endophthalmitis. Endophthalmitis Research Group. *Am J Ophthalmol*, Vol.128, pp. 242-244, ISSN: 0002-9394

Kvist, M.; Hancock, V. & Klemm, P. (2008). Inactivation of efflux pumps abolishes bacterial biofilm formation. *Appl Environ Microbiol*, Vol.74, pp. 7376-7382, ISSN: 0099-2240

Kwon, AS.; Park, GC.; Ryu, SY.; Lim, DH.; Lim, DY.; Choi, CH.; Park, Y. & Lim, Y. (2008). Higher biofilm formation in multidrug-resistant clinical isolates of *Staphylococcus aureus*. *Int J Antimicrob Agents*, Vol.32, pp. 68-72, ISSN: 0924-8579

Lane, SS.; Osher, RH.; Masket, S. & Belani, S. (2008). Evaluation of the safety of prophylactic intracameral moxifloxacin in cataract surgery. *J Cataract Refract Surg*, Vol.34, pp. 1451-1459, ISSN: 0886-3350

Laplante, KL. (2007). In vitro activity of lysostaphin.; mupirocin.; and tea tree oil against clinical methicillin-resistant *Staphylococcus aureus*. *Diagn Microbiol Infect Dis*, Vol.57, pp. 413-418, ISSN: 0732-8893

Larkin, EA.; Carman, RJ.; Krakauer, T. & Stiles, BG. (2009). *Staphylococcus aureus*: the toxic presence of a pathogen extraordinaire. *Curr Med Chem*, Vol.16, pp. 4003-4019, ISSN: 0929-8673

Larkin, EA.; Stiles, BG. & Ulrich, RG. (2010). Inhibition of toxic shock by human monoclonal antibodies against staphylococcal enterotoxin B. *PLoS One*, Vol.5, e13253, ISSN: 1932-6203

Levin, BR. & Rozen, DE. (2006). Non-inherited antibiotic resistance. *Nat Rev Microbiol*, Vol.4, pp. 556-562, ISSN: 1740-1526

Lewis, K. (2010). Persister cells. *Annu Rev Microbiol*, Vol.64, pp. 357-372, ISSN: 0066-4227

Lewis, K. (2008). Multidrug tolerance of biofilms and persister cells. *Curr Top Microbiol Immunol*, Vol.322, pp. 107-131, ISSN: 0070-217X

Lewis, K. & Ausubel, FM. (2006). Prospects for plant-derived antibacterials. *Nat Biotechnol*, Vol.24, pp. 1504-1507, ISSN: 1087-0156

Liesegang, TJ. & Forster, RK. (1980). Spectrum of microbial keratitis in South Florida. *Am J Ophthalmol*, Vol.90, pp. 38-47, ISSN: 0002-9394

Locke, JB.; Hilgers, M. & Shaw, KJ. (2009). Novel ribosomal mutations in *Staphylococcus aureus* strains identified through selection with the oxazolidinones linezolid and torezolid (TR-700). *Antimicrob Agents Chemother*, Vol.53, pp. 5265-5274, ISSN: 1502-2307

Loessner, MJ.; Gaeng, S.; Wendlinger, G.; Maier, SK. & Scherer, S. (1998). The two-component lysis system of *Staphylococcus aureus* bacteriophage Twort: a large TTG-start holin and an associated amidase endolysin. *FEMS Microbiol Lett*, Vol.162, pp. 265-274, ISSN: 0378-1097

Lorenz, U.; Ohlsen, K.; Karch, H.; Hecker, M.; Thiede, A. & Hacker, J. (2000). Human antibody response during sepsis against targets expressed by methicillin resistant *Staphylococcus aureus*. *FEMS Immunol Med Microbiol*, Vol.29, pp. 145-153, ISSN: 0928-8244

Lu, TK. & Collins, JJ. (2007). Dispersing biofilms with engineered enzymatic bacteriophage. *Proc Natl Acad Sci U S A*, Vol.104, pp. 11197-11202, ISSN: 1091-6490

Mamo, W.; Froman, G. & Muller, HP. (2000). Protection induced in mice vaccinated with recombinant collagen-binding protein (CnBP) and alpha-toxoid against intramammary infection with *Staphylococcus aureus*. *Microbiol Immunol*, Vol.44, pp. 381-384, ISSN: 0385-5600

Mann, NH. (2008). The potential of phages to prevent MRSA infections. *Res Microbiol*, Vol.159, pp. 400-405, ISSN: 0923-2508

Manoharadas, S.; Witte, A. & Blasi, U. (2009). Antimicrobial activity of a chimeric enzybiotic towards *Staphylococcus aureus*. *J Biotechnol*, Vol.139, pp. 118-123, ISSN: 0168-1656

Martinez, JL.; Fajardo, A.; Garmendia, L.; Hernandez, A.; Linares, JF.; Martinez-Solano, L. & Sanchez, MB. (2009a). A global view of antibiotic resistance. *FEMS Microbiol Rev*, Vol.33, pp. 44-65, ISSN: 0168-6445

Martinez, JL.; Sanchez, MB.; Martinez-Solano, L.; Hernandez, A.; Garmendia, L.; Fajardo, A. & Alvarez-Ortega, C. (2009b). Functional role of bacterial multidrug efflux pumps in microbial natural ecosystems. *FEMS Microbiol Rev*, Vol.33, pp. 430-449, ISSN: 0168-6445

McCallum, N.; Berger-Bachi, B. & Senn, MM. (2010). Regulation of antibiotic resistance in *Staphylococcus aureus*. *Int J Med Microbiol*, Vol.300, pp. 118-129, ISSN: 0022-2615

McClellan, KA.; Bernard, PJ. & Billson, FA. (1989). Microbial investigations in keratitis at the Sydney Eye Hospital. *Aust N Z J Ophthalmol*, Vol.17, pp. 413-416, ISSN: 0814-9763

McCulley, JP.; Dougherty, JM. & Deneau, DG. (1982). Classification of chronic blepharitis. *Ophthalmology*, Vol.89, pp. 1173-1180, ISSN: 0161-6420

McDonald, M. & Blondeau, JM. (2010). Emerging antibiotic resistance in ocular infections and the role of fluoroquinolones. *J Cataract Refract Surg*, Vol.36, pp. 1588-1598, ISSN: 0886-3350

Merabishvili, M.; Pirnay, JP.; Verbeken, G.; Chanishvili, N.; Tediashvili, M.; Lashkhi, N.; Glonti, T.; Krylov, V.; Mast, J.; Van Parys, L.; Lavigne, R.; Volckaert, G.; Mattheus, W.; Verween, G.; De Corte, P.; Rose, T.; Jennes, S.; Zizi, M.; De Vos, D. & Vaneechoutte, M. (2009). Quality-controlled small-scale production of a well-defined bacteriophage cocktail for use in human clinical trials. *PLoS One*, Vol.4, e4944, ISSN: 1932-6203

Morar, M. & Wright, GD. (2010). The genomic enzymology of antibiotic resistance. *Annu Rev Genet*, Vol.44, pp. 25-51, ISSN: 0066-4197

Morel, C.; Stermitz, FR.; Tegos, G. & Lewis, K. (2003). Isoflavones as potentiators of antibacterial activity. *J Agric Food Chem*, Vol.51, pp. 5677-5679, ISSN: 0021-8561

O'Flaherty, S.; Coffey, A.; Meaney, W.; Fitzgerald, GF. & Ross, RP. (2005a). The recombinant phage lysin LysK has a broad spectrum of lytic activity against clinically relevant staphylococci.; including methicillin-resistant *Staphylococcus aureus. J Bacteriol*, Vol.187, pp. 7161-7164, ISSN: 0021-9193

O'Flaherty, S.; Ross, RP. & Coffey, A. (2009). Bacteriophage and their lysins for elimination of infectious bacteria. *FEMS Microbiol Rev*, Vol.33, pp. 801-819, ISSN: 0168-6445

O'Flaherty, S.; Ross, RP.; Meaney, W.; Fitzgerald, GF.; Elbreki, MF. & Coffey, A. (2005b). Potential of the polyvalent anti-Staphylococcus bacteriophage K for control of antibiotic-resistant staphylococci from hospitals. *Appl Environ Microbiol*, Vol.71, pp. 1836-1842, ISSN: 0099-2240

Ohlsen, K. & Lorenz, U. (2010). Immunotherapeutic strategies to combat staphylococcal infections. *Int J Med Microbiol*, Vol.300, pp. 402-410, ISSN: 0022-2615

Ohshita, Y.; Hiramatsu, K. & Yokota, T. (1990). A point mutation in *norA* gene is responsible for quinolone resistance in *Staphylococcus aureus*. *Biochem Biophys Res Commun*, Vol.172, pp. 1028-1034, ISSN: 0006-291X

Oluwatuyi, M.; Kaatz, GW. & Gibbons, S. (2004). Antibacterial and resistance modifying activity of *Rosmarinus officinalis*. *Phytochemistry*, Vol.65, pp. 3249-3254, ISSN: 0031-9422

Ormerod, LD.; Hertzmark, E.; Gomez, DS.; Stabiner, RG.; Schanzlin, DJ. & Smith, RE. (1987). Epidemiology of microbial keratitis in southern California. A multivariate analysis. *Ophthalmology*, Vol.94, pp. 1322-1333, ISSN: 0161-6420

Patron, RL.; Climo, MW.; Goldstein, BP. & Archer, GL. (1999). Lysostaphin treatment of experimental aortic valve endocarditis caused by a *Staphylococcus aureus* isolate with reduced susceptibility to vancomycin. *Antimicrob Agents Chemother*, Vol.43, pp. 1754-1755, ISSN: 1502-2307

Patti, JM. (2005). Vaccines and immunotherapy for staphylococcal infections. *Int J Artif Organs*, Vol.28, pp. 1157-1162, ISSN: 0391-3988

Polak, J.; Della Latta, P. & Blackburn, P. (1993). In vitro activity of recombinant lysostaphin-antibiotic combinations toward methicillin-resistant *Staphylococcus aureus*. *Diagn Microbiol Infect Dis*, Vol.17, pp. 265-270, ISSN: 0732-8893

Proctor, RA.; Balwit, JM. & Vesga, O. (1994). Variant subpopulations of *Staphylococcus aureus* as cause of persistent and recurrent infections. *Infect Agents Dis*, Vol.3, pp.302-312, ISSN: 1056-2044

Proctor, RA.; Kahl, B.; von Eiff, C.; Vaudaux, PE.; Lew, DP. & Peters, G. (1998). Staphylococcal small colony variants have novel mechanisms for antibiotic resistance. *Clin Infect Dis*, Vol.27 Suppl 1, pp. S68-74, ISSN: 1058-4838

Proctor, RA. (2006). Respiration and small-colony variants of *Staphylococcus aureus*, In: *Gram Positive Pathogens*, V.A. Fischetti, VA., Novick, RP., Ferretti, DA., Portnoy, DA. & Rood, JI. (Ed.)., pp. 434-442, ASM Press, ISSN: 978-1-55581-343-7, Washington, DC, USA

Rashel, M.; Uchiyama, J.; Ujihara, T.; Uehara, Y.; Kuramoto, S.; Sugihara, S.; Yagyu, K.; Muraoka, A.; Sugai, M.; Hiramatsu, K.; Honke, K. & Matsuzaki, S. (2007). Efficient elimination of multidrug-resistant *Staphylococcus aureus* by cloned lysin derived from bacteriophage phi MR11. *J Infect Dis*, Vol.196, pp. 1237-1247, ISSN: 0022-1899

Reddy, AK.; Garg, P.; Alam, MR.; Gopinathan, U.; Sharma, S. & Krishnaiah, S. (2010). Comparison of in vitro susceptibilities of Gram-positive cocci isolated from ocular infections against the second and fourth generation quinolones at a tertiary eye care centre in South India. *Eye (Lond)*, Vol.24, pp. 170-174, ISSN: 0950-222X

Resch, A.; Fehrenbacher, B.; Eisele, K.; Schaller, M. & Gotz, F. (2005). Phage release from biofilm and planktonic *Staphylococcus aureus* cells. *FEMS Microbiol Lett*, Vol. 252, pp. 89-96, ISSN: 0378-1097

Rohde, H.; Knobloch, JK.; Horstkotte, MA. & Mack, D. (2001). Correlation of biofilm expression types of *Staphylococcus epidermidis* with polysaccharide intercellular adhesin synthesis: evidence for involvement of *icaADBC* genotype-independent factors. *Med Microbiol Immunol*, Vol.190, pp. 105-112, ISSN: 0300-8584

Romanowski, EG.; Mah, FS.; Yates, KA.; Kowalski, RP. & Gordon, YJ. (2005). The successful treatment of gatifloxacin-resistant *Staphylococcus aureus* keratitis with Zymar (gatifloxacin 0.3%). in a NZW rabbit model. *Am J Ophthalmol*, Vol.139, pp. 867-877, ISSN: 0002-9394

Ruiz, J. (2003). Mechanisms of resistance to quinolones: target alterations.; decreased accumulation and DNA gyrase protection. *J Antimicrob Chemother*, Vol.51, pp. 1109-1117, ISSN: 0305-7453

Sass, P. & Bierbaum, G. (2007). Lytic activity of recombinant bacteriophage phi11 and phi12 endolysins on whole cells and biofilms of *Staphylococcus aureus*. *Appl Environ Microbiol*, Vol.73, pp. 347-352, ISSN: 0099-2240

Schaffer, AC.; Solinga, RM.; Cocchiaro, J.; Portoles, M.; Kiser, KB.; Risley, A.; Randall, SM.; Valtulina, V.; Speziale, P.; Walsh, E.; Foster, T. & Lee, JC. (2006). Immunization with *Staphylococcus aureus* clumping factor B.; a major determinant in nasal carriage.; reduces nasal colonization in a murine model. *Infect Immun*, Vol.74, pp. 2145-2153. ISSN: 0019-9567

Schwalbe, RS.; Stapleton, JT. & Gilligan, PH. (1987). Emergence of vancomycin resistance in coagulase-negative staphylococci. *N Engl J Med*, Vol.316, pp. 927-931, ISSN: 0028-4793

Shah, A.; Mond, J.& Walsh, S. (2004). Lysostaphin-coated catheters eradicate *Staphylococccus aureus* challenge and block surface colonization. *Antimicrob Agents Chemother*, Vol.48, pp.2704-277, ISSN: 1502-2307

Shanmuganathan, VA.; Armstrong, M.; Buller, A. & Tullo, AB. (2005). External ocular infections due to methicillin-resistant *Staphylococcus aureus* (MRSA). *Eye (Lond)*, Vol.19, pp. 284-291, ISSN: 0950-222X

Sharma, S.; Kunimoto, DY.; Rao, NT.; Garg, P. & Rao, GN. (1999). Trends in antibiotic resistance of corneal pathogens: Part II. An analysis of leading bacterial keratitis isolates. *Indian J Ophthalmol*, Vol. 47, pp. 101-109, ISSN: 0301-4738

Sharma, V.; Sharma, S.; Garg, P. & Rao, GN. (2004). Clinical resistance of *Staphylococcus keratitis* to ciprofloxacin monotherapy. *Indian J Ophthalmol*, Vol.52, pp. 287-292, ISSN: 0301-4738

Shinefield, H.; Black, S.; Fattom, A.; Horwith, G.; Rasgon, S.; Ordonez, J.; Yeoh, H.; Law, D.; Robbins, JB.; Schneerson, R.; Muenz, L.; Fuller, S.; Johnson, J.; Fireman, B.; Alcorn, H. & Naso, R. (2002). Use of a *Staphylococcus aureus* conjugate vaccine in patients receiving hemodialysis. *N Engl J Med*, Vol.346, pp. 491-496, ISSN: 0028-4793

Sillankorva, S.; Neubauer, P. & Azeredo, J. (2010). Phage control of dual species biofilms of *Pseudomonas fluorescens* and *Staphylococcus lentus*. *Biofouling*, Vol.26, pp. 567-575, ISSN: 0892-7014

Singh, R.; Ray, P.; Das, A. & Sharma, M. (2010). Enhanced production of exopolysaccharide matrix and biofilm by a menadione-auxotrophic *Staphylococcus aureus* small-colony variant. *J Med Microbiol*, Vol.59, pp. 521-527, ISSN: 0022-2615

Singh, R.; Ray, P.; Das, A. & Sharma, M. (2009). Role of persisters and small-colony variants in antibiotic resistance of planktonic and biofilm-associated *Staphylococcus aureus*: an in vitro study. *J Med Microbiol*, Vol.58, pp. 1067-1073, ISSN: 0022-2615

Skurnik, D.; Merighi, M.; Grout, M.; Gadjeva, M.; Maira-Litran, T.; Ericsson, M.; Goldmann, DA.; Huang, SS.; Datta, R.; Lee, JC. & Pier, GB. (2010). Animal and human antibodies to distinct *Staphylococcus aureus* antigens mutually neutralize opsonic killing and protection in mice. *J Clin Invest*, Vol.120, pp. 3220-33, ISSN: 0021-9738

Speaker, MG.; Milch, FA.; Shah, MK.; Eisner, W. & Kreiswirth, BN. (1991). Role of external bacterial flora in the pathogenesis of acute postoperative endophthalmitis. *Ophthalmology*, Vol.98, pp. 639-649, discussion 650, ISSN: 0161-6420

Spearman, P.; Lakey, D.; Jotte, S.; Chernowitz, A.; Claycomb, S. & Stratton, C. (1996). Sternoclavicular joint septic arthritis with small-colony variant *Staphylococcus aureus*. *Diagn Microbiol Infect Dis*, Vol.26, pp. 13-15, ISSN: 0732-8893

Srinivasan, R.; Tiroumal, S.; Kanungo, R. & Natarajan, MK. (2002). Microbial contamination of the anterior chamber during phacoemulsification. *J Cataract Refract Surg*, Vol.28, pp. 2173-2176, ISSN: 0886-3350

Stavri, M.; Piddock, LJ. & Gibbons, S. (2007). Bacterial efflux pump inhibitors from natural sources. *J Antimicrob Chemother*, Vol.59, pp. 1247-1260, ISSN: 0305-7453

Stermitz, FR.; Lorenz, P.; Tawara, JN.; Zenewicz, LA. & Lewis, K. (2000). Synergy in a medicinal plant: antimicrobial action of berberine potentiated by 5'-methoxyhydnocarpin.; a multidrug pump inhibitor. *Proc Natl Acad Sci U S A*, Vol.97, pp. 1433-1437, ISSN: 1091-6490

Stranger-Jones, YK.; Bae, T. & Schneewind, O. (2006). Vaccine assembly from surface proteins of *Staphylococcus aureus*. *Proc Natl Acad Sci U S A*, Vol.103, pp. 16942-16947, ISSN: 1091-6490

Sudano Roccaro, A.; Blanco, AR.; Giuliano, F.; Rusciano, D. & Enea, V. (2004). Epigallocatechin-gallate enhances the activity of tetracycline in staphylococci by inhibiting its efflux from bacterial cells. *Antimicrob Agents Chemother*, Vol.48, pp. 1968-1973, ISSN: 1502-2307

Sulakvelidze, A.; Alavidze, Z. & Morris, JG Jr. (2001). Bacteriophage therapy. *Antimicrob Agents Chemother*, Vol.45, pp. 649-659, ISSN: 1502-2307

Tenover, FC.; Weigel , LM.; Appelbaum, PC.; McDougal, LK.; Chaitram, J.; McAllister, S.; Clark, N.; Killgore, G.; O'hara, CM.; Jevitt, L.; Patel, JB. & Bozdogan, B. (2004). Vancomycin-resistant *Staphylococcus aureus* isolate from a patient in Pennsylvania. *Antimicrob Agents Chemother*, Vol.48, pp. 275-280, ISSN: 1502-2307

Tomar, VP.; Sharma, OP. & Joshi, K. (1971). Bacterial and fungal flora of normal conjunctiva. *Ann Ophthalmol*, Vol.3, pp. 669-671, ISSN: 0042-465x

Truong-Bolduc, QC.; Strahilevit, J. & Hooper, DC. (2006). NorC, a new efflux pump regulated by MgrA of *Staphylococcus aureus*. *Antimicrob Agents Chemother*, Vol.50, pp. 1104-1107, ISSN: 1502-2307

Tsubakishita, S.; Kuwahara-Arai, K.; Sasaki, T. & Hiramatsu, K. (2010). Origin and molecular evolution of the determinant of methicillin resistance in staphylococci. *Antimicrob Agents Chemother*, Vol.54, pp. 4352-4359, ISSN: 1502-2307

Uttley, AH.; Collins, CH.; Naidoo, J. & George, RC. (1988). Vancomycin-resistant enterococci. *Lancet*, Vol.1, pp. 57-58, ISSN: 0140-6736

Varshney, AK.; Wang, X.; Cook, E.; Dutta, K.; Scharff, MD.; Goger, MJ. & Fries, BC. (2010). Generation.; characterization and epitope mapping of neutralizing and protective monoclonal antibodies against staphylococcal enterotoxin B induced lethal shock. *J Biol Chem*, Vol.286, pp. 9737-9747, ISSN: 0021-9258

von Eiff, C.; Becker, K.; Machka, K.; Stammer, H. & Peters, G. (2001). Nasal carriage as a source of *Staphylococcus aureus* Bacteremia Study Group. *N Engl J Med*, Vol.344, pp. 11-16, ISSN: 0028-4793

Walencka, E.; Sadowska, B.; Rozalska, S.; Hryniewicz, W. & Rozalska, B. (2005). Lysostaphin as a potential therapeutic agent for staphylococcal biofilm eradication. *Pol J Microbiol*, Vol. 54, pp. 191-200, ISSN: 1733-1331

Walsh, S.; Shah, A. & Mond, J. (2003). Improved pharmacokinetics and reduced antibody reactivity of lysostaphin conjugated to polyethylene glycol. *Antimicrob Agents Chemother*, Vol.47, pp. 554-558, ISSN: 1502-2307

Wang, J.; Kodali, S.; Lee, SH.; Galgoci, A.; Painter, R.; Dorso, K.; Racine, F.; Motyl, M.; Hernandez, L.; Tinney, E.; Colletti, SL.; Herath, K.; Cummings, R.; Salazar, O.; Gonzalez, I.; Basilio, A.; Vicente, F.; Genilloud, O.; Pelaez, F.; Jayasuriya, H.; Young, K.; Cully, DF. & Singh, SB. (2007). Discovery of platencin.; a dual FabF and FabH inhibitor with in vivo antibiotic properties. *Proc Natl Acad Sci U S A*, Vol.104, pp. 7612-7616, ISSN: 1091-6490

Wang, J.; Soisson, SM.; Young, K.; Shoop, W.; Kodali, S.; Galgoci, A.; Painter, R.; Parthasarathy, G.; Tang, YS.; Cummings, R.; Ha, S.; Dorso, K.; Motyl, M.; Jayasuriya, H.; Ondeyka, J.; Herath, K.; Zhang, C.; Hernandez, L.; Allocco, J.; Basilio, A.; Tormo, JR.; Genilloud, O.; Vicente, F.; Pelaez, F.; Colwell, L.; Lee, SH.; Michael, B.; Felcetto, T.; Gill, C.; Silver, LL.; Hermes, JD.; Bartizal, K.; Barrett, J.; Schmatz, D.; Becker, JW.; Cully, D. & Singh, SB. (2006). Platensimycin is a selective FabF inhibitor with potent antibiotic properties. *Nature*, Vol.441, pp. 358-361, ISSN: 0028-0836

Weigel, LM.; Clewell, DB.; Gill, SR.; Clark, NC.; McDougal, LK.; Flannagan, SE.; Kolonay, JF.; Shetty, J.; Killgore, GE. & Tenover, FC. (2003). Genetic analysis of a high-level vancomycin-resistant isolate of *Staphylococcus aureus*. *Science*, Vol.302, pp. 1569-1571, ISSN: 1095-9203

Wertheim, HF.; Vos, MC.; Ott, A.; van Belkum, A.; Voss, A.; Kluytmans, JA.; van Keulen, PH.; Vandenbroucke-Grauls, CM.; Meester, MH. & Verbrugh, HA. (2004). Risk and outcome of nosocomial *Staphylococcus aureus* bacteraemia in nasal carriers versus non-carriers. *Lancet*, Vol.364, pp. 703-705, ISSN: 0140-6736

Wong, TY. & Chee, SP. (2004). The epidemiology of acute endophthalmitis after cataract surgery in an Asian population. *Ophthalmology*, Vol.111, pp. 699-705, ISSN: 0161-6420

Wu, JA.; Kusuma, C.; Mond, JJ. & Kokai-Kun, JF. (2003). Lysostaphin disrupts *Staphylococcus aureus* and *Staphylococcus epidermidis* biofilms on artificial surfaces. *Antimicrob Agents Chemother*, Vol.47, pp. 3407-3414, ISSN: 1502-2307

Zhou, H.; Xiong, ZY.; Li, HP.; Zheng, YL. & Jiang, YQ. (2006). An immunogenicity study of a newly fusion protein Cna-FnBP vaccinated against *Staphylococcus aureus* infections in a mice model. *Vaccine*, Vol.24, pp. 4830-4837, ISSN: 0264-410X

10

Prevalence of Carbapenemases in *Acinetobacter baumannii*

M.M. Ehlers, J.M. Hughes and M.M. Kock
University of Pretoria/NHLS
South Africa

1. Introduction

Acinetobacter baumannii (A. baumannii) is an important opportunistic pathogen and causes a variety of nosocominal infections especially in Intensive Care Units (ICU's) (Bergogne-Berezin & Towner, 1996; Villegas & Harstein, 2003). These infections include bacteraemia, surgical-site infections, secondary meningitis, urinary tract infections and ventilator associated pneumonia (Bergogne-Berezin & Towner, 1996; Villegas & Harstein, 2003). *Acinetobacter baumannii* has multiresistant phenotypes, including resistance to broad-spectrum β-lactams, fluoroquinolones, aminoglycosides and carbapenems and therefore treatment of this pathogen is complicated (Coelho et al., 2004; Dalla-Costa et al., 2003; Jeon et al., 2005; Landman et al., 2002; Naas et al., 2005; Vahaboglu et al., 2006; Zarrilli et al., 2004). The multiresistant phenotypes of *A. baumannii* also contributed to the emergence of multi drug resistant *Acinetobacter baumannii* (MDRAB), which have become more prevalent within the past decade (Coelho et al., 2004) and has also caused an increase in the number of nosocomial infections in the past decade (Joly-Guillou, 2005).

Over the last 20 years, there has been an increase in the interest of the *Acinetobacter* species (Giamarellou et al., 2008). The increase in interest is due to i) worldwide expansion of ICU's, leading to a change in the types of infections caused by *Acinetobacter spp* and ii) due to the emergence of MDRAB and cases of pan-drug resistant *A. baumannii* (PDRAB) have also been reported (Giamarellou et al., 2008).

The acquired carbapenem resistance in *A. baumannii* is often associated with carbapenemase production; IMP, VIM and SIM-type metallo-β-lactamase production or the OXA-24, OXA-23 and OXA-58 type class D carbapenemases (Brown & Amyes, 2006; Poirel & Nordmann, 2006). Also associated with acquired carbapenem resistance in *A. baumannii* is the over production of natural oxacillinase (OXA-51) (Poirel & Nordmann, 2006).

Carbapenemases are the most versatile of all β-lactamases and many of them recognize almost all hydrolysable β-lactams (Livermore & Woodford, 2006; Nordmann & Poirel 2002; Walther-Rasmussen & Hoiby, 2006). Most carbapenemases are resistant to commercial β-lactamase inhibitors (Livermore & Woodford, 2006; Nordmann & Poirel, 2002; Walther-Rasmussen & Hoiby, 2006). Carbapenemases are divided into three subclasses on the basis of their hydrolysis characteristics (Frere et al., 2005). The first carbapenemases described were from Gram-positive bacilli and were inhibited by EDTA (Frere et al., 2005). These carbapenemases were described as metalloenzymes and have one zinc atom in the active site (Frere et al., 2005). This zinc atom facilitates hydrolysis of a bicyclic β-lactam ring (Frere et al., 2005). The second form of carbapenemases use serine at the active sites and are inactivated by clavulanic acid and tazobactam (β-lactamase inhibitors) (Rasmussen et al., 1996; Yang et al., 1990). Molecular classes A, C and D have serine in the active site and form part of the β-lactamases (Bush, 1988). The molecular class B of the β-lactamases are metalloenzymes and have zinc in the active site (Bush, 1988). The enzymes from the molecular classes A, B and D have the ability to hydrolyse carbapenems, which results in an elevated carbapenem minimum inhibitory concentration (Bush, 1988).

The aim of this study was to optimise and evaluate multiplex polymerase chain reaction (PCR) assays to rapidly differentiate the four subgroups of the oxacillinase (OXA) genes and the five subgroups of the metallo-β-lactamase (MBL) antibiotic resistant genes. The PCR assays results were compared to the phenotypic tests i) Hodge test and ii) Double disk synergy test. Antibiotic resistance testing is important to decrease the spread of antibiotic resistant strains of A. baumannii in clinical settings.

2. History of Acinetobacter baumannii

Acinetobacter baumannii (Figure 1) was first isolated in 1911 from a soil sample by MW Beijerink (Kuo et al., 2004). *Acinetobacter spp* were first thought to be non-virulent saprophytes (Bergogne-Berezin & Towner, 1996). In the 1970s the widespread use and misuse of antibiotics started (Kuo et al., 2004). In 1986 *Acinetobacter baumannii* was taxonomically classified (Bouvet et al., 1986). The first carbapenem resistant A. baumannii (CRAB) isolates were discovered in 1991 (Kuo et al., 2004). The first carbapenem hydrolyzing oxacillinase (CHDL's) was identified in 1995 (Scaife et al., 1995). It was initially named ARI-1 and was later renamed OXA-23 (Scaife et al., 1995).

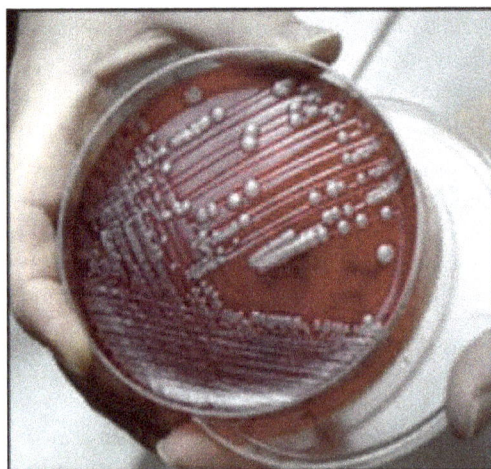

Fig. 1. *Acinetobacter baumannii* isolates (www.acinetobacter.org)

The first reported outbreak of CRAB occurred in the USA in 1991 (Go et al., 1994). Carbapenem Resistant *A. baumannii* isolates were isolated from a leukaemia patient in the oncology ward of a Taiwanese hospital in May 1998 (Hsueh et al., 2002). These isolates were observed to be resistant to almost all antibiotics e.g. cephalosporins, aztreonam, aminoglycosides and ciprofloxacin and were therefore named pan-drug resistant *A. baumannii* (PDRAB) (Hsueh et al., 2002). The rise in the number of multi drug resistant *A. baumannii* (MDRAB) strains has been due to the extensive use of antimicrobial chemotherapy against bacterial infections (Hsueh et al., 2002).

3. Classification of *Acinetobacter baumannii*

In 1986 *Acinetobacter baumannii* was taxonomically classified (Bouvet et al., 1986). *Acinetobacter* are grouped into three main complexes: i) *Acinetobacter calcoaceticus-baumannii* complex, which is glucose oxidizing and non-haemolytic; ii) *Acinetobacter lwoffii*, which are glucose negative and non-haemolytic and iii) *Acinetobacter haemolyticus*, which is haemolytic (Euzeby, 2008). The full classification of *A. baumannii* is listed in Table 1.

Domain	*Bacteria*
Phylum	*Proteobacteria*
Class	*Gammaproteobacteria*
Order	*Pseudomonadales*
Family	*Moraxellaceae*
Genus	*Acinetobacter*
Species	*A. baumannii* *A. baylyi* *A. beijerinckii* *A. bouvetii* *A. calcoaceticus* *A. gerneri* *A. grimontii* *A. gyllenbergii* *A. haemolyticus* *A. johnsonnii* *A. junnii* *A. lwoffii* *A. parvus* *A. radioresistens* *A. schindleri* *A. soli* *A. tandoii* *A. tjernbergiae* *A. towneri* *A. ursingii* *A. venetianus* 14 species are still unnamed

Table 1. Nomenclature of *Acinetobacter baumannii* (Euzeby, 2008)

There are 21 recognized genomic species of the genus *Acinetobacter* and 14 unnamed genomic species (Euzeby, 2008).

4. General characteristics of *Acinetobacter baumannii*

Acinetobacter baumannii are Gram-negative, non-fermentative, non-motile, oxidase-negative, aerobic coccobacilli that are ubiquitous in nature and commonly found within the hospital environment causing a variety of opportunistic nosocomial infections (Bergogne-Berezin et al., 1996). The bacteria can be isolated from water, soil and the environment and from human skin (Bergogne-Berezin et al., 1996). The morphology of *Acinetobacter* spp is variable in Gram-stained human clinical specimens and thus cannot be used to differentiate *Acinetobacter* from other causes of common nosocomial infections (http://microbewiki.kenyon.edu/index.php/Acinetobacter_baumannii). *Acinetobacter baumannii* are non-lactose fermenting bacteria, however they partially ferment lactose on MacConkey agar (http://microbewiki.kenyon.edu/index.php/Acinetobacter_baumannii). All the species of the *Acinetobacter* genus grow well on MacConkey agar (except for *A. lwoffii*), when salt is absent (http://microbewiki.kenyon.edu/index.php/Acinetobacter_baumannii). *Acinetobacter baumannii* are strict aerobes and grow well on nutrient agar (http://microbewiki.kenyon.edu/index.php/Acinetobacter_baumannii). Infection by *A. baumannii* is difficult to combat due to the Gram-negative nature of the cell wall as the outer wall provides a barrier so that the antimicrobial agent is unable to enter the bacterial cell (Projan, 2004).

Acinetobacter baumannii is an opportunistic pathogen that is successful in colonizing and persisting in the hospital environment and is able to resist desiccation (Getchell-White et al., 1989; Jawad et al., 1996). The bacterium is also able to survive on inanimate surfaces for months (Kramer et al., 2006). *Acinetobacter baumannii* is among the most common causes of device related nosocomial infections (Dima et al., 2007; Thongpiyapoom et al., 2004), resulting when the bacterium is able to resist both physical and chemical disinfection, by forming a biofilm (Cappelli et al., 2003; Loukili et al., 2006; Pajkos et al., 2004). Biofilm associated proteins (BAP's) were first characterized in *S. aureus* (Cucarella et al., 2001) and have been found in a number of other Gram-positive and Gram-negative pathogenic bacteria.

4.1 Optimal Growth conditions for *Acinetobacter baumannii*

Acinetobacter baumannii form part of the natural flora of the skin and mucous membranes of humans (Seifert et al., 1997). *Acinetobacter baumannii* are ubiquitous in clinical and natural environments and commonly colonises the skin, oropharynx secretions, respiratory secretions, urine, irrigating and intravenous solutions (Seifert et al., 1997). *Acinetobacter baumannii* can be cultured from sputum or respiratory secretions, wound and urine (Go & Cuhna, 1999). The pathogen colonises the gastro-intestinal tract and is associated with nosocomial meningitis, nosocomial pneumonia and bacteraemia (Go & Cuhna, 1999).

Acinetobacter baumannii grown on trypticase soy agar produce circular, convex, smooth and slightly opaque colonies, which are 1.5 to 2.0 mm in diameter after 24 hours at 30°C or 3.0 to 4.0 mm after 48 hours (Garrity et al., 2005). *Acinetobacter baumannii* do neither haemolyse horse blood nor sheep blood when grown on blood agar plates (Garrity et al., 2005). Seasonal variations have been reported for nosocomial *A. baumannii* infections and bacteraemia, with increased incidences occurring in the summer months (McDonald et al., 1999).

5. Risk factors for *Acinetobacter baumannii* infections

Acinetobacter baumannii can survive on various surfaces within hospitals, including catheters and other medical equipment (http://microbewiki.Kenyon.edu/index.php/Acinetobacter_baumannii). Thus environmental contamination is an important source of infection as pathogens are spread directly from surfaces or through the hands of healthcare workers to patients (Corbella et al., 1996). Infected or colonized patients are important reservoirs of *A. baumannii*. *Acinetobacter baumannii* is passed from patient to patient via direct and indirect contact (D'Agata et al., 2000). The main risk factors of *Acinetobacter baumannii* bacteraemia are invasive procedures e.g. central venous catheterization, mechanical ventilation and surgery (Seifert et al., 1995b). Another major risk factor for *A. baumannii* infections is the widespread use of broad-spectrum antibiotics (Cisneros & Rodriguez-Bano, 2002). Other risk factors include prolonged hospital stay, ICU stay, enteral feeding, previous administration to another unit and previous use of third generation cephalosporins (Mulin et al., 1995; Scerpella et al., 1995).

The risk factors within the ICU's concern the immunosuppressed patients, patients previously exposed to antimicrobial therapy, patients who underwent high invasive procedures and patients who suffered from previous sepsis (Garcia-Garmendia et al., 2001). Other risk factors include pneumonia as a source of infection, inappropriate empirical treatment and prior treatment with carbapenems (Robenshtok et al., 2006). Surgical procedures performed within the emergency operating theatre is another major risk factor contributing to the spread of epidemic cases of *A. baumannii*, however the main risk factor was the previous use of fluoroquinolones (Villers et al., 1998).

5.1 Pathogenesis of Acinetobacter baumannii

Acinetobacter baumannii infections are associated with systems of high fluid content e.g. lungs, cerebrospinal fluid, peritoneal fluid and the urinary tract and usually only occur in the immunocompromised patients (Cuhna, 2007). Patients with *A. baumannii* bacteraemia usually have signs and symptoms that are related to the organ system involved (Cuhna, 2007). Symptoms include wound infections, outbreaks of nosocomial pneumonia, catheter associated bacteriuria, urethritis and continuous ambulatory peritoneal dialysis (CAPD) associated peritonitis (Cuhna, 2007). Bacteraemia results in septic shock in 25-30% of all cases and disseminated intravascular coagulation frequently occurs (Cisneros et al., 1996: Seifert et al., 1997). Colonisation may occur after an invasive infection (Corbella et al., 1996), especially in burn patients (Wisplinghoff et al., 2004). Problems rarely associated with *A. baumannii* infections include meningitis, endocarditis, urinary tract infections, pneumonia and cholangitis (Cuhna, 2007). Other problems that rarely occur are soft tissue infections and complicated skin, abdominal infections and central nervous system (CNS) infections (Fournier & Richet, 2006). Allen and Green documented the first report of airborne spread of *A. baumannii* in 1987. *Acinetobacter baumannii* survives much better on fingertips or on dry surfaces when tested under stimulated hospital environmental conditions (Jawad et al., 1996). The skin of patients and medical personnel is involved in the transmission of *A. baumannii* strains and in some outbreaks; molecular typing has identified the epidemic strain on the skin of the patients (Gerner-Smidt, 1987; Patterson et al., 1991). Contaminated reusable medical equipment e.g. ventilator tubing, respirometers and arterial pressure monitoring devices are used for the management of severely ill patients serve as another route of transmission to patients (Beck-Sague et al., 1990; Cefai et al., 1990). Fomites e.g. bed mattresses (Sheretz & Sullivan., 1985), pillows (Weernink et al., 1995), a tape recorder, television set and a fan (Jawad et al., 1994) were found to be contaminated with *Acinetobacter* and served as reservoirs during nosocomial outbreaks.

The mortality rate within the hospitals is high, with a 23% mortality recorded for hospitalized patients and a 43% mortality rate among patients in intensive care (Falagas et al., 2006). The Antimicrobial Availability Task Force (AATF) of the Infectious Disease Society of America identified *Acinetobacter baumannii, Aspergillus* spp, extended spectrum β-lactamase producing *Enterobacteriaceae, Pseudomonas aeruginosa, Staphylococcus aureus* as "particularly problematic pathogens" and there is a desperate need for new drug development (Talbot et al., 2006).

It is difficult to distinguish between colonization and infection regarding *A. baumannii* (Joly-Guillou, 2005). There is controversy over whether infections caused by *A. baumannii* result in unfavourable outcomes (Blot et al., 2003; Falagas et al., 2006). The isolation of *A. baumannii* in hospitalized patients is an indicator of severe illness with an associated mortality of approximately 30% (Wilson et al., 2004).

Community acquired *A. baumannii* (CAAB) occurs within an individual with one or more cultures of blood, collected within 48 hours of admission, that is positive for *A. baumannii* complex and is identified by a biochemical method (API 20NE system) (bioMerieux, France) (Schreckenberger & Von Graevenitz, 2000). Patients with CAAB associated pneumonia had an increased mortality rate and presented with a more severe disease than the patients without pneumonia (Wang et al., 2002). The development of CAAB is associated with underlying malignancies e.g. lung cancer, lymphoma and thymic carcinoma (Wang et al., 2002). *Acinetobacter baumannii* genomic species were responsible for CAAB; however there is no evidence of clonal spread of *A. baumannii* in the community (Wang et al., 2002). Carbapenems, cefopirome, cefepime, ceftazidime, aminoglycosides and fluoroquinolones are the antimicrobials of choice for treating CAAB (Wang et al., 2002).

5.2 Virulence factors of *Acinetobacter baumannii* strains

Acinetobacter baumannii have very few virulence factors (Cisneros & Rodriguez-Bano, 2002), however some strains have virulence factors associated with invasiveness, transmissibility or the enhanced ability to colonise immunocompromised patients (Dijkshoorn et al., 1996). Ethanol stimulates the virulence of *A. baumannii* (Smith et al., 2004), which led to the identification of a number of genes, affecting virulence towards *Caenorhabditis elegans* and *Dictyostelium discoideum* (Smith et al., 2007).

A new strain (OXA-23 clone II) was identified in a military hospital and was found to be a particularly virulent strain, which is very difficult to eliminate from medical facilities (promedmail). There are three major European clones of *A. baumannii* (Giamarellou et al., 2008) Clone I, found in South Africa, Czech Republic, Poland, Italy and Spain; Clone II, found in South Africa, Spain, Turkey, Greece and France and clone III is found in the Netherlands, Italy, France and Spain (Van Dessel et al., 2004). Clones I and II are responsible for the outbreaks of

A. baumannii bacteraemia in South Africa and Northern Europe (Van Dessel et al., 2004). *Acinetobacter* can efficiently transfer genes horizontally (only observed and analysed in *A. baylyi*), especially the genes encoding antibiotic resistance (Gerischer, 2008).

A large portion of the *A. baumannii* genome is dedicated to pathogenesis, with a large number of genes occurring within virulence islands (Perez et al., 2007). *Acinetobacter baumannii* together with *Acinetobacter* DNA group13TU is involved in the majority of *Acinetobacter* hospital outbreaks (Bergogne-Berezin & Towner, 1996). Strains of the *Acinetobacter* DNA group 3 and *A. junii* have only occasionally been implicated in outbreaks of nosocomial infections (Bernards et al., 1997). *Acinetobacter baumannii* has environmental resilience and a wide range of resistance determinants, therefore making it a successful nosocomial pathogen (Nordmann, 2004). *Acinetobacter baumannii* has caused numerous global outbreaks and displayed ever increasing rates of resistance (Villegas & Harstein, 2003). In hospital outbreaks the emergence of imipenem-resistant strains has been documented (Brown et al., 1996; Go et al, 1994).

6. Clinical manifestations of *Acinetobacter baumannii* infections

The clinical manifestations of *A. baumannii* are non-specific and present as a trans-maculopapular rash affecting the palms of the hands and the soles of the feet of endocarditis patients, or necrotic lesions of the skin and soft tissue (Seifert et al., 1995). *Acinetobacter baumannii* bacteraemia is polymicrobial, and is often associated with *Klebsiella pneumoniae* (Seifert et al., 1995).

6.1 Treatment of *Acinetobacter baumannii* infections

Acinetobacter baumannii are Gram-negative bacteria and therefore are particularly difficult to treat due to the presence of an outer membrane (Projan, 2004). The recommended treatment therefore is a limited spectrum active β-lactam e.g. ceftazidime or imipenem the most active agent against *A. baumannii* and an aminoglycoside (Cisneros & Rodriguez-Bano, 2002).

There is incomplete current knowledge of the clinical response and bacterial mechanisms of resistance to antimicrobials (Kahlmeter et al., 2006). The reliability and comparability of different methods of susceptibility testing e.g. disc diffusion and broth microdilution have not been consistent for *A. baumannii* (Swenson et al., 2004). The persistence of subtle growth beyond an obvious end point by broth microdilution is of great concern in the case of β-lactams, which therefore explains its poor reaction with the disc diffusion method (Swenson et al., 2004). Doripenem, a novel carbapenem is active against susceptible *A. baumannii* (Fritsche et al., 2005; Jones et al., 2004; Jones et al., 2005; Mushtaq et al., 2004). Doripenem was not effective against *A. baumanni* isolates producing bla$_{OXA-23}$ or bla$_{IMP-4}$ or metallo-β-lactamases (Mushtaq et al., 2004).

6.2 Carbapenems as treatment for *Acinetobacter baumannii* infections

Carbapenems are structurally related to the penicillins ("penams"), differing only by the substitution of carbon ("carba") for the sulfur atom at position 1 and the presence of a double bond between C2 and C3 (Bradley, 1997; Wise, 1986). A hydroxyethyl side chain instead of the acylamino group found in penicillins and cephalosporins is present and provides resistance to most β-lactamases (Bradley, 1997; Wise, 1986).

Carbapenems were introduced into clinical practice in the 1970's and the 1980's marked the emergence of Gram-negative bacterial resistance to carbapenems (Nordmann & Poirel, 2002; Walsh, 2005). Carbapenems were derived from the naturally occurring antibiotic, thienamycin, which is produced by the soil microorganism *Streptomyces cattleya* (Jacobs, 1986). The first carbapenemases described were from Gram-positive bacilli and were inhibited by EDTA (Frere et al., 2005). Carbapenems are recognised as the gold standard for treating infections caused by resistant Gram-negative bacteria (Rahal, 2006).

6.3 Combination therapy as a strategy for the treatment of multiple drug resistant *Acinetobacter baumannii*

Sulbactam is an inhibitor of β-lactamases and has *in vitro* bactericidal activity against *Acinetobacter spp* (Cisneros & Rodriguez-Bano, 2002). The efficacy of sulbactam against susceptible *A. baumannii* is similar to imipenem (Rodriguez-Hernandez, 2000). Sulbactam exhibits bacteriostatic action against *A. baumannii* (Corbella et al., 1998). Sulbactam is also used to treat meningitis caused by multiple drug resistant *Acinetobacter baumannii* (MDRAB) (Cisneros & Rodriguez-Bano, 2002). Combinations of sulbactam with aminoglycosides, rifampin and azithromycin have demonstrated synergy against imipenem susceptible strains (Appleman et al., 2000; Savov et al., 2002). There is little or no advantage to the combination sulbactams with cephalosporins (Appleman et al., 2000; Savov et al., 2002).

Polymyxins (colistimethate and polymyxin B) are the only alternative treatment for sulbactam resistant *A. baumannii* strains (Wood & Reboli, 1993). Colistin was used in the 1960's and the 1970's, but had many adverse side effects, including nephrotoxicity, neuro-muscular blockage (Cisneros & Rodriguez-Bano, 2002). Colistin disrupts the outer cell membranes of many Gram-negative bacilli by changing the permeability of the membrane and causing a bactericidal effect (Cisneros & Rodriguez-Bano, 2002). Colistin is only recommended for patients who have no other treatment alternatives (Cisneros & Rodriguez-Bano, 2002). Rifampicin combined with colistin or sulbactam acts synergistically against MDRAB (Hogg et al., 1998).

7. Mechanisms of antibiotic resistance in *Acinetobacter baumannii*

The general mechanisms of resistance are enzyme-mediated resistance, genetic adaption, efflux pumps and changes in the structure of outer membrane components (Cloete, 2003). Enzyme mediated resistance is the ability of the bacteria to produce enzymes that transform the antibiotics into non-toxic or inactivated forms (Ma et al., 1998). Efflux pumps involve a large number of seemingly unrelated (structurally) compounds, pumped out of the cell, which lowers the concentration of the drug within the cell and therefore prohibits the drug to take proper effect (Nikaido, 1996). Changes in the structure of the outer membrane and its components e.g. porins and alterations in the penicillin binding proteins (PBP's), allows for the cells to develop resistance to antimicrobials on the basis of exclusion because the drugs are no longer able to penetrate the cells and therefore the drugs can't reach their intended site of action in the cell (Cloete, 2003).

Acinetobacter baumannii has become resistant to many classes of antibiotics and is well suited for genetic exchange (Lorenz & Wackernagel, 1994; Metzgar et al., 2004). *Acinetobacter baumannii* are among a unique class of Gram-negative bacteria that are described as "naturally transformable" (Lorenz & Wackernagel, 1994; Metzgar et al., 2004). *Acinetobacter* strains lack the *mutS* gene, which is part of the mismatch repair system that preserves genetic stability and exhibits increased mutation rates (Young & Ornston, 2001). It is unknown whether *A. baumannii* are naturally competent or whether through the alteration of environmental conditions facilitates pathogenicity or antibiotic resistance gene acquisition (Fournier et al., 2006). The key resistance genes identified were those coding for VEB-1, AmpC, and OXA-10 beta-lactamases, various amino glycoside-modifying enzymes (AME) and those genes encoding for the tetracycline efflux pumps (Fournier *et al.*, 2006).

Plasmids, transposons and the bacterial chromosome are involved in antibiotic resistance within *A. baumannii* (Bergogne-Berezin & Towner, 1996). Carbapenemases occurring within *A. baumannii* belong to the class D family of serine-β-lactamases or the imipenemase (IMP)/Verona integrase (VIM) class B family of metallo-β-lactamases (Brown & Amyes, 2006). Imipenem is the most active drug against *A. baumannii* (Cisneros & Rodriguez-Bano, 2002). Resistance to carbapenems is associated with reduced drug uptake due to porin deficiency and reduced affinity for the drug due to modification of the PBP's by mutations (Clark, 1996).

Acinetobacter baumannii's largest virulence island contains genetic elements, which are homologous to the type IV secretion systems of *Legionella* and *Coxiella burnetti* (Goldstein et al., 1983). Over 25 years ago *A. baumannii* was observed to acquire antimicrobial resistance factors through conjugation of plasmids (Goldstein et al., 1983). Transposons are important in the dissemination of genetic determinants of resistance in *Acinetobacter* spp (Devaud et al., 1982; Palmen & Hellingwerf, 1997) and many of the transposons contain integrons, predominantly from class I. Integrons contain an *int* gene and gene cassettes that can be mobilized to other integrons or to secondary sites in the bacterial genome (Poirel et al., 2005).

A multi drug resistant (MDR) phenotype in *A. baumannii* occurs when integron-born resistance determinants acting against different classes of antibiotics co-exist, giving rise to MDR gene cassettes (Seward, 1999; Yum et al., 2002). Insertion sequences (IS), which promote gene expression, have played an important role in explaining the regulation of resistance (Segal et al., 2005). The IS$_{Aba1}$ element found in *A. baumannii* but not in *Enterobacteriaceae* or in *Pseudomonas aeruginosa* (Segal et al., 2005), results in the over expression of Amp C and OXA-51/OXA-69-like beta–lactamases and in decreased levels of susceptibility to ceftazidime and carbapenems (Heritier et al., 2006).

7.1 Oxacillinase (OXA) genes in *Acinetobacter baumannii*

Carbapenemases are classified into four major functional groups (groups 1 to 4) with multiple subgroups of group 2 that are differentiated according to a group specific inhibitor or substrate profiles (Bush et al., 1995). According to this classification scheme carbapenemases are found primarily in group's 2f and 3 (Nordmann et al., 1993; Yang et al., 1990).

Class D carbapenemases are classified into four subgroups (Vahaboglu et al., 2006). Subgroup 1, the OXA-23 group (including OXA-27 and OXA-49), are the plasmid encoded genes (Vahaboglu et al., 2006). The OXA extended spectrum beta-lactamases are able to hydrolyze extended spectrum cephalosporins (Aubert, 2001; Walther-Rasmussen & Hoiby, 2006). The OXA-23 was the first OXA carbapenemase (OXA β-lactamases that inactivate carbapenems) within *A. baumannii* obtained from a clinical isolate (Aubert, 2001; Walther-Rasmussen & Hoiby, 2006). The OXA-23 genes originated in *A. radioresistens* (Turton et al., 2005). This plasmid-encoded enzyme was found in 1985 in Scotland before the introduction of carbapenems (Paton et al., 1993). It was initially named "*Acinetobacter* resistant to imipenem" (ARI-1) and has been discovered in Brazil, England, Polynesia, Singapore, Korea and China (Brown & Amyes, 2006; Jeon et al., 2005). Subgroup 2 is the OXA-24 group (including OXA-25, OXA-26 and OXA-40), which is chromosomally encoded (Vahaboglu et al., 2006). The OXA-24 carbapenemase has a crystal structure and therefore suggests a novel catalytic role for Tyr112 and Met223 side chains (Santillana et al., 2007). Subgroup 1 and 2 share 60% identity (Heritier et al., 2005b).

Subgroup 3 consists of OXA-51 and its variants, which are chromosomally encoded (Vahaboglu et al., 2006). The OXA-51/69 expression varies according to the presence of IS$_{Aba1}$ (Poirel & Nordmann, 2006). The OXA-51 gene was first detected in Argentina in 2005, within genetically distinct *A. baumannii* isolates (Brown & Amyes, 2005). Subgroup 3 has 56% identity with subgroup 1 and 61% to 62% identity with subgroup 2 (Brown et al., 2005). Subgroup 4 contains OXA-58, which is a plasmid-encoded gene (Vahaboglu et al., 2006) and was first detected in Toulouse (France) in 2003 (Heritier et al., 2005a; Poirel et al., 2005). Subgroup 4 shares less than 50% homology with the other three groups (Poirel et al., 2005). The OXA-58 gene is rapidly disseminating and those isolates, which contain both OXA-51-type and OXA-58 genes, are pandrug-resistant *A. baumannii* (PDRAB) (Coelho et al., 2006). The plasmid borne carbapenemase, OXA-58, was found in France, England, Argentina, Spain, Turkey, Romania, Austria, Greece, Scotland and Kuwait (Coelho et al., 2006; Marque et al., 2005; Pournaras et al., 2006). It is uncertain whether these genes are acquired or occur naturally in *A. baumannii* (Brown & Amyes, 2006). In *A. baumannii* isolates with OXA-51 as the sole carbapenemase, carbapenem resistance was associated with an insertion sequence IS$_{Aba1}$ and it is thought that this might be the promoter for the hyper-production of β-lactamase genes (Turton et al., 2006).

Bacteria producing carbapenemase enzymes have a reduced susceptibility to imipenem (Ambler et al., 1991). However, the minimum inhibitory concentration (MIC) of imipenem can range from mildly elevated to fully resistant (Ambler et al., 1991). Therefore, these β-lactamases may not be recognised following routine susceptibility testing (Ambler et al., 1991). Beta-lactamases have the ability to hydrolyse carbapenems, resist commercially available β-lactamase inhibitors and are susceptible to inhibition by metal ion chelators (Lim et al., 1988). The widespread presence of oxacillinases and their division into distinct subgroups, indicates that these enzymes are an essential component of the genetic makeup of *Acinetobacter* spp (Walther-Rasmussen & Hoiby, 2006). The OXA enzymes as emerging carbapenemases are increasingly associated with outbreaks of *A. baumannii containing OXA-40 and OXA-58* in the United States (Hujer et al., 2006; Lolans et al., 2006). The OXA-51/69-like beta-lactamase is a "naturally occurring" chromosomal enzyme in *Acinetobacter baumannii* and has been found in isolates from four continents (Heritier et al., 2005a).

7.2 Metallo-β-lactamase (MBL) genes in Acinetobacter baumannii

Metallo-β-lactamases form part of the class B β-lactamases, capable of hydrolyzing carbapenems and other β-lactam antibiotics except for aztreonam (Walsh et al., 2005; Walsh,

2005). Class B β-lactamases differ from class A and class D carbapenemases by having a metal ion, zinc, in their active site, which participates in catalysis (Walsh et al., 2005; Walsh, 2005). There are five types of metallo-β-lactamases (MBL's) that have been identified in *A. baumannii* (Brown & Amyes, 2006). The most common metallo-β-lactamases include "Verona integron-encoded metallo-β-lactamases" (VIM), "Imipenem hydrolyzing β-lactamase"(IMP), "German Imipenemase" (GIM), Seoul imipenemase (SIM) and Sao Paulo metallo-β-lactamases (SPM-1) enzymes, which are located on a variety of integron structures and are incorporated as gene cassettes (Brown & Amyes, 2006). The integration of the integron on the plasmids or transposons allows for facilitated transfer between bacteria (Watanabe et al., 1991).

Imipenem (IMP) metallo-β-lactamases were first described in a *P. aeruginosa* strain found in Japan in 1988 (Watanabe et al., 1991). Metallo-β-lactamases is not the predominant carbapenemases found within *A. baumannii* however the following carbapenemases have been described: IMP-1, IMP-2, IMP-4, IMP-5, IMP-6, and IMP-11 (Walsh et al., 2005; Walsh, 2005). The IMP type MBL's have stronger carbapenem-hydrolysing activity than the OXA-type-β-lactamases (Laraki et al., 1999). The VIM, IMP, SPM, and GIM genes are found on cassettes in class 1 integrons, although IMP genes have also been found on class 3 integrons (Collis et al., 2002). Watanabe et al. (1991) reported the detection of IMP-1, located on an integron situated on a conjugative plasmid, in *Serratia marcescens* and other *Enterobacteriaceae* in Japan. The imipenem-hydrolyzing β-lactamase has been detected in rare clinical isolates of *Enterobacter cloacae* in Argentina, the USA and France (Nordmann et al., 1993; Pottumarthy et al., 2003; Radice et al., 2004; Rasmussen et al., 1996).

Imipenem hydrolyzing β-lactamase contains the conserved active site motifs S-X-X-K, S-D-N and K-T-G of the class A β-lactamases (Aubron, 2005; Yu et al., 2006). The carbapenemases have conserved cysteine residues at positions 238 and 69 that form a disulfide bridge (Aubron, 2005; Yu et al., 2006). Genes encoding IMP-2 β-lactamases were found on plasmids in *Enterobacter asburiae* isolated from river water in the US and on plasmids from an *E. cloacae* isolated from China (Aubron, 2005; Yu et al., 2006). The disulfide bond is necessary for the hydrolytic activity and is used to stabilize the enzyme structurally (Majiduddin & Palzkill, 2003; Sougakoff et al., 2002). The mechanism of cleavage of the β-lactam ring is different for MBL's as compared to β-lactamases, however, both gene products still share a unique αββα fold in the active sites of the enzymes (Ullah et al., 1998). The bla_{IMP} is a foreign gene that is introduced from another species of bacteria and *A. baumannii* only retain the gene in environments where there is selective pressure in the form of the presence of imipenem (Takhashi et al., 2000).

Pandrug-resistant *A. baumannii* (PDRAB) are resistant to nearly all the commercially available antibiotics including amikacin, aztreonam, cefepime, ceftazidime, ciprofloxacin, gentamycin, imipenem, meropenem, ofloxacin, ticarcillin-clavulanate and piperacillin-tazobactam (Hsueh et al., 2002). Carbapenem-resistant *A. baumannii* are usually susceptible to ciprofloxacin, ofloxacin, gentamycin or amikacin (Hsueh et al., 2002). Increasing the use of carbapenems and ciprofloxacin has contributed to the development and spread of PDRAB strains (Hsueh et al., 2002).

Verona integron-encoded MBL (VIM-1) was first identified in Italy in 1997 in a *P. aeruginosa* isolate (Lauretti et al., 1999). *Acinetobacter baumannii* containing the VIM-2 gene has been reported only in Korea (Yum et al., 2002). *Acinetobacter baumannii* isolates producing metallo-β-lactamases from Korea were reported to be incredibly diverse, containing Seoul imipenemase (SIM-1), which is a novel metallo-β-lactamase (Lee et al., 2005).

7.3 Non-enzymatic mechanisms of antibiotic resistance

In *A. baumannii* isolates from Madrid the loss of the 22-kDa and 33-kDa outer membrane proteins combined with the production of OXA-24, resulted in resistance to carbapenems (Bou et al., 2000). A homologue of OprD, a 43-kDa protein was identified in *A. baumannii* (Dupont et al., 2005). The 43-kDa protein is a well studied porin, which is frequently associated with imipenem resistance in *P. aeruginosa* (Dupont et al., 2005). Confirming resistance to imipenem and meropenem in *A. baumannii* is the channel formation of CarO, a 29-kDa outer membrane protein (Limansky et al., 2002; Mussi et al., 2005; Siroy et al., 2005). Reduced expression of PBP-2 within isolates from Seville, Spain explained the resistance of *A. baumannii* to carbapenems (Fernandez-Cuenca et al., 2003).

7.3.1 Efflux pumps as mechanisms of resistance in *Acinetobacter baumannii*

Efflux pumps cause resistance against several different classes of antibiotics and mediate the efflux of compounds that are toxic to the bacterial cell, including antibiotics, in a coupled exchange with protons (Poole, 2005). The distinct families of efflux pumps the major facilitator superfamily, the small multidrug resistance superfamily, the multidrug and toxic compound extrusion superfamily and the resistance-nodulation-cell division family are found in various species of bacteria (Poole, 2005). Over expression of the AdeABC efflux pump, which forms part of the resistance-nodulation-cell division family, confers high-level resistance to carbapenems, together with carbapenem-hydrolyzing oxacillinase (Marque et al., 2005). The mechanism, which controls the expression of the efflux pump, functions as a two-step regulator (adeR) and sensor (adeS) system (Marchand et al., 2004). A single point mutation within the *ade*R and *ade*S genes results in increased expression and increased efflux (Marchand et al., 2004).

8. Resistance of *Acinetobacter baumannii* to various antibiotics

Resistance to aminoglycosides is mediated by aminoglycoside-modifying enzymes (AME's) (Perez et al., 2007). Examples of such enzymes include aminoglycoside phosphotransferases (aph), aminoglycoside acetyltransferases (acc) and aminoglycoside adenyltransferase (aad) (Perez et al., 2007). *Acinetobacter baumannii* have transposon mediated efflux pumps, which involves tetracycline A (Tet) and TetB (Guardabassi et al., 2000). Tetracycline A allows for the efflux of tetracycline, while TetB allows for the efflux of both tetracycline and minocycline (Huys et al., 2005). The other mechanism of resistance to the tetracyclines is due to the ribosomal protection protein (Perez et al., 2007). The ribosomal protection protein is encoded by the tetracycline M gene and protects the ribosome from the action of tetracycline, minocycline and doxycline (Ribera et al., 2003).

Modification in the structure of the DNA gyrase decreases the affinity of the enzyme to quinolones (Seward & Towner, 1998); therefore *A. baumannii* becomes resistant to quinolones (Perez et al., 2007). Modifications of the lipopolysaccharides (LPS's) in A. *baumannii* cause the bacterium to become resistant to polymyxins (Perez et al., 2007).

Modifications to the LPS in *A. baumannii* include acylation, presence of antigens and acidification, which all interfere with the binding of the polymyxins to the cell membrane (Peterson et al., 1987).

9. Spread and control of *Acinetobacter baumannii*

Infection control is critical concerning *A. baumannii* given its ability to cause outbreaks (Boyce & Pittet, 2002; Pittet, 2004). Contact precautions, hand washing and alcohol hand decontamination are rarely applied however are universally encouraged and important (Boyce & Pittet, 2002; Pittet, 2004). However, the applications of meticulous environmental decontamination and aggressive chlorhexidine baths as temporary measures to control outbreaks are the favourable approach (Maragakis et al., 2004; Wilks et al., 2006). However these methods are expensive, labour-intensive and must be clinically proven through trials (Maragakis et al., 2004; Wilks et al., 2006). The key to infection control measures lies within preventing dissemination of MDR clones (Maragakis et al., 2004; Wilks et al., 2006). The use of molecular tools for investigation of outbreaks to establish clonality among isolates allows for a more effective implementation of infection control measures and aids in the identification of environmental sources (Maragakis et al., 2004; Wilks et al., 2006). Polymerase Chain Reaction followed by electronspray ionization mass spectrometry and base composition analysis are used to determine clonality (Ecker et al., 2006; Hujer et al., 2006). Restriction of the use of especially broad-spectrum activity antibiotics is necessary for infection control strategies (Chakravarti et al., 2000; Hughes, 2003). The refinement of genomic and proteomic techniques represents hope for the discovery of new antimicrobials active against MDR organisms and for the development of vaccines (Chakravarti et al., 2000; Hughes, 2003). The success of these and other approaches for the containment of MDR *A. baumannii* depends on the commitment of clinical practitioners, scientists, hospitals and public health administrators and on the support of the informed public (Chakravarti et al., 2000; Hughes, 2003).

10. Diagnosis and detection of *Acinetobacter baumannii*

Monitoring the geographical spread of virulent or epidemic pathogens is achieved through the identification and typing of bacteria (Grundmann et al., 1997). Traditional methods for the identification of *A. baumannii* are unsatisfactory (Gerner-Smidt et al., 1991), due to the difficulty in distinguishing *A. baumannii* from *A. calcoaceticus* phenotypically (Giamarellou et al., 2008). *Acinetobacter baumanni* is predominantly diagnosed from sputum, blood, central venous catheter tips, pleural fluid, wound pus, bronchial washing and urine (Hsueh et al., 2002).

10.1 Direct phenotypic detection of *Acinetobacter baumannii*

Phenotypic methods of detecting *A. baumannii* include growing the isolates on fluorescence-lactose-denitrification media (FLN) in order to determine the amount of acid produced by the metabolism of glucose (http://microbewiki.kenyon.edu/index.php/Acinetobacter baumannii). This method is used to differentiate the respective species within the *Acinetobacter* genus (http://microbewiki.kenyon.edu/index.php/Acinetobacter_baumannii). Crude enzyme extracts and β-lactamase activity assays are other phenotypic methods used to detect antibiotic resistant strains of *A. baumannii* (Takahashi et al., 2000). Biochemical tests used to differentiate *A. baumannii* from other species of the *Acinetobacter* genus include the following: haemolysis test (-), histamine assimilation test (-), glucose oxidation test, citrate assimilation test (+), gelatin liquefaction test (-) (Prashanth & Badrinath, 2000).

10.1.1 Automated detection of *Acinetobacter baumannii*

A Vitek GNI card (bio Mérieux, France) is used for the detection of carbapenemase activity in clinical isolates. The results of the Vitek test are confirmed using the API 20NE system (bio Mérieux, France) (Clinical and Laboratory Standards Institute, 2009).

10.1.2 Manual methods of detection of *Acinetobacter baumannii*

The E-test (AB Biodisk, Sweden) is used to identify metallo-β-lactamase production by determining the minimum inhibitory concentration (MIC), which allows for the detection of the production of VIM or IMP enzymes (Walsh, 2005). Susceptibility testing can be performed using broth microdilution according to Clinical and Laboratory Standards Institute standards (2009) and the Kirby-Bauer double disk synergy test (Peleg et al., 2005). The disk approximation test with 2-mercaptopropionic acid or EDTA is used to screen for metallo-β-lactamase producers (Arakawa, 2000; Yong et al., 2006). Ethylenediaminetetraacetic acid (EDTA) is a chelator of Zn^{2+} and other divalent cations and therefore inhibits the metallo-β-lactamases that have zinc ions in their active sites (Lim et al., 1988).

The imipenem (IMP)-EDTA double-disk synergy test (DDST) can distinguish metallo-β-lactamase producing from metallo-β-lactamase non-producing Gram-negative bacilli (Lee et al., 2001). However, occasional isolates show false negative results due to a deficiency of zinc within the isolate's active site (Yigit et al., 2001). The test can be improved by using an IMP disk to which 10 µl of 50 mM zinc sulfate (140 µg/disk) has been added, to compensate for the lack of zinc or by using Mueller-Hinton agar to which zinc sulfate has been added to a final concentration of 70 µg.ml^{-1} (Yigit et al., 2001).

The Hodge test is a simple method for screening metallo-β-lactamase producing isolates of Gram-negative bacilli (Lee et al., 2001). The Hodge test/cloverleaf test is a microbiological assay of carbapenemase activity, where an extract of the whole cell or the suspected isolates are tested against imipenem on an agar plate (Hornstein et al., 1997). It is unnecessary to test an isolate for a carbapenemase using the modified Hodge test when all of the carbapenems that are reported by a laboratory test are either intermediate or resistant (Clinical and Laboratory Standards Institute, 2009). However, the modified Hodge test is used for infection control and epidemiological purposes (Clinical and Laboratory Standards Institute, 2009). The imipenem disk test is a poor screening method for carbapenemases (Clinical and Laboratory Standards Institute, 2009).

10.2 Molecular detection of *Acinetobacter baumannii*

Molecular methods based on PCR for the detection of carbapenemase producing genes are used due to the problems with the direct phenotypic detection methods e.g. difficulty in distinguishing between species of the *Acinetobacter* genus (Vaneechoutte, 1996). The molecular methods include a PCR with primers for detecting OXA-23, OXA-24, OXA-51,

OXA-58, IMP-1, IMP-2, IMP-4, VIM-1, VIM-2, SPM-1, GIM-1, and SIM-1 genes can be used to detect all families and subgroups of the presumed carbapenemases (Petropoulou et al., 2006). The genotypic tests used to determine the clonal relatedness of the isolates include, Random amplified polymorphism DNA (RAPD PCR)-fingerprinting with the primers M13, Enterobacterial Repetitive Intergenic Consensus (ERIC2) and Pulsed Field Gel Electrophoresis (PFGE) using the *ApaI* enzyme can be performed (Seifert et al., 2005). The main advantages of the molecular techniques in comparison with the traditional phenotypic methods are high reproducibility and applicability to a wide variety of bacteria and time saving (Grundmann et al., 1997).

10.3 Indirect diagnosis of *Acinetobacter baumannii*

Gram-negative bacteria contain lipopolysaccharides (LPS's) on their outer membranes, which consist of covalently linked lipid A (anchors the LPS into the outer membrane) and the core polysaccharide (O-polysaccharide or O-antigen), which is linked to the lipid A (Pantophlet et al., 1999). The type of LPS found within *A. baumannii* has the smooth or S-form phenotype and can be used in clinical microbiology laboratories for clinical research purposes (Pantophlet et al., 1999).

11. Materials and methods

Ninety-seven imipenem/meropenem resistant *A. baumannii* isolates were collected between March and April 2009 from a Tertiary Academic hospital. These isolates were all given a unique number. The *A. baumannii* isolates were analysed by the Diagnostic Division of the department of Medical Microbiology, National Health Laboratory service (NHLS) at the University of Pretoria. The isolates were identified as *A. baumannii* and underwent susceptibility testing. The Vitek 2 (bioMérieux, France) automated system was used to phenotypically test for the presence of carbapenemases within the *A. baumannii* isolates. Ninety-seven imipenem/meropenem resistant isolates were streaked out onto 5% sheep blood agar plates (Diagnostics Media Products, NHLS, South Africa). The plates were incubated (Horo incubator) overnight at 37°C. Gram-staining was performed for each isolate. (2002). Brain-Heart infusion broth (Biolab, Wadeville, South Africa) was prepared and aliquoted into Bijou culture bottles before sterilization. The broth bottles were inoculated from overnight plate cultures of *A. baumannii* grown on 5% sheep blood agar (Diagnostic Media Products, NHLS, South Africa) by adding 3 to 4 colonies of an isolate into the broth. The inoculated broths were incubated in a Labcon shake incubator at 37°C overnight. A volume of 900 µl of the inoculated turbid broth and 900 µl of sterile glycerol was added to a sterilized cryotube and were stored at -70°C. The CLSI (2009) guidelines for the performance of the modified Hodge test and for the double disk synergy test were followed for the detection of carbapenemase production.

A MagNA Pure Compact Nucleic Acid Isolation Kit 1 (Roche, Germany) was used to perform automated whole cell DNA extraction according to the manufacturer's guidelines. A volume of 400 µl of each of the *A. baumannii* broth culture samples was added to a Magna Pure sample tube for automated DNA extraction. Sealed cartridges with the necessary reagents were added to each lane. The purified nucleic acids (100 µl of pure *A. baumannii*

DNA) were eluted and stored at -20°C for further analysis. The Nanodrop Spectrophotometer ND-1000 instrument was used to measure the DNA concentration for each of the samples.

Two multiplex PCR assays: 1) Multiplex PCR I reaction of OXA-23, OXA-24, OXA-51 and OXA-58 genes (Woodford et al., 2006) and 2) Multiplex PCR II reaction of IMP, VIM, GIM-1, SPM-1 and SIM-1 genes (Ellington et al., 2007) were performed using the QIAGEN Multiplex PCR 1000 kit (Promega, Madison, USA), which was set up according to the manufacturer's guidelines. The QIAGEN Multiplex PCR 1000 kit contains Multiplex PCR Master mix, RNAse free water and Q solution. The thermocycling was performed using the Eppendorf, Mastercycler epgradient S (Hamburg, Germany). The DNA gel electrophoresis (Elite 300 power pack, Wealtec, South Africa) was performed on a 2% agarose gel (Whitehead Scientific, Brackenfell, Cape Town), which contained 0.5 µg.ml^{-1} ethidium bromide (Promega, Madison, USA). The loading dye used was Fermentas 6X orange loading dye solution (Fermentas UAB, Lithuania). The ready to use 100 bp ladder (Promega, Madison, USA) was used as a molecular size marker. A 10% solution of TBE buffer 10X (Promega, Madison. USA) was used for the preparation and running of the gels.

12. Prevalence of antibiotic resistance genes in *Acinetobacter baumannii* isolates in a clinical setting in the Pretoria area, South Africa

The origins of the *Acinetobacter baumannii* isolates collected in this study were 58% (56/97) from sputum specimens, 7% (7/97) from urine specimens, 11% (11/97) from blood cultures and 24% (23/97) from diverse specimens. The *A. baumannii* isolates collected for this study were both imipenem and meropenem resistant with a minimum inhibitory concentration (MIC) of >=16. The 97 *A. baumannii* isolates were subjected to susceptibility testing using the Vitek 2 instrument. The panel consisted of 18 antibiotics to determine the overall pattern of resistance. The selection of *A. baumannii* isolates used in this study was based on the Vitek 2 instrument. Both imipenem and meropenem resistant *A. baumannii* isolates were included in this study. All of the *A. baumannii* isolates showed 100% resistance to the following antibiotics in the panel: ampicillin; amoxicillin/clavulanic acid; cefuroxime; cefuroxime axetil; cefepime; imipenem; meropenem; nitrofurantoin and trimethoprim/sulfamethoxazole. The *A. baumannii* clinical isolates were all susceptible (0% resistance) to colistin (Table 2).

The Hodge test showed that 74% (72/97) of the *A. baumannii* isolates were positive for carbapenemase production and 26% (25/97) of the *A. baumannii* isolates were negative for carbapenemase production (Figure 2). These results are similar to the findings of the study conducted in Korea by Lee et al. (2003), which reported a prevalence of 66% positive for carbapenemase production, 26% negative for carbapenemase production and 8% data unknown.

The Cloverleaf or Hodge test is cumbersome and imperfect. False positives occur due to AmpC and impermeability, not due to β-lactamase production. Weak false positives occur due to AmpC hyperproducers. AmpC hydrolysing β-lactams are produced by Gram-negative bacteria [Presentation by David Livermore on "Detecting carbapenemases" at the 49th Interscience conference on antimicrobial agents and chemotherapy (ICAAC)]. Some *A. baumannii* isolates are resistant to ertapenem, but are rarely resistant to any of the other

Antibiotic Tested	Percentage resistance
Ampicillin	100% (97/97)
Amoxicillin/Clavulanic acid	100% (97/97)
Piperacillin/Tazobactam	99% (96/97)
Cefuroxime	100% (97/97)
Cefuroxime Axetil	100% (97/97)
Cefotaxime	99% (96/97)
Ceftazidime	49% (48/97)
Cefepime	100% (97/97)
Imipenem	100% (97/97)
Meropenem	100% (97/97)
Amikacin	25% (24/97)
Gentamicin	89% (86/97)
Tobramycin	5% (5/97)
Nalidixic acid	95% (92/97)
Ciprofloxacin	91% (88/97)
Nitrofurantoin	100% (97/97)
Colistin	0% (0/97)
Trimethoprim/sulfamethoxazole	100% (97/97)

Table 2. Antibiotic resistance patterns in *Acinetobacter baumannii* isolates from a Tertiary Academic Hospital

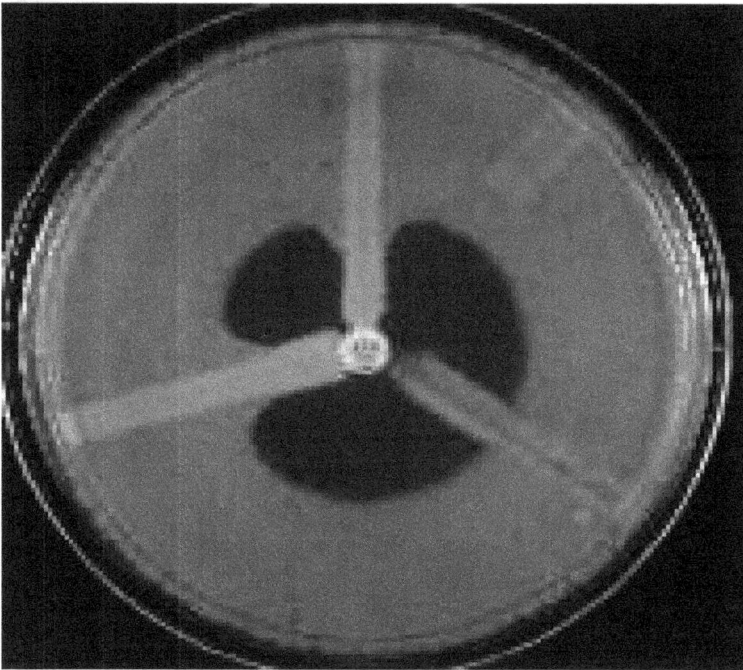

Fig. 2. Hodge or cloverleaf test of three *Acinetobacter baumannii* isolates

carbapenems. The Hodge test is very time consuming to set up and the reading of the results is subjective. Some strains produce bacteriocins, which kill the indicator organism [Presentation by David Livermore on "Detecting carbapenemases" at the 49th Interscience conference on antimicrobial agents and chemotherapy (ICAAC)]. Beta-lactamase production affects the porins of the outer membrane, thus making *A. baumannii* impermeable to antibiotics and therefore resistant to antibiotics e.g. carbapenems [Presentation by David Livermore on "Detecting carbapenemases" at the 49th Interscience conference on antimicrobial agents and chemotherapy (ICAAC)]. The class of carbapenemase cannot be determined by the results of the Modified Hodge test. Some isolates show a slight indentation, but do not produce carbapenemase (Standard operating procedure of the Department of Health and Human Services, Centres for Disease Control and Prevention: "Modified Hodge Test for Carbapenemase Detection in Enterobacteriaceae").

The double disk synergy test showed that 33% (32/97) of the *A. baumannii* isolates were susceptible to both ertapenem and EDTA and 19% (18/97) of the isolates did not grow (Figure 3). A prevalence of 45% (44/97) was recorded for *A. baumannii* isolates that were ertapenem resistant and EDTA susceptible and a prevalence of 3% (3/97) was recorded for both ertapenem and EDTA resistance. These findings are lower than the results of the study conducted in Korea by Lee et al. (2003), which reported a prevalence of 94% (75/80) of *A. baumannii* isolates susceptible for both imipenem and EDTA; all the isolates grew in that study; 5% (5/97) of the *A. baumannii* isolates were resistant to imipenem and susceptible to EDTA and 0% (0/97) isolates were resistant to both imipenem and EDTA.

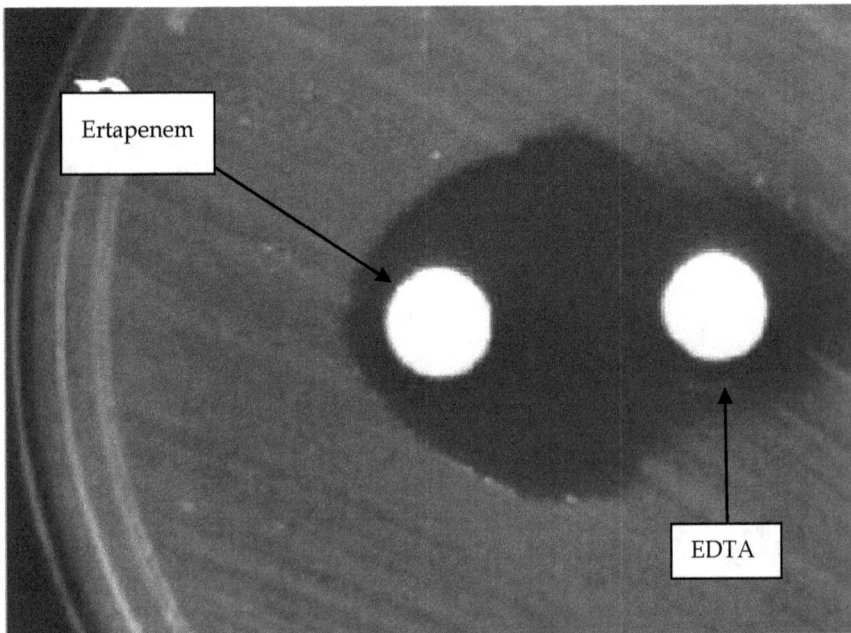

Fig. 3. Double disk synergy test of one *Acinetobacter baumannii* isolate

EDTA permeabilizes the bacterial cell, is a chelator of zinc and disrupts OXA dimers, which may be stabilized by zinc [Presentation by David Livermore on "Detecting carbapenemases" at the 49th Interscience conference on antimicrobial agents and chemotherapy (ICAAC)]. Therefore EDTA disrupts the function of the carbapenemase producing genes and hence the *A. baumannii* isolates are more susceptible to ertapenem in the presence of EDTA than without EDTA. The discrepancies in the results of this study compared to the results of the study conducted by Lee et al. (2003) were due to the use of different carbapenems. Ertapenem was used in this study, while Lee et al. used imipenem in their study conducted in 2003. Imipenem disks perform poorly as a screen for carbapenemases (Clinical and Laboratory Standards Institute, 2009) and thus ertapenem was used in this study.

The *A. baumannii* clinical specimens were cultured and two different multiplex PCR assays were performed on the extracted DNA sample of each isolate. The first multiplex PCR assay (Multiplex PCR I) was performed to screen for the presence of the OXA-group genes (OXA-23, OXA-24, OXA-51 and OXA-58). The second Multiplex PCR assay (Multiplex PCR II) screened for the presence of the Metallo-β-lactamase genes (IMP, VIM, SIM, SPM and GIM). Multiplex PCR I showed that 80% (78/97) of the *A. baumannii* isolates were positive for OXA-51, 52% (50/97) were positive for OXA-23, 1% (1/97) were positive for OXA-58 and 2% (2/97) were positive for OXA-24 (Figure 4). Figure 5 showed the gel electrophoresis pattern of the OXA-51, OXA-23, OXA-58 and OXA-24 genes.

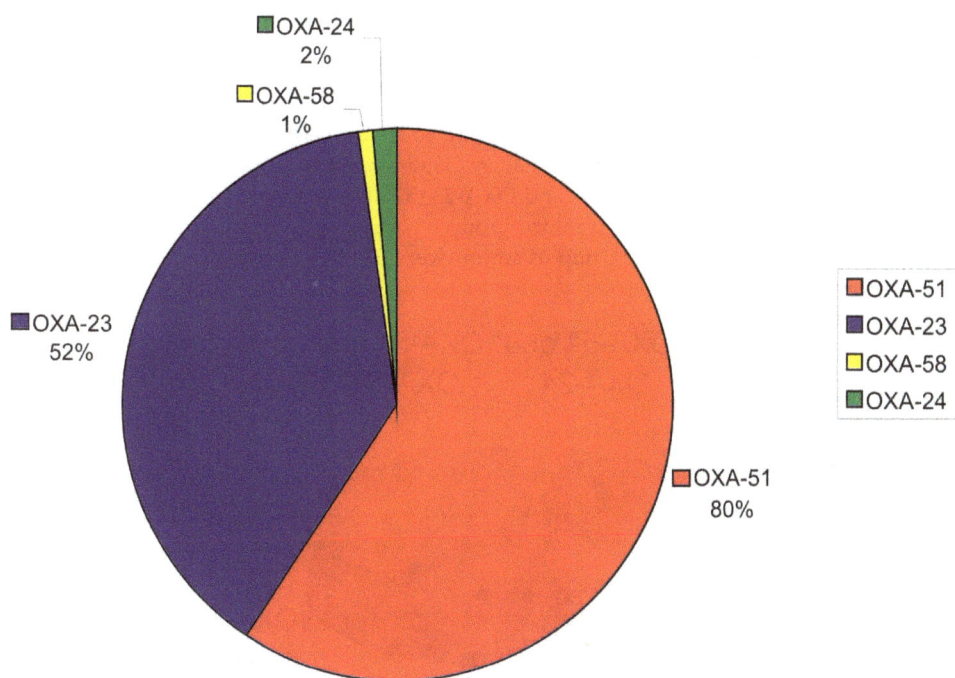

Fig. 4. Pie chart showing the results of the Multiplex PCR I for the prevalence of the OXA genes in the 97 *Acinetobacter baumannii* isolates obtained from a Tertiary Academic Hospital

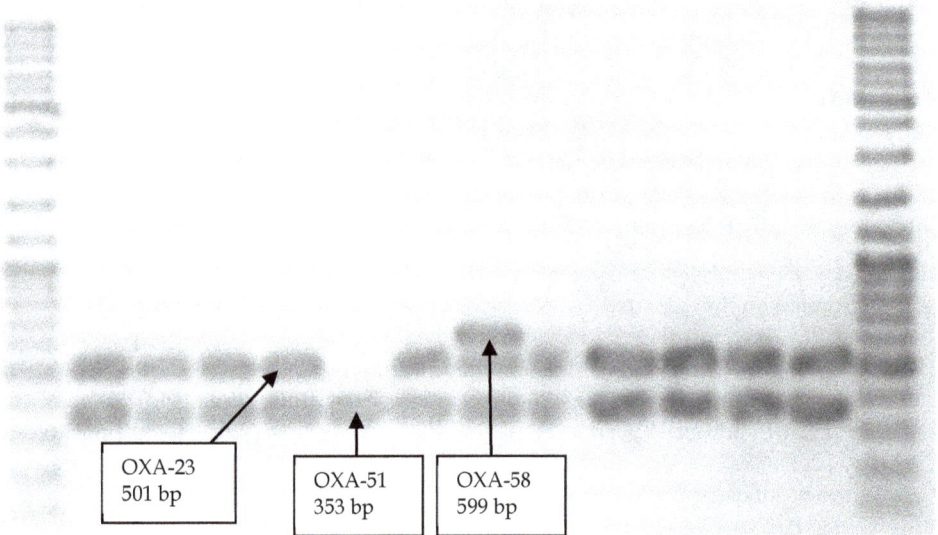

Fig. 5. Results obtained after Multiplex PCR I was performed, using a 2% agarose gel for the detection of OXA genes in the *Acinetobacter baumannii* isolates. Lanes 2, 3, 4, 5, 7, 9, 10, 11, 12 and 13 were positive for both OXA 51 and OXA-23. Lane 6 was positive only for OXA-51. Lane 8 was positive for OXA-23, OXA-51 and OXA-58. Lanes 1 and 14 contain the molecular weight markers (100 bp DNA ladder).

The multiplex PCR I results showed there were four distinctive strains of *A. baumannii* circulating in a Tertiary Academic hospital in Gauteng, South Africa. The first group of strains were positive for both OXA-51 and OXA-23 (52%). The second group of strains was positive for OXA-51 (26%) alone. The third group of strains were positive for both OXA-51 and OXA-24 (2%) and the fourth group of strains were positive for both OXA-51 and OXA-58 (1%) (Figure 6).

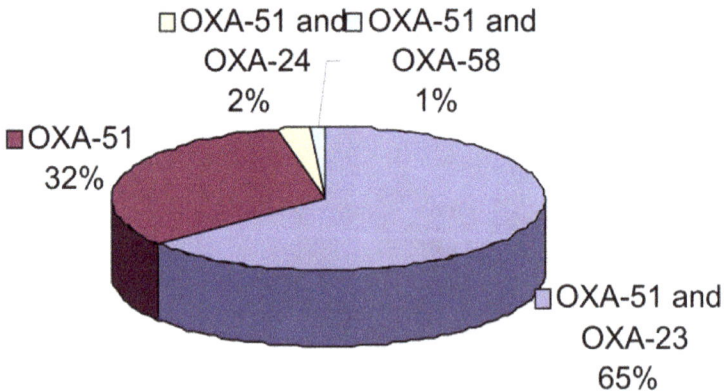

Fig. 6. Pie chart showing the results of the Multiplex PCR I for the four strains of *Acinetobacter baumannii* circulating in a Tertiary Academic Hospital

OXA-51 is an abiquitous or naturally occurring gene within *A. baumannii* (Merkier & Centron, 2006). OXA-51 is a chromosomally located gene, which needs to be regulated upstream by IS_{Aba1} to provide resistance [Presentation by David Livermore on "Detecting carbapenemases" at the 49th Interscience conference on antimicrobial agents and chemotherapy (ICAAC)]. The prevalence of OXA-51 in clinical isolates of *A. baumannii* in this study was 80% (78/97). This figure is lower than the findings of a study conducted in Iran by Feizabadi and colleagues (2008), which reported a 100% prevalence of the OXA-51 gene in clinical isolates of *A. baumannii*.

The prevalence of OXA-23 in clinical isolates of *A. baumannii* in this study was 52% (50/97). This finding was similar to the OXA-23 prevalence of 66.5% in the Asia Pacific nations (India, China, Thailand, Singapore, Hong kong and Korea) (Mendes et al., 2009). However, based on other studies conducted in Iran by Feizabadi and colleagues (2008) who reported a prevalence of 36.5% in clinical isolates of *A. baumannii* the prevalence of OXA-23 varies worldwide. OXA-23 forms part of the class D metallo-β-lactamases and is an acquired carbapenemase gene, thus a varied prevalence is observed as not all *A. baumannii* isolates will obtain the gene compared to OXA-51 which is a chromosomal carbapenemase gene occuring naturally in *A. baumannii* (Merkier & Centron, 2006). The carbapenemase gene occurs in widespread clones and contributes to the multidrug resistant nature of *A. baumannii* [Presentation by David Livermore on "Detecting carbapenemases" at the 49th Interscience conference on antimicrobial agents and chemotherapy (ICAAC)].

The OXA-24 genes also form part of the class D metallo-β-lactamases and are acquired carbapenemase genes, which occur within widespread clones [Presentation by David Livermore on "Detecting carbapenemases" at the 49th Interscience conference on antimicrobial agents and chemotherapy (ICAAC)]. The prevalence of OXA-24 in *A. baumannii* in this study was 2% (2/97). This finding was similar to the OXA-24 prevalence of 5.6% in *A. baumannii* clinical isolates from a study conducted in Thailand, Taiwan and Indonesia in 2008 (Mendes et al., 2008). However, a prevalence of 26% of OXA-24 was reported in the study conducted by Feizabadi and colleagues in Iran in 2008. The varied prevalence results are due to OXA-24 being an acquired gene within *A. baumannii* and thus not all isolates will contain the gene (Merkier & Centron, 2006).

The prevalence of OXA-58 in clinical isolates of *A. baumannii* in this study was 1% (1/97). This finding was lower than the OXA-58 prevalence of 15% in *A. baumannii* isolates in the study conducted by Feizabadi and colleagues in Iran in 2008. The differences in the results of this study and other studies are due to OXA-58 being an acquired carbapenemase gene and the presence of this gene within widespread clones Presentation by David Livermore on "Detecting carbapenemases" at the 49th Interscience conference on antimicrobial agents and chemotherapy (ICAAC)].

No metallo-β-lactamase genes were detected in any of the *A. baumannii* isolates. IMP, VIM, SIM, SPM and GIM genes belong to the class B metallo-β-lactamases and are acquired carbapenemase genes. IMP (primarily detected in South Korea) and VIM (previously detected in China) are the two metallo-β-lactamase genes, which are the most frequently detected genes in *A. baumannii* isolates (Coelho et al., 2006). The prevalence of the metallo-β-lactamase genes is generally low within *A. baumannii* isolates as illustrated in a study by Mendes and colleagues (2009) where the prevalence was 0.8% in Taiwan. VIM, SIM, SPM, IMP and GIM have not been detected in South Africa yet. Therefore the results of this study compared with the literature in that the selected *A. baumannii* isolates were negative for all metallo-β-lactamase genes.

13. Conclusions

Acinetobacter baumannii is an important opportunistic pathogen and causes a variety of nosocomial infections especially within the ICU of the Tertiary Academic Hospital in Gauteng, South Africa. The results of the phenotypic analysis in the form of the Hodge test and Double disk synergy test were similar to the results obtained from the study conducted by Lee et al. in Korea in 2003. The discrepancies with the results of the two studies can be largely due to the use of different carbapenem antibiotic disks. The Hodge test is imperfect as false positives occur due to AmpC production and impermeability of the bacterium to antibiotics due to β-lactamase ability to affect the porins of the outer membrane.

After completion of this study it is evident that the OXA group of genes (class D carbapenemases) are a problem in clinical isolates of *A. baumannii* from the Tertiary Academic Hospital. It was found that OXA-51 genes (80%) and OXA-23 genes (52%) were highly prevalent in this study and these prevalence rates were similar to the worldwide prevalence of OXA genes, which are widespread in *A. baumannii* throughout the world (Feizabadi et al., 2008). Metallo-β-lactamase (MBL) genes were not prevalent in the selected clinical isolates of *A. baumannii* due to the contained spread of the genes and thus no metallo-β-lactamase has been detected in South Africa thus far. According to Livermore molecular tests are definitive, but a few isolates with strong carbapenemase activity were negative in all molecular tests [Presentation by David Livermore on "Detecting carbapenemases" at the 49th Interscience conference on antimicrobial agents and chemotherapy (ICAAC)].

The multiplex PCR assays proved to be a rapid technique for antimicrobial susceptibility testing, however, there is much work to be done in order to investigate the possibilities of multiplex PCR assays as an alternative to current antimicrobial susceptibility testing. Continuous research and surveillance is necessary to monitor the prevalence of antibiotic resistance genes associated with *A. baumannii* in clinical settings. The ability of *A. baumannii* to grow in biofilms poses a threat concerning the possibilities of the spread of both the bacteria and the antibiotic resistance genes, which should be investigated in future research.

14. References

Allen KD & Green HT (1987) Hospital outbreak of multi-resistant *Acinetobacter anitratus*: an airborne mode of spread? *Journal of Hospital Infections* 9:110-119

Ambler R P, Coulson A F W, Frere J M, Ghuysen J M, Joris B, Forsman M, Levesque R C, Tiraby G & Waley S G (1991) A standard numbering scheme for the class A -β-lactamases. *Biochemistry Journal* 276:269-270

Appleman MD, Belzberg H, Citron DM, Heseltine PN, Yellin AE, Murray J & Berne TV (2000) In vitro activities of nontraditional antimicrobials against multiresistant *Acinetobacter baumannii* strains isolated in an intensive care unit outbreak. *Antimicrobial Agents and Chemotherapy* 44:1035-1040

Arakawa Y, Shibata N, Shibayama K, Kurokawa H, Yagi T, Fujiwara H & Goto M (2000) Convenient test for screening metallo-β-lactamase-producing gram-negative bacteria by using thiol compounds. *Journal of Clinical Microbiology* 38:40-43

Aubert D, Poirel L, Chevalier J, Leotard S, Pages JM & Nordmann P (2001) Oxacillinase-mediated resistance to cefepime and susceptibility to ceftazidime in *Pseudomonas aeruginosa*. *Antimicrobial Agents and Chemotherapy* 45:1615–1620

Aubron C, Poirel L, Ash RJ & Nordmann P (2005) Carbapenemase-producing *Enterobacteriaceae*, U.S rivers. *Emerging Infectious Diseases* 11:260–264

Beck-Sagué CM, Jarvis WR, Brook JH, Culver DH, Potts A, Gay E, Shotts BW, Hill B, Anderson RL & Weinstein MP (1990) Epidemic bacteremia due to *Acinetobacter baumannii* in five intensive care units. *American Journal of Epidemiology* 132: 723-733

Bergogne-Berezin E & KJ Towner (1996) *Acinetobacter* spp. as nosocomial pathogens: microbiological, clinical, and epidemiological features. *Clinical Microbiology Reviews* 9:148–165

Bernards AT, Beauford AJ, Dijkshoorn L and van Boven CPA (1997) Outbreak of septicemia in neonates caused by *Acinetobacter junii* investigated by amplified ribosomal DNA restriction analysis (ARDRA) and four typing methods. *Journal of Hospital Infections* 35: 129-140

Blot S, Vandewoude K & Colardyn F (2003) Nosocomial bacteremia involving *Acinetobacter baumannii* in critically ill patients: a matched cohort study. *Intensive Care Medicine* 29:471-475

Bou G, Cervero G, Dominguez MA, Quereda C & Martinez-Beltran J (2000) Characterization of a nosocomial outbreak caused by a multiresistant *Acinetobacter baumannii* strain with a carbapenem-hydrolyzing enzyme: high-level carbapenem resistance in *A. baumannii* is not due solely to the presence of beta-lactamases. *Journal of Clinical Microbiology* 38:3299–3305

Bouvet PJM & Grimont PAD (1986) Taxonomy of the genus *Acinetobacter* with the recognition of *Acinetobacter baumannii* sp. nov., *Acinetobacter haemolyticus* sp. nov., *Acinetobacter johnsonii* sp. nov,. *Acinetobacter junii* sp. nov. & emended description of *Acinetobacter calcoaceticus* and *Acinetobacter lwoffii*. *International Journal of Systematic Bacteriology* 36: 228-240

Boyce JM & Pittet D (2002) Guideline for hand hygiene in health-care settings: recommendations of the Healthcare Infection Control Practices Advisory Committee and the HICPAC/SHEA/APIC/IDSA Hand Hygiene Task Force. *Infection Control and Hospital Epidemiology* 23:S3–40

Bradley JS (1997) Meropenem: A new, extremely broad-spectrum beta-lactam antibiotic for serious infections in pediatrics. *The Pediatric Infectious Disease Journal* 16:263-268

Brown S, Bantar C, Young H & Amyes S (1996) An outbreak of imipenem resistance in *Acinetobacter* strains from Buenos Aires, Argentina, abstract C-122, p 56 In Abstracts of the 36th Interscience Conference on Antimicrobial Agents and Chemotherapy. American Society for Microbiology, Washington, DC

Brown S & Amyes SG (2005) The sequences of seven class D β-lactamases isolated from carbapenem-resistant *Acinetobacter baumannii* from four continents. *Clinical Microbiology and Infectious Diseases* 11:326-329

Brown S, Young HK & Amyes SG (2005) Characterisation of OXA-51, a novel class D carbapenemase found in genetically unrelated clinical strains of *Acinetobacter baumannii* from Argentina. *Clinical Microbiology and Infectious Diseases* 11: 15-23

Brown S & Amyes S (2006) OXA-β-lactamases in *Acinetobacter*: the story so far. *Journal of Antimicrobial Chemotherapy* 57:1-3

Bush K (1988) Recent developments in lactamase research and their implications for the future. *Reviews of Infectious Diseases* 10:681–690; 739–743

Bush K, Jacoby GA & Medeiros AA (1995) A functional classification scheme for beta-lactamases and its correlation with molecular structure. *Antimicrobial Agents and Chemotherapy*. 39:1211-1233

Cappelli G, Sereni L, Scialoja MG, Morselli M, Perrone S, Ciuffreda A, Bellesia M, Inguaggiato P, Albertazzi A & Tetta C (2003) Effects of biofilm formation on haemodialysis monitor disinfection. *Nephrology Dialysis Transplantation* 18:2105–2111.

Cefai C, Richards J, Gould FK & McPeake P (1990) An outbreak of *Acinetobacter* respiratory tract infection resulting from incomplete disinfection of ventilatory equipment. *Journal of Hospital Infections* 15: 177-182

Chakravarti DN, Fiske MJ, Fletcher LD, & Zagursky RJ (2000) Application of genomics and proteomics for identification of bacterial gene products as potential vaccine candidates. *Vaccine* 19:601–612

Cisneros JM, Reyes MJ & Pachón J (1996) Bacteremia due to *Acinetobacter baumannii*: Epidemiology, clinical and prognostic features. *Clinical Infectious Diseases* 22: 1026-1032

Cisneros JM & Rodriguez-Bano J (2002) Nosocomial bacteremia due to *Acinetobacter baumannii*: epidemiology, clinical features and treatment. *Clinical Microbiology and Infection* 8: 687-693

Clark RB (1996) Imipenem resistance among *Acinetobacter baumannii*: association with reduced expression of a 33-36-kDa outer membrane protein. *Journal of Antimicrobial Chemotherapy* 38: 245-51

Clinical and Laboratory Standards Institute (2009) Performance standards for antimicrobial susceptibility testing, Nineteenth informal supplement. CLSI document M100-S-19. Clinical and Laboratory Standards Institute, Wayne, Pennsylvania

Cloete TE (2003) Resistance mechanisms of bacteria to antimicrobial compounds. *International Biodeterioration and Biodegradation* 51: 277-282

Coelho J, Woodford N, Turton J & Livermore D M (2004) Multiresistant *Acinetobacter* in the UK: how big a threat? *Journal of Hospital Infections* 58:167–169

Coelho J, Woodford N, Afzal-Shah M & Livermore D (2006) Occurrence of OXA-58-like carbapenemases in *Acinetobacter* spp. collected over 10 years in three continents. *Antimicrobial Agents and Chemotherapy* 50:756–758

Collis CM, Kim JM, Stokes HW & Hall RM (2002) Integron-encoded Intl integrases preferentially recognize the adjacent cognate attl site in recombination with a 59-be site. *Molecular Microbiology* 46: 1415-1427

Corbella X, Pujol M & Ayats J (1996) Relevance of digestive tract colonization in the epidemiology of nosocomial infections due to multiresistant *Acinetobacter baumannii*. *Clinical Infectious Diseases* 23:329-334

Corbella X, Ariza J, Ardanuy C, Vuelta M, Yubau F, Sora M, Pujol M & Gudiol F (1998) Efficacy of sulbactam alone and in combination with ampicillin in nosocomial infections caused by multiresistant *Acinetobacter baumannii*. *Journal of Antimicrobial Chemotherapy* 42: 793-802

Cucarella C, Solano C, Valle J, Amorena B, Lasa I & Penades JR (2001) Bap, a *Staphylococcus aureus* surface protein involved in biofilm formation. *Journal of Bacteriology* 183:2888–2896

Cuhna BA. *Acinetobacter* (2007) http://www.emedicine.com/MED/topic3456.htm

Dalla-Costa LM, Coelho JM, Souza HAPHM, Castro MES, Stier CJN, Bragagnolo KL, Rea-Neto A, Penteado-Filho SR, Livermore DM & Woodford N (2003) Outbreak of carbapenem-resistant *Acinetobacter baumannii* producing the OXA-23 enzyme in Curitiba, Brazil. *Journal of Clinical Microbiology* 41:3403–3406

D'Agata EMC, Thayer V & Schaffner W (2000) An outbreak of *Acinetobacter baumannii*: the importance of cross-transmission. *Infection Control of Hospital Epidemiology* 21: 588-591

Devaud M, Kayser FH & Bachi B (1982) Transposon-mediated multiple antibiotic resistance in *Acinetobacter* strains. *Antimicrobial Agents and Chemotherapy* 22:323–329

Dijkshoorn L, Aucken HM, Gerner-Smidt P, Janssen P, Kaufmann ME, Garaizar J, Ursing J & Pitt TL (1996) Comparison of outbreak and non-outbreak *Acinetobacter baumannii* strains by genotypic and phenotypic methods. *Journal of Clinical Microbiology* 34: 1519-1525

Dima S, Kritsotakis EI, Roumbelaki M, Metalidis S, Karabinis A, Maguina N, Klouva F, Levidiotou S, Zakynthinos E, Kioumis J & Gika A (2007) Device-associated nosocomial infection rates in intensive care units in Greece. *Infection Control and Hospital Epidemiology* 28:602–605

Dupont M, Pages JM, Lafitte D, Siroy A & Bollet C (2005) Identification of an OprD homologue in *Acinetobacter baumannii*. *Journal of Proteome Research* 4:2386–2390

Ecker JA, Massire C, Hall TA, Ranken R, Pennella TT, Ivy CA, Blyn LB, Hofstadler SA, Endy TP, Scott PT, Lindler L, Hamilton T, Gaddy C, Snow K, Pe M, Fishbain J, Craft D, Deye G, Riddell S, Milstrey E, Petruccelli B, Brisse S, Harpin V, Schink A, Ecker DJ, Sampath R & Eshoo MW (2006) Identification of *Acinetobacter* species and genotyping of *Acinetobacter baumannii* by multilocus PCR and mass spectrometry. *Journal of Clinical Microbiology* 44:2921–2932

Ellington MJ, Kistler J, Livermore DM and Woodford N (2007) Multiplex PCR for rapid detection of genes encoding acquired metallo-β-lactamases. *Journal of Antimicrobial Chemotherapy* 59: 321-322

Euzéby JP (2008) List of prokaryotic names with standing in nomenclature http://www.bacterio.cict.fr/classificationac.html#*Acinetobacter*

Falagas ME, Bliziotis IA, & Siempos II (2006) Attributable mortality of *Acinetobacter baumannii* infections in critically ill patients: a systematic review of matched cohort and case-control studies. *Critical Care* 10:R48

Feizabadi MM, Fathollahazadeh B, Taherikalani M, Rasoolinejad M, Sadeghifard N, AligholiM, Soroush S & Mohammadi-Yegane S (2008) Antimicrobial susceptibility patterns and distribution of bla$_{OXA}$ genes among *Acinetobacter* spp isolated from patients at Tehran hospitals. *Japanese Journal of Infectious Diseases* 61: 274-278

Fernandez-Cuenca F, Martinez-Martinez L, Conejo MC, Ayala JA, Perea EJ & Pascual A (2003) Relationship between beta-lactamase production, outer membrane protein and penicillin-binding protein profiles on the activity of carbapenems against clinical isolates of *Acinetobacter baumannii*. *Journal of Antimicrobial Chemotherapy* 51:565–574

Fournier PE, Vallenet D, Barbe V, Audic S, Ogata H, Poirel L, Richet H, Robert C, Mangenot S, Abergel C, Nordmann P, Weissenbach J, Raoult D & Claverie JM (2006) Comparative genomics of multidrug resistance in *Acinetobacter baumannii*. *PLoS Genetics*. 2:e7

Frere J M, Galleni M, Bush K & Dideberg O (2005) Is it necessary to change the classification of lactamases? *Journal of Antimicrobial Chemotherapy* 55:1051–1053

Fritsche TR, Stilwell MG, and Jones RN (2005) Antimicrobial activity of doripenem (S-4661): a global surveillance report (2003). *Clinical Microbiology and Infections* 11:974–984

Garcia-Garmendia JL, Ortiz-Leyba C, Garnacho-Montero J, Jimenez-Jimenez FJ, Perez-Paredes C, Barrero-Almodovar AE & Gili-Miner M (2001) Risk factors for *Acinetobacter baumannii* nosocomial bacteremia in critically ill patients: a cohort study. *Clinical Infectious Diseases*. 33:939–946

Garrity GM, Brenner DJ, Krieg RN & Staley JT (2005) Bergey's Manual of Systematic Bacteriology, Volume 2: The Proteobacteria, Part B: The Gammaproteobacteria, pg 415-435. Springer, New York, USA

Gerischer U (2008) *Acinetobacter* Molecular Biology 1st edition, Caister Academic Press ISBN 987-1-904455-20-2

Gerner-Smidt P (1987) Endemic occurrence of *Acinetobacter calcoaceticus* biovar anitratus in an intensive care unit. *Journal of Hospital Infections*. 10: 265-272

Gerner-Smidt P, Tjernberg I & Usring J (1991) Reliability of phenotypic tests for identification of *Acinetobacter species*. *Journal of Clinical Microbiology* 29: 277-282

Getchell-White SI; Donowitz LG & Groeschel DHM (1989) The inanimate environment of an intensive care unit as a potential source of nosocomial bacteria: evidence for long survival of *Acinetobacter calcoaceticus*. *Infection Control and Hospital Epidemiology* 10: 402-407

Giamarellou H, Antoniadou A & Kanellakopoulou (2008) Review: *Acinetobacter baumannii*: a universal threat to public health? *International Journal of Antimicrobial Agents* 32: 106-119

Go ES, Urban C, Burns J, Kreiswirth B, Eisner W & Mariano NF (1994) Clinical and molecular epidemiology of *Acinetobacter* infections sensitive only to polymyxin B and sulbactam. *Lancet* 12:1329-1332

Go J and Cuhna BA (1999) *Acinetobacter baumannii:* Infection control implications. *Infectious Disease Practices* 23: 65-68

Goldstein FW, Labigne-Roussel A, Gerbaud G, Carlier C, Collatz E & Courvalin P (1983) Transferable plasmid-mediated antibiotic resistance in *Acinetobacter*. *Plasmid* 10:138-147

Grundmann HJ, Towner KJ, Dijkshoorn L, Gerner-Smidt P, Maher M, Seifert H & Vaneechoutte M (1997) Multicenter study using standardized protocols and reagents for evaluation of reproducibility of PCR-based fingerprinting of *Acinetobacter* spp. *Journal of Clinical Microbiology* 35: 3071-3077

Guardabassi L, Dijkshoorn L, Collard JM, Olsen JE & Dalsgaard A (2000) Distribution and *in vitro* transfer of tetracycline resistance determinants in clinical and aquatic *Acinetobacter* strains. *Journal of Medical Microbiology* 49: 929-936

Heritier C, Dubouix A, Poirel L, Marty N & Nordmann P (2005a) A nosocomial outbreak of *Acinetobacter baumannii* isolates expressing the carbapenem-hydrolysing oxacillinase OXA-58. *Journal of Antimicrobial Chemotherapy* 55: 115-118

Heritier C, Poirel L, Fournier, Claverie J, Raoult D & Nordmann P (2005b) Characterization of the naturally occurring oxacillinase of *Acinetobacter baumannii*. *Antimicrobial Agents and Chemotherapy* 49: 4174-4179

Heritier C, Poirel L & Nordmann P (2006) Cephalosporinase overexpression resulting from insertion of IS*Aba1* in *Acinetobacter baumannii*. *Clinical Microbiology and Infection* 12:123-130

Hogg GM, Barr JG & Webb CH (1998) *In-vitro* activity of the combination of colistin and rifampicin against multidrug-reistant strains of *Acinetobacter baumannii*. *Journal of Antimicrobial Chemotherapy* 41: 494-495

Hornstein M, Sautjeau-Rostoker C, Peduzzi J, Vessieres A, Hong LT, Barthelemy M, Scavizzi M & Labia R (1997) Oxacillin-hydrolyzing lactamase involved in resistance to imipenem in *Acinetobacter baumannii*. *FEMS Microbiology Letters* 153:333–339

Hsueh P-R, Teng L-J, Chen C-Y, Chen W-H, Yu C-J, Ho S-W & Luh K-T (2002) Pandrug-Resistant *Acinetobacter baumannii* causing nosocomial infections in a University in Taiwan. *Emerging Infectious Diseases* 8: 827-832

Hughes D (2003) Exploiting genomics, genetics and chemistry to combat antibiotic resistance. *Nature Reviews Genetics* 4:432–441

Hujer KM, Hujer AM, Hulten EA, Bajaksouzian S, Adams JM, Donskey CJ, Ecker DJ, Massire C, Eshoo MW, Sampath R, Thomson JM, Rather PN, Craft DW, Fishbain JT, Ewell AJ, Jacobs MR, Paterson DL & Bonomo RA (2006) Analysis of antibiotic resistance genes in multidrug-resistant *Acinetobacter* sp. isolates from military and civilian patients treated at the Walter Reed Army Medical Center. *Antimicrobial Agents and Chemotherapy* 50:4114–4123

Huys G, Cnockaert M, Vaneechoutte M, Woodford N, Nemec A, Dijkshoorn L & Swings J (2005) Distribution of tetracycline resistance genes in genotypically related and unrelated multiresistant *Acinetobacter baumannii* strains from different European hospitals. *Research in Microbiology* 156: 348-355

Jacobs RF: Imipenem-cilastatin (1986) The first thienamycin antibiotic *The Pediatric Infectious Disease Journal* 5:444-448

Jawad A, Hawkey PM, Herritage J & Snelling AM (1994) Description of Leeds *Acinetobacter* Medium, a new selective and differential medium for isolation of clinically important *Acinetobacter* spp and comparison with Herellea agar and Holton's agar. *Journal of Clinical Microbiology*. 32: 2353-2358

Jawad A, Heritage J, Snelling AM, Gascoyne-Binzi DM & Hawkey PM (1996) Influence of relative humidity and suspending menstrual on survival of *Acinetobacter* spp on dry surfaces. *Journal of Clinical Microbiology* 34: 2881-2887

Jeon B, Jeong SH, Bae IK, Kwon SB, Lee K, Young D, Lee JH, Song JS & Lee SH (2005) Investigation of a nosocomial outbreak of imipenem- resistant *Acinetobacter baumannii* producing the OXA-23-lactamase in Korea. *Journal of Clinical Microbiology* 43:2241–2245

Joly-Guillou ML (2005) Clinical impact and pathogenicity of *Acinetobacter*. *Clinical Microbiology and Infection* 11:868–873

Jones RN, Huynh HK, Biedenbach DJ, Fritsche TR & Sader HS (2004) Doripenem (S-4661), a novel carbapenem: comparative activity against contemporary pathogens including bactericidal action and preliminary in vitro methods evaluations. *Journal of Antimicrobial Chemotherapy* 54:144– 154

Jones RN, Sader HS & Fritsche TR (2005) Comparative activity of doripenem and three other carbapenems tested against Gram-negative bacilli with various beta-lactamase resistance mechanisms. *Diagnostic Microbiology and Infectious Disease* 52:71-74

Kahlmeter G., Brown DF, Goldstein FW, MacGowan AP, Mouton JW, Odenholt I, Rodloff A, Soussy CJ, Steinbakk M, Soriano F & Stetsiouk O (2006) European Committee on Antimicrobial Susceptibility Testing (EUCAST) technical notes on antimicrobial susceptibility testing. *Clinical Microbiology and Infection* 12:501–503

Kramer A, Schwebke I & Kampf G (2006) How long do nosocomial pathogens persist on inanimate surfaces? A systematic review. *BMC Infectious Diseases* 6:130

Kuo L, Teng L, Yu C, Ho S and Hsueh P (2004) Dissemination of a clone of unusual phenotype of pandrug-resistant *Acinetobacter baumannii* at a University Hospital in Taiwan. *Journal of Clinical Microbiology* 42: 1759-1763

Landman D, Quale J M, Mayorga D, Adedeji A, Vangala K, Ravishankar J, Flores C & Brooks S (2002) Citywide clonal outbreak of multiresistant *Acinetobacter baumannii* and *Pseudomonas aeruginosa* in Brooklyn, NY: the preantibiotic era has returned. *Archives of Internal Medicine* 162:1515–1520

Laraki N, Franceschini N, Rossolini GM, Santucci P, Meunier C, de Pauw, Amicosante G, Frère JM & Galleni (1999) Biochemical characterization of the *Pseudomonas aeruginosa* 101/1477 metallo-β-lactamase IMP-1 produced by *Escherichia coli*. *Antimicrobial Agents and Chemotherapy* 43: 902-906

Lauretti L, Riccio ML, Mazzariol A, Cornaglia G, Amicosante G, Fontana R & Rossolini GM (1999) Cloning and characterization of bla_{VIM}, a new integron-borne metallo-lactamase gene from a *Pseudomonas aeruginosa* clinical isolate. *Antimicrobial Agents and Chemotherapy* 43:1584– 1590

Lee K, Chong Y, Shin HB, Kim YA, Yong D & Yum JH (2001) Modified Hodge test and EDTA-disk synergy tests to screen metallo-ß-lactamase-producing strains of *Pseudomonas* and *Acinetobacter* species. *Clinical Microbiology and Infection* 7:88-91

Lee K, Lee WG, Uh Y, Ha GY, Cho J, Chong Y & the Korean Nationwide Surveillance of Antimicrobial Resistance group (2003) VIM- and IMP-Type Metallo-β-lactamase-Producing *Pseudomonas* spp. and *Acinetobacter* spp. in Korean Hospitals. *Emerging Infectious Diseases* 9: 868–871

Lee K, Yum JH, Yong D, Lee HM, Kim HD, Docquier JD, Rossolini GM & ChongY (2005) Novel acquired metallo-beta-lactamase gene, bla_{SIM-1}, in a class 1 integron from *Acinetobacter baumannii* clinical isolates from Korea. *Antimicrobial Agents and Chemotherapy* 49:4485–4491

Lim HM, Pene JJ & Shaw RW (1988) Cloning, nucleotide sequence, and expression of the *Bacillus cereus* 5/B/6-lactamase II structural gene. *Journal of Bacteriology* 170:2873–2878

Limansky AS, Mussi MA & Viale AM (2002) Loss of a 29-kilodalton outer membrane protein in *Acinetobacter baumannii* is associated with imipenem resistance. *Journal of Clinical Microbiology* 40:4776–4778

Livermore DM & Woodford N (2006) The lactamase threat in *Enterobacteriaceae*, *Pseudomonas* and *Acinetobacter*. *Trends in Microbiology* 14:413–420

Lolans K, Rice TW, Munoz-Price LS & Quinn JP (2006) Multicity outbreak of carbapenem-resistant *Acinetobacter baumannii* isolates producing the carbapenemase OXA-40. *Antimicrobial Agents and Chemotherapy* 50:2941– 2945

Loukili NH, Granbastien B, Faure K, Guery B, and Beaucaire G (2006) Effect of different stabilized preparations of peracetic acid on biofilm. *Journal of Hospital Infections* 63:70-72

Lorenz MG & Wackernagel W (1994) Bacterial gene transfer by natural genetic transformation in the environment. *Microbiological Reviews* 58:563– 602

Ma JF, Hager PW, Howell ML, Phibbs PV & Hasset D (1998) Cloning and characterization of *Pseudomonas aeruginosa* zwf gene encoding glucose-6-phosphate dehydrogenase, an enzyme important in resistance to methyl viologen (paraquat). *Journal of Bacteriology* 180: 1741-1749

Majiduddin FK & Palzkill T (2003) Amino acid sequence requirements at residues 69 and 238 for the SME-1-lactamase to confer resistance to-lactam antibiotics. *Antimicrobial Agents and Chemotherapy* 47:1062–1067

Maragakis LL, Cosgrove SE, Song X, Kim D, Rosenbaum P, Ciesla N, Srinivasan A, Ross T, Carroll K & Perl TM (2004) An outbreak of multidrug-resistant *Acinetobacter baumannii* associated with pulsatile lavage wound treatment. *Journal of the American Medical Association* 292:3006–3011

Marchand I, Damier-Piolle L, Courvalin P & Lambert T (2004) Expression of the RND-type efflux pump AdeABC in *Acinetobacter baumannii* is regulated by the AdeRS two-component system. *Antimicrobial Agents and Chemotherapy* 48:3298–3304

Marque S, Poirel L, Heritier C, Brisse S, Blasco MD, Filip R, Coman G, Naas T & Nordmann P (2005) Regional occurrence of plasmid mediated carbapenem-hydrolyzing oxacillinase OXA-58 in *Acinetobacter* spp. in Europe. *Journal of Clinical Microbiology* 43:4885–4888

McDonald LC, Banerjee SN, Jarvis WR & the National Nosocomial Infections Surveillance System (1999) Seasonal variation of *Acinetobacter* infections: 1987-96. *Clinical Infectious Diseases* 29: 1133-1137

Mendes RE, Bell JM, Turnidge JD, Castanheira M & Jones RN (2009) Emergence and widespread dissemination of OXA-23, -24/40 and –58 carbapenemases among *Acinetobacter* spp in Asia-Pacific nations: report from the SENTRY Surveillance Program. *Journal of Antimicrobial Chemotherapy* 63: 55-59

Merkier AK & Centrón D (2006) *bla*$_{OXA-51}$-type β-lactamase genes are ubiquitous and vary within a strain in *Acinetobacter baumannii*. *International Journal of Antimicrobial Agents* 28: 110-113

Metzgar D, Bacher JM, Pezo V, Reader J, Doring V, Schimmel P, Marliere P & de Crecy-Lagard V (2004) *Acinetobacter* sp. ADP1: an ideal model organism for genetic analysis and genome engineering. *Nucleic Acids Research* 32:5780–5790

Mulin B, Talon D & Viel JF (1995) Risk factor for nosocomial colonization with multiresistant *Acinetobacter baumannii*. *European Journal of Clinical Microbiology and Infectious Diseases* 14: 569-576

Mushtaq S, Ge Y & Livermore DM (2004) Comparative activities of doripenem versus isolates, mutants, and transconjugants of *Enterobacteriaceae* and *Acinetobacter* spp. with characterized beta-lactamases. *Antimicrobial Agents and Chemotherapy* 48:1313–1319

Mussi MA, Limansky AS & Viale AM (2005) Acquisition of resistance to carbapenems in multidrug-resistant clinical strains of *Acinetobacter baumannii*: natural insertional inactivation of a gene encoding a member of a novel family of beta-barrel outer membrane proteins. *Antimicrobial Agents and Chemotherapy* 49:1432–1440

Naas T, Levy M, Hirschauer C, Marchandin H & Nordmann P (2005) Outbreak of carbapenem-resistant *Acinetobacter baumannii* producing the carbapenemase OXA-23 in a tertiary care hospital of Papeete, French Polynesia. *Journal of Clinical Microbiology* 43:4826-4829

Nikaido H (1996) Multidrug efflux pumps of Gram-negative bacteria. *Journal of Bacteriology* 178: 5853-5859

Nordmann P, Mariotte S, Naas T, Labia R & Nicolas M-H (1993) Biochemical properties of a carbapenem-hydrolyzing-lactamase for *Enterobacter cloacae* and cloning of the gene into *Escherichia coli*. *Antimicrobial Agents and Chemotherapy* 37:939–946

Nordmann, P & Poirel L (2002) Emerging carbapenemases in Gram negative aerobes. *Clinical Microbiology and Infection* 8:321–331

Nordmann, P (2004) *Acinetobacter baumannii*, the nosocomial pathogen par excellence. *Pathologie Biologie* 52:301–303

Pajkos A, Vickery K & Cossart Y (2004) Is biofilm accumulation on endoscope tubing a contributor to the failure of cleaning and decontamination? *Journal of Hospital Infections* 58:224–229

Palmen R & Hellingwerf KJ (1997) Uptake and processing of DNA by *Acinetobacter calcoaceticus* – a review. *Gene* 192:179–190

Pantophlet R, Brade L & Brade H (1999) Identification of *Acinetobacter baumannii* strains with monoclonal antibodies against the O antigens of their lipopolysaccharides. *Clinical and Diagnostic Laboratory Immunology* 6: 323-329

Paton R, Miles RS and Hood J (1993) ARI-1: β-lactamase mediated imipenem resistance in *Acinetobacter baumannii*. *International Journal of Antimicrobial Agents* 2: 81-88

Patterson JE, Vecchio J, Pantelick EL, Farrel P, Mazon D, Zervos MJ & Heirholzer WJ Jr (1991) Association of contaminated gloves with transmission of *Acinetobacter calcoaceticus* var *anitratus* in an intensive care unit. *American Journal of Medicine* 91: 479-483

Peleg AY, Franklin C, Bell J & Spelman DW (2005) Dissemination of the metallo-β-lactamase gene bla_{IMP-4} amongst Gram negative pathogens in a clinical setting in Australia. *Clinical Infectious Diseases* 41:1549-1556

Perez F, Hujer AM, Hujer KM, Decker BK, Rather PN & Bonomo RA (2007) Minireview: Global challenge of mulidrug-resistant *Acinetobacter baumannii*. *Antimicrobial Agents and Chemotherapy* 51: 3471-3484

Peterson AA, Fesik SW & McGroarty EJ (1987) Decreased binding of antibiotics to lipopolysaccharides from polymyxin-resistant strains of *Escherichia coli* and *Salmonella typhimurium*. *Antimicrobial Agents and Chemotherapy* 31: 230-237

Petropoulou D, Tzanetou K, Syriopoulou VP, Daikos GL, Ganteris G & Malamou-Lada E (2006) Evaluation of imipenem/imipenem EDTA disk method for detection of metallo-lactamase-producing *Klebsiella pneumoniae* isolated from blood cultures. *Microbial Drug Resistance* 12:39–43

Pittet D (2004) The Lowbury lecture: behaviour in infection control. *Journal of Hospital Infection* 58:1–13

Poirel L, Cabanne L, Vahaboglu H, & Nordmann P (2005) Genetic environment and expression of the extended-spectrum Beta-lactamase bla_{PER-1} gene in gram-negative bacteria. *Antimicrobial Agents and Chemotherapy* 49:1708–1713

Poirel L & Nordmann P (2006) Carbapenem resistance in *Acinetobacter baumannii*: mechanisms and epidemiology. *Clinical Microbiology and Infection* 12:826–836

Poole K (2005) Efflux-mediated antimicrobial resistance. *Journal of Antimicrobial Chemotherapy* 56:20–51

Pottumarthy S, Moland ES, Jeretschko S, Swanzy SR, Thomson KS and Fritsche TR (2003) NmcA carbapenem-hydrolyzing enzyme in *Enterobacter cloacae* in North America. *Emerging Infectious Diseases* 9:999–1002

Pournaras S, Markogiannakis A, Ikonomidis A, Kondyli L, Bethimouti K, Maniatis AN, Legakis NJ & Tsakris A (2006) Outbreak of multiple clones of imipenem-resistant *Acinetobacter baumannii* isolates expressing OXA-58 carbapenemase in an intensive care unit. *Journal of Antimicrobial Chemotherapy* 57:557–561

Prashanth K & Badrinath S (2000) Simplified phenotypic tests for identification of *Acinetobacter spp* and their antimicrobial susceptibility status. *Journal of Medical Microbiology* 49: 773-778

Projan SJ (2004) Small molecules for small minds? The case for biologic pharmaceuticals. *Expert Opinion on Biological Therapy* 4: 1345-1350

Radice M, Power P, Gutkind G, Fernandez K, Vay C, Famiglietti A, Ricover N & Ayala J (2004) First class A carbapenemase isolated from *Enterobacteriaceae* in Argentina. *Antimicrobial Agents and Chemotherapy* 48:1068– 1069

Rahal J (2006) Novel antibiotic combinations against infections with almost completely resistant *Pseudomonas aeruginosa* and *Acinetobacter* species. *Clinical Infectious Diseases* 43: 95-99

Rasmussen B A, Bush K, Keeney D, Yang Y, Hare R, O'Gara C & Medeiros A A (1996) Characterization of IMI-1 β-lactamase, a class A carbapenem-hydrolyzing enzyme from *Enterobacter cloacae*. *Antimicrobial Agents and Chemotherapy* 40:2080–2086

Ribera A, Ruiz J & Vila J (2003) Presence of the Tet M determinant in a clinical isolate of *Acinetobacter baumannii*. *Antimicrobial Agents and Chemotherapy* 47: 2310-2312

Robenshtok E, Paul M, Leibovici L, Fraser A, Pitlik S, Ostfeld I, Samra Z, Perez S, Lev B & Weinberger M (2006) The significance of *Acinetobacter baumannii* bacteraemia compared with *Klebsiella pneumoniae* bacteraemia: risk factors and outcomes. *Journal of Hospital Infection* 64: 282-287

Rodriguez-Hernández MJ, Pachoń J & Pichardo C (2000) Imipenem, doxycycline and amikacin in monotherapy and in combination in *Acinetobacter baumannii* experimental pneumonia. *Journal of Antimicrobial Chemotherapy* 45: 493-501

Santillana E, Beceiro A, Bou G & Romero A (2007) Crystal structure of the carbapenemase OXA-24 reveals insights into the mechanism of carbapenem hydrolysis. *Proceedings of the National Academy of Science USA* 104:5354–5359

Savov E, Chankova D, Vatcheva R & Dinev N (2002) In vitro investigation of the susceptibility of *Acinetobacter baumannii* strains isolated from clinical specimens to ampicillin/sulbactam alone and in combination with amikacin. *International Journal of Antimicrobial Agents* 20:390–392

Scaife W, Young HK, Paton RH & Amyes SG (1995) Transferable imipenem-resistance in *Acinetobacter* species from a clinical source. *Journal of Clinical Microbiology* 36: 585-586

Scerpella EG, Wanger AR, Armitige L, Anderlini P and Ericsson CD (1995) Nosocomial outbreak caused by a multiresistant clone of *Acinetobacter baumannii*: results of the case control and molecular epidemiologic investigations. *Infection Control and Hospital Epidemiology* 16: 92-97

Schreckenberger PC & Von Graevenitz A (2000) *Acinetobacter, Achromobacter, Acaligenes, Moraxella, Methylobacterium* and other non-fermentative Gram-negative rods, pg 539-560. In Murray PR, Baron EJ, Pfaller MA, Tenover FC and Yolken RH (ed), Manual of clinical Microbiology, 7th ed. ASM Press, Washington DC, USA

Seifert H, Strate A & Pulverer G (1995) Nosocomial bacteremia due to *Acinetobacter baumannii*, clinical features, epidemiology and predictors of mortality. *Medicine* 74: 340-349

Seifert H, Dijkshoorn L, Gerner-Smidt P, Pelzer N, Tjernberg I & Vaneechoutte A (1997) Distribution of *Acinetobacter* species on human skin: comparison of phenotypic and genotypic identification methods. *Journal of Clinical Microbiology* 35: 2819-2825

Seifert H, Dolzani L & Bressan R (2005) Standardization and interlaboratory reproducibility assessment of pulsed-field gel electrophoresis-generated fingerprints of *Acinetobacter baumannii*. *Journal of Clinical Microbiology* 43:4328–35

Segal H, Garny S & Elisha BG (2005) Is IS (ABA-1) customized for *Acinetobacter*. *FEMS Microbiology Letters* 243:425–429

Seward, R. J (1999) Detection of integrons in worldwide nosocomial isolates of *Acinetobacter* spp. *Clinical Microbiology and Infection* 5:308–318

Seward RJ & Towner KJ (1998) Molecular epidemiology of quinolone resistance in *Acinetobacter spp. Clinical Microbiology and Infection* 4: 248-254

Sheretz RJ & Sullivan ML (1985) An outbreak of infections with *Acinetobacter calcoaceticus* in burn patients: contamination of patients' mattresses. *Journal of Infectious Diseases* 151: 252-258

Siroy A, Molle V, Lemaitre-Guillier C, Vallenet D, Pestel-Caron M, Cozzone AJ, Jouenne T & De E (2005) Channel formation by CarO, the carbapenem resistance-associated outer membrane protein of *Acinetobacter baumannii*. *Antimicrobial Agents and Chemotherapy* 49:4876–4883

Smith MG, Des Etages SG & Snyder M (2004) Microbial synergy via an ethanol-triggered pathway. *Molecular and Cellular Biology* 24:3874–3884

Smith MG, Gianoulis TA, Pukatzki S, Mekalanos JJ, Ornston LN, Gerstein M & Snyder M (2007) New insights into *Acinetobacter baumannii* pathogenesis revealed by high-density pyrosequencing and transposon mutagenesis. *Genes and Development* 21:601–614

Sougakoff W, L'Hermite G, Pernot L, Naas T, Guillet V, Nordmann P, Jarlier V & Delettre J (2002) Structure of the imipenem-hydrolyzing class A-lactamase SME-1 from *Serratia marcescens*. *Acta Crystallographica Section D Biological Crystallography Journal* 58:267–274

Swenson JM, Killgore GE & Tenover FC (2004) Antimicrobial susceptibility testing of *Acinetobacter* spp. by NCCLS broth microdilution and disk diffusion methods. *Journal of Clinical Microbiology* 42:5102–5108

Takahashi A, Yomoda S, Kobayashi I, Okubo T, Tsunoda M & Iyobe S (2000) Detection of carbapenemase-producing *Acinetobacter baumannii* in a hospital. *Journal of Clinical Microbiology* 38: 526-529

Talbot GH, Bradley J, Edwards JE Jr, Gilbert D, Scheld M, & Bartlett JG (2006) Bad bugs need drugs: an update on the development pipeline from the Antimicrobial Availability Task Force of the Infectious Diseases Society of America. *Clinical Infectious Disease* 42:657–668

Thongpiyapoom S, Narong MN, Suwalak N, Jamulitrat S, Intaraksa P, Boonrat J, Kasatpibal N & Unahalekhaka A (2004) Device-associated infections and patterns of antimicrobial resistance in a medical-surgical intensive care unit in a university hospital in Thailand. *Journal of the Medical Association of Thailand* 87:819–824

Turton JF, Kaufmann ME, Glover J, Coelho JM, Warner M, Pike R & Pitt TL (2005) Detection and typing of integrons in epidemic strains of *Acinetobacter baumannii* found in the United Kingdom. *Journal of Clinical Microbiology* 43:3074–3082

Turton JF, Woodford N, Glover J, Yarde S, Kaufmann ME & Pitt TL (2006) Identification of *Acinetobacter baumannii* by detection of the $bla_{\text{OXA-51-like}}$ carbapenemase gene intrinsic to this species. *Journal of Clinical Microbiology* 44: 2974-2976

Ullah JH, Walsh TR, Taylor IA, Emery DC, Verma CS & Gamblin SJ (1998) The crystal structure of the L1 metallo-β-lactamase from *Stenotrophomonas maltophilia* at 1.7 resolution. *Journal of Molecular Biology* 284: 125-136

Vahaboglu H, Budak F, Kasap M, Gacar G, Torol S, Karadenizli A, Kolayli F & Eroglu C (2006) High prevalence of OXA-51-type class D Beta-lactamases among ceftazidime-resistant clinical isolates of *Acinetobacter* spp.: co-existence with OXA-58 in multiple centers. *Journal of Antimicrobial Chemotherapy* 58:537-542

Van Dessel H, Dijkshoorn L, Van der Reijden T, Bakker N, Paauw A & Van de Broek E (2004) Identification of a new geographically widespread multiresistant *Acinetobacter baumannii* clone from European hospitals. *Research in Microbiology* 155: 105-112

Vaneechoutte M (1996) DNA fingerprinting techniques for microorganisms. A proposal for classification and nomenclature. *Molecular Biotechnology* 6: 115-142

Villegas MV & Hartstein AI (2003) *Acinetobacter* outbreaks, 1977–2000. *Infection Control and Hospital Epidemiology* 24:284–295

Villers D, Espaze E, Coste-burel M, Giauffret F, Ninin E, Nicolas F & Richet H (1998) Nosocomial *Acinetobacter baumannii* infections: Microbiological and clinical epidemiology. *Annals of Internal Medicine* 129: 182-189

Walsh T, Toleman M, Poirel L & Nordmann P (2005) Metallo-β-lactamases: the quiet before the storm? *Clinical Microbiological Reviews* 18:306-325

Walsh TR (2005) The emergence and implications of metallo-beta-lactamases in Gram-negative bacteria. *Clinical Microbiology and Infection* 11(Suppl. 6):2–9.

Walther-Rasmussen J & Hoiby N (2006) OXA-type carbapenemases. *Journal of Antimicrobial Chemotherapy* 57:373–383

Wang JT, McDonald LC, Chang SC & Ho M (2002) Community-Acquired *Acinetobacter baumannii* bacteremia in adult patients in Taiwan. *Journal of Clinical Microbiology* 40: 1526-1529

Watanabe M, Iyobe S, Inoue M & Mitsuhashi S (1991) Transferable imipenem resistance in *Pseudomonas aeruginosa*. *Antimicrobial Agents and Chemotherapy* 35:147–151

Weernink A, Severin WPJ, Tjernberg I & Dijkshoorn L (1995) Pillows an unexpected source of *Acinetobacter*. *Journal of Hospital Infections*. 29: 189-199

Wilks M, Wilson A, Warwick S, Price E, Kennedy D, Ely A & Millar MR (2006) Control of an outbreak of multidrug-resistant *Acinetobacter baumannii-calcoaceticus* colonization and infection in an intensive care unit (ICU) without closing the ICU or placing patients in isolation. *Infection Control and Hospital Epidemiology* 27:654–658

Wilson SJ, Knipe CJ, Zieger MJ, Gabehart KM, Goodman JE, Volk HM & Sood R (2004) Direct costs of multidrug-resistant *Acinetobacter baumannii* in the burn unit of a public teaching hospital. *American Journal of Infection Control* 32:342–344

Wise R (1986) In vitro and Pharmacokinetic properties of the carbapenems. *Antimicrobial Agents and Chemotherapy* 30:343-349

Wisplinghoff H, Bischoff T, Tallent SM, Seifert H, Wenzel RP & Edmond MB (2004) Nosocomial bloodstream infections in US hospitals: analysis of 24 179 cases from a prospective nationwide surveillance study. *Clinical Infectious Diseases* 39: 309-317

Wood CA & Reboli AC (1993) Infections caused by carbapenem-resistant *Acinetobacter calcoaceticus* biotype anatraus. *Journal of Infectious Diseases* 167: 448-451

Woodford N, Ellington MJ, Coehlo JM, Turton JF, Ward ME, Brown S, Amyes SGB & Livermore DM (2006) Multiplex PCR for genes encoding prevalent OXA carbapenemases in *Acinetobacter spp. International Journal of Antimicrobial Agents* 27: 351-353

Yang Y, Wu P & Livermore D M (1990) Biochemical characterization of a lactamase that hydrolyzes penems and carbapenems from two *Serratia marcescens* isolates. *Antimicrobial Agents and Chemotherapy* 34:755–758

Yigit H, Queenan AM, Anderson GJ, Domenech-Sanchez A, Biddle JW, Steward CD, Alberti S, Bush K & Tenover F C (2001) Novel carbapenem-hydrolyzing-lactamase, KPC-1, from a carbapenem-resistant strain of *Klebsiella pneumoniae. Antimicrobial Agents and Chemotherapy* 45:1151– 1161

Yong D, Choi YS, Roh KH, Kim CK, Park YH, Yum JH, Lee K and Chong Y (2006) Increasing prevalence and diversity of metallo-β-lactamases in *Pseudomonas* spp., *Acinetobacter* spp., and *Enterobacteriaceae* from Korea. *Antimicrobial Agents and Chemotherapy* 50:1884–1886

Young DM. & Ornston LN (2001) Functions of the mismatch repair gene *mut*S from *Acinetobacter* sp. strain ADP1. *Journal of Bacteriology* 183: 6822–6831

Yu Y-S, Du X-X, Zhou Z-H, Chen Y-G & Li L-J (2006) First isolation of *bla*IMI-2 in an *Enterobacter cloacae* clinical isolate from China. *Antimicrobial Agents and Chemotherapy* 50:1610–1611

Yum JH, Yi K, Lee H, Yong D, Lee K, Kim JM, Rossolini GM & Chong Y (2002) Molecular characterization of metallo-beta-lactamase-producing *Acinetobacter baumannii* and *Acinetobacter* genomospecies 3 from Korea: identification of two new integrons carrying the *bla*VIM-2 gene cassettes. *Journal of Antimicrobial Chemotherapy* 49:837–840.

Zarrilli R, Crispino M, Bagattini M, Barretta E, Popolo A. D, Triassi M & Villari P (2004) Molecular epidemiology of sequential outbreaks of *Acinetobacter baumannii* in an intensive care unit shows the emergence of carbapenem resistance. *Journal of Clinical Microbiology* 42:946–953

11

Antibiotic Resistance in *Staphylococcus* Species of Animal Origin

Miliane Moreira Soares de Souza[1], Shana de Mattos de Oliveira Coelho[1],
Ingrid Annes Pereira[2], Lidiane de Castro Soares[3],
Bruno Rocha Pribul[1] and Irene da Silva Coelho[1]
[1]Institute of Veterinary, Microbiology and Immunology Department,
Federal Rural University of Rio de Janeiro,
[2]Institute Osvaldo Cruz Foundation, Rio de Janeiro,
[3]University Severino Sombra, Rio de Janeiro,
Brazil

1. Introduction

Staphylococcus is a genus of worldwide distributed bacteria correlated to several infectious of different sites in human and animals. Its importance is not only because of its distribution and pathogenicity but especially due to its ability to overcome antimicrobial effects. The goal of this chapter is to report data obtained from a decade of research in animal science field concerning to staphylococci antimicrobial resistance.

2. Characteristics and distribution of Staphylococci species in animals: An overview

The genus *Staphylococcus* is in the bacterial family Staphylococcaceae (Ludwig, 2009). Staphylococci are Gram-positive spherical bacteria that occur in clusters resembling grapes due to its perpendicular division planes where cells remains attached to one another following each successive division.

The genotypic standards for assigning an organism to the genus *Staphylococcus* include determination of guanine plus cytosine (G+C) content of 30-39mol% and phylogenetic trees constructed by comparison of 16S rRNA or 23R rRNA sequences (Takahashi et al., 1999). The phenotypic criteria is based on the ultrastructure and chemical composition of the cell wall, typical form Gram positive bacteria and catalase reaction positive for all species, except for *S. aureus* subsp *anaerobius* and *S. saccharolyticus*, which are strictly anaerobic. This genus comprises more than 50 species separated into two distinct groups based on their ability to produce coagulase. This topic approaches *Staphylococcus* spp distribution considering that different animal species have specific staphylococcal microbiota. Otherwise some clonal strains can colonize different animal species as is the case of methicillin-resistant *Staphylococcus aureus* (MRSA). Molecular techniques have been used to relate clonal groups of MRSA isolated from different animal species in order to understand its model of dissemination.

2.1 Coagulase-positive Staphylococci

This group includes the major pathogenic *Staphylococcus* species. *Staphylococcus aureus* is considered the most pathogenic one, especially due to its ability to produce a large range of virulence factors that enables it to colonize different tissues of a large range of animal species. The coagulase protein has the ability to turn fibrinogen into fibrin threads by a mechanism different from natural clotting (Palma et al., 1999). This protein is codified by the gene *coa* which possess a conserved and a repeated polymorphic region that can be used to measure relatedness among *Staphylococcus* coagulase positive isolates (Reinoso et al., 2006). The variable region of *coa* is comprised of 81-bp tandem short sequence repeats (SSRs) that are variable in both number and sequence, as determined by restriction fragment length polymorphism analysis of PCR products (Goh et al., 1992).

Staphylococcal protein A is a membrane-bound exoprotein characterized and well known for its ability to bind to the Fc region of immunoglobulins of most mammalian species. This protein is encoded by the *spaA* gene with a polymorphic (X) and a conserved region. The polymorphic X region consists of a variable number of repeated 24 pairs of bases located in the coding region for the cellular wall C-terminal extremity (Koreen et al., 2004). The diversity of the *spaA* short sequence repeat region seems to arise from deletion and duplication of the repetitive units and also by point mutation and this variation can be used in epidemiological studies. Frenay et al. (1994) reported epidemic MRSA strains with more than seven repeats and Montesinos et al. (2002) described isolates with 11 repeats as the most common type involved in an epidemic human outbreak caused by MRSA. The *coa* typing can be used to enhance the value of *spa* typing by providing more supported inferences on strain lineage and clonality among isolates with similar or identical *spa* repeat organization (Tenover et al., 1994). The use of more than one genetic marker for relating strains is desirable and likely to become increasingly important because recombination will eventually diversify resistant staphylococcal species to the extent that clonal types within a given region can no longer be distinguished by a single locus.

Staphylococcus aureus also produces others exoproteins that contribute to its ability to colonize host tissues such as slime and hemolysins. The adherence and fixation of *S. aureus* on biological surfaces represent the fundamental step in the development of infections. The production of slime mediates adhesion to implanted surfaces acting as a cementing matrix making bacteria less accessible to the host's defense system (Coelho et al, 2009). Slime production is controlled by the *ica* operon (*icaADBC*) and the co-expression of the *icaA* and *icaD* genes leads to a significant increase in such production (Arciola et al., 2001).

The alpha and beta hemolysins are important factors in the pathogenesis of Staphylococcal infections. The beta-toxin is an Mg^{2+}-dependent sphingomyelinase C which degrades sphingomyelin in the outer phospholipid layer of the membrane (Linehan et al., 2003).

The *agr* (*accessory gene regulator*) operon (*agrA, agrB, agrC agrD* and *hld*) is recognized as a quorum-sensing gene cluster that up-regulates production of secreted virulence factors such as alpha and beta-hemolysins, proteases, DNAses and sphingomyelinase. This same cluster also down-regulates the production of cell-associated virulence factors in a cell density-dependent manner in *S. aureus* (Lyon et al., 2000). The *agr* locus comprises two divergent transcriptional units under the control of the promoters P2 (RNA II) and P3 (RNA III). The

P3 transcript, an RNA III molecule, mediates the up-regulation of secreted virulence factors as well as the down-regulation of surface proteins (Novick, 2000).

Coelho et al. (2011) evaluated the presence of some *Staphylococcus aureus* virulence genes, including *coa*, *spaA*, *hla* e *hlb* in order to understand the distribution of *S. aureus* strains in dairy farms at Rio de Janeiro, Brazil, and contribute to the establishment of preventive strategies to reduce the spread of infection.

In veterinary medicine, others coagulase-positive staphylococci are reported as important pathogens, such as *Staphylococcus intermedius*, whose reclassification was proposed by Devriese et al. (2005), creating the *S. intermedius* group (SIG) including *S. intermedius*, a new specie *S. pseudintermedius* and *S. delphini*. Like *S. aureus*, the *S. intermedius* strains isolated from animals have been reported to produce an array of virulence factors, including leukotoxin, enterotoxin, and hemolysins, together with elements essential for biofilm formation (Futagawa-Saito et al., 2006). Besides SIG, others significative coagulase-positive in animals are *S. schleiferi* subsp. *coagulans*, *S. aureus* subsp. *anaerobius*.

2.2 Coagulase-negative Staphylococci

This group comprises the majority of *Staphylococcus* species. Coagulase-negative staphylococci (CNS), which were traditionally considered to be minor infectious pathogens, have become more common (Huxley et al., 2002). Several CNSs have been isolated from animal clinical specimens such as *Staphylococcus epidermidis*, *Staphylococcus simulans*, *Staphylococcus xylosus*, *Staphylococcus chromogenes*, *Staphylococcus warneri*, *Staphylococcus haemolyticus*, *Staphylococcus sciuri*, *Staphylococcus saprophyticus*, *Staphylococcus hominis*, *Staphylococcus caprae*, *Staphylococcus cohnii* subsp. *cohnii*, *Staphylococcus cohnii* subsp. *urealyticus*, *Staphylococcus capitis* subsp. *capitis* and *Staphylococcus capitis* subsp. *urealyticus* (Lilenbaum et al., 2000; Pereira et al., 2009; Pyörälä et al., 2009; Soares et al., 2008).

The conventional methods for CNS identification were primarily developed for human strains and their poor performance for identifying strains of animal origin seems to be related to a limited number of veterinary strains in databases (Bes et al., 2000). Additionally, the reference method developed by Bannerman (2003) is costly and too time consuming to be used in a clinical laboratory. Several molecular targets have been exploited for the molecular identification of *Staphylococcus* species, including the *groEL* gene (Goh et al., 1996). This gene, which encodes a 60-kDa polypeptide (known as GroEL, 60-kDa chaperonin, or HSP60 for heat shock protein 60) has the potential to serve as a general phylogenic marker because of its ubiquity and conservation in nature (Segal & Ron, 1996). Also it was proven to be an ideal universal DNA target for identification to the species level because it has well-conserved DNA sequences within a given species, but with sufficient sequence variations to allow for species-specific identification (Goh et al., 1996). Santos et al., (2008) had successfully used the *groEL* gene as a tool for the identification of the main *Staphylococcus* coagulase-negative species by PCR restriction fragment length polymorphism (RFLP). This group investigated 54 cows from 23 dairy herds located in the Brazilian States of Minas Gerais, Rio de Janeiro and São Paulo, between 1995 and 2003 and concluded that this gene constitutes a reliable and reproducible molecular method for identification of CNS species responsible for bovine mastitis.

2.3 Staphylococcal infections in animals

Reports of the importance of *Staphylococcus* species as pathogens in animal infections have been described and appear to be increasing. Among coagulase-positive species, *Staphylococcus aureus* is a cause of mastitis, dermatitis and suppurative conditions in several animal species. *S. aureus* causing mastitis is widely distributed in cattle, goats and sheep. The infection is often subclinical in cattle, leading to reduced milk production and milk quality, but acute catarrhal or even gangrenous inflammation may also occur.

For a long time, *S. intermedius* had been majorly considered a primary cause of pyoderma in dogs. It has also been reported to be involved in other diseases, such as pyometra, otitis externa and purulent infections of the joints, eyelids and conjunctiva (Werckenthin et al., 2001). Nowadays, a new classification was proposed by Devriese et al. (2005), creating the *S. intermedius* group (SIG) including *S. intermedius*, a new specie *S. pseudintermedius* and *S. delphini*. According to Sasaki et al. (2007), *S. pseudintermedius* is actually the major specie involved in this pathology. Futhermore, according to these authors, *S. intermedius* is restricted to feral pigeons and *S. delphini* which was usually described as the cause of suppurative skin lesions in dolphins is now considered to be involved in a larger spectrum of infectious animal diseases. *S. aureus* subsp. *anaerobius* has been implicated in lymphadenitis in sheep and *S. schleiferi* subsp. *coagulans* in external otitis in dogs.

Coagulase Negative Staphylococci (CNSs) have also been studied considering its potential pathogenicity for human and animals. Nowadays these bacteria are of great interest in veterinary medicine because they are currently considered emerging pathogens of bovine mastitis. Although CNS are not as pathogenic as the other principal mastitis pathogens and infection mostly remains subclinical, they can cause persistent infections, which result in increased milk somatic cell count (SCC) and decreased milk quality (Pyorala & Taponen, 2009). The prevalence of CNS mastitis is higher in primiparous cows than in older cows. Also this agent is implicated in the etiology of infectious diseases in household pets (Pereira et al., 2009). The most frequently isolated CNS species vary according to the geographical region under scrutiny and sample origin. In Brazil, Soares et al. (2008) detected prevalence of *S.xylosus* in mastitic milk samples, despite *S. chromogenes*, *S. simulans* and *S. epidermidis*, in general, appear to be the most frequently isolated CNS from mammary secretion samples worldwide (De Vliegher et al., 2003; Taponen et al., 2006).

Besides, *S. hyicus*, a variable coagulase producer, but mainly coagulase-negative, causes exudative epidermitis ("greasy pig disease") and an often acute generalized skin infection in piglets. Systemic forms of the disease which result in the death of the animals are also seen. Poor hygienic conditions as well as ec

toparasitic infestations favour the onset of the *S. hyicus* infection. Surviving piglets show retarded growth rates. In adult pigs, subacute skin infections, mastitis or metritis, but also septic arthritis may be caused by *S. hyicus* (Brückler et al., 1994). In goats and sheep however, enzootic acute gangrenous mastitis is commonly seen.

3. Antimicrobial resistance in Staphylococci of animal origin

Antibiotic resistance is the most puzzling question of public healthy in the earlier decade of this 21st century. Among bacteria this question seems to be more alarming due to its short generation time and efficient gene recombination mechanisms. *Staphylococcus aureus* is the most representative example of how antibiotic resistance is a serious threatening worldwide. Nevertheless, all others coagulase-positive staphylococci are also able to develop resistance mechanisms to a large range of antimicrobials. Furthermore, the strains of several CNS species were also found to have high levels of resistance to various antibiotics.

This topic will discuss features of the resistance of staphylococci to antimicrobials, specially methicillin (oxacillin) and vancomicin, its mechanisms and epidemiology. Crucial questions about the use or abolishment of antibiotics used as "growth promoters" to food animal production will also be discussed.

3.1 Methicillin resistance

ß-lactamic antibiotics are the most frequently used in anti-staphylococcal infection therapy. Bacterial resistance mechanisms to this class of antibiotics include production of ß-lactamases and low-affinity penicillin-binding protein 2a (PBP2a) determined by the presence of the chromosomal genes *bla* and *mecA*, respectively. The latter, designated for methicillin resistance, precludes therapy with any of the currently available ß-lactam antibiotics, and may predict resistance to several classes of antibiotics (Moon et al., 2007). The isolation of *Staphylococcus aureus* methicillin- resistant (MRSA) from animals was first reported in 1972 following its detection in milk from mastitic cows (Devriese et al., 1972). Recent works reports a low incidence of MRSA mastitis and low prevalence of methicillin resistance among bovine *S. aureus* isolates (Juhász-Kaszanyitzky et al., 2007; Lee, 2003; Moon et al., 2007) so clinically it can be concluded that MRSA does not appear to be an important bovine mastitis pathogen. Nevertheless, the importance of epidemiological data concerns about MRSA in animals is reasonable and requires careful study in order to understand its emergence and dissemination. The long-term low prevalence of MRSA mastitis is quite surprising given the number of years since the first identification of MRSA in cattle and the close contact of humans with the udders of dairy cattle. Otherwise, several reports have been published showing MRSA infection in domestic animals, including dogs, cats, cattle, sheep, chickens, rabbits, and horses as an increasing trend (Goni et al., 2004; Hartmann et al., 1997; Lee, 2003; O'Mahony et al. 2005; Rich & Roberts 2004; Weese, 2005; Weese et al., 2006).

It is certain that animals are a source of human MRSA infection in some circumstances, but humans may also serve as sources of infection in animals. Exposure of household pets to MRSA was probably inevitable due to its increasingly prevalence in humans. Changes in the epidemiology of MRSA in unique specie may be reflected in changes in other species. The true scope of MRSA in animals and its impact on human health are still only superficially understood, but it is clear that MRSA is a potentially important veterinary and public health concern that requires a great deal more study to enhance understanding and effective response (Weese & Van Duijkeren, 2010). While most animals with MRSA are merely colonized, a wide range of clinical infections can occur. As would be expected with staphylococci, most MRSA infections in pets affect the skin and soft tissue. Wound infections, surgical site infections, pyoderma, otitis, and urinary tract infections are most common, but various other opportunistic infections have been reported (Baptiste et al., 2005; Griffeth & Morris, 2008). In a research developed by our team, 8% of MRSA was detected in a hundred of clinical specimens from different sites of household pets evaluated (Pereira et al., 2009).

Recently, a new MRSA was identified using high throughput DNA microarray screening. Complete genome sequencing revealed that this strain is distinctly different to previously described MRSA. It carries a new type of SCC*mec* encoding highly divergent genes that are very different to any described previously in MRSA or in any other organism. It was found to belong to the genetic lineage clonal complex 130 (CC130), which has previously only been associated with MSSA from cows and other animals, but not humans, strongly suggesting that the new MRSA originated in animals. (Gárcia-Alvarez et al., 2011)

Staphylococcal cassette chromosome *mec* (SCC*mec*) is a mobile genetic element composed by *mec* and *ccr* genes complex, which encodes methicillin resistance and the recombinases responsible for its mobility, respectively (Katayama et al., 2000). The expression of PBP-2a is controlled by regulator elements encoded by *mecR1* and *mecI* which are located adjacent to *mecA* on the chromosome. Deletion or mutation which occurred in *mec* regulator gene is considered to be associated with constitutive production of PBP-2a. Hence *Staphylococcus* spp possessing intact *mecRI* and *mecI* as well as *mecA* are phenotypically methicillin susceptible because of the repression of PBP-2a production by *mec* regulator elements. Such genomic changes in *mec* regulator genes are considered to alter or remove their repressor function on *mecA* gene transcription, which may lead to constitutive production of PBP-2a. The *mec* gene complex has been classified into four classes, and the *ccr* gene complex has been classified into three allotypes. Different combinations of *mec* and *ccr* gene complex types have so far defined six types of SCC*mec* elements (type I, II, III, IV, V) (Ito et al., 2004). It is important to analyze the genomic diversity found in *mec* regulator genes of staphylococci in order to understand the molecular basis for methicillin resistance.

The detection of methicillin resistance in routine clinical laboratories has been problematic ever since the emergence of MRSA during the 1960s and the difficulties are associated mainly with heterogeneous expression of resistance in most staphylococal strains currently prevalent (Witte et al., 2007). Misidentification of methicillin resistance can have serious adverse clinical consequences. False-susceptibility may result in treatment failure and in the spread of resistant *Staphylococcus* spp making it difficult to apply control measures and leading to the increasing of healthcare costs and may lead to overuse of glycopeptides (Velasco et al., 2005).

3.2 Vancomycin resistance

The glycopeptide vancomycin was first released in 1958. Vancomycin is an inhibitor of cell wall synthesis in *S. aureus* and other gram-positive organisms. While beta-lactam antibiotics inhibit cell wall synthesis by binding to the transpeptidase active site of penicillin binding proteins, vancomycin acts by a completely different mechanism so it has been the treatment of choice for serious infections caused by MRSA (Howden et al., 2010), but increase in vancomycin use has led to the emergence of two types of glycopeptide-resistant *S. aureus*. The first one, designated vancomycin intermediate resistant *S. aureus* (VISA) and the vancomycin-resistant S. aureus (VRSA).

The first report of clinical *S.aureus* isolate with reduced vancomycin susceptibility (VISA) was made by Hiramatsu et al. (1997) and generated great concern in the medical community. From there on, reports of strains of *S. aureus* (predominately MRSA) demonstrating the heterogeneous VISA (hVISA) or VISA phenotype have now been reported for many countries including the United States, Japan, Australia, France, Scotland, Brazil, South Korea, Hong Kong, South Africa, Thailand, Israel, and others (Bierbaum et al. 1999; Chang et al., 2003; Denis et al. 2002; Ferraz et al., 2000 Gemmell, 2004; Howden et al., 2010; Kim et al., 2000; Perichon & Courvalin, 2006; Sng et al.,2005; Song et al., 2004; Tenover et al., 2004; Weigel et al., 2007)

Nowadays it is conceivable that VISA phenotype is related to the bacterial cell wall thickening, a passive resistance mechanism that reduces vancomycin access to its active site, which is localized in the cytoplasmic membrane in the division septum (Howden et al., 2010). It results in accumulation of acyl-D-alanyl-D-alanine (X-DAla-D-Ala) targets in the periphery that sequester glycopeptides (Cui et al., 2003).

Since 2002, nine methicillin-resistant *Staphylococcus aureus* (MRSA) strains that are also resistant to vancomycin (VRSA) have been reported in the United States. The fully vancomicin-resistant *Staphylococcus aureus* phenotype (VRSA) is due to acquisition from *Enterococcus* spp. of the *vanA* operon, carried by transposon Tn1546, resulting in high-level resistance (Arthur et al., 1993, Patel et al., 1997).

The emergence of enterococci vancomicin-resistant strains has been related to the use of avoparcin as growth promoter in swine culture (Aarestrup et al., 1996). Studies report the transfer of glycopeptide- and macrolide-resistance genes by transconjugation among enterococci and from *Enterococcus faecalis* to *S. aureus* (Młynarczyk et al., 2002). The vancomycin-resistance gene acquisition by *S. aureus* from *E. faecium* in the clinical environment has also been reported by Weigel et al. (2007). Recently, Tiwari & Sen (2006) have reported a VRSA which is *van* gene-negative.

In veterinary medicine, vancomycin-resistant enterococci were isolated from the feces of poultry and pig herds. It has significant impact in public healthy cause dissemination via contaminated animal food products possible (Aarestrup, 1995). These vancomycin-resistant *E. faecium* isolates from animals had decreased susceptibilities to avoparcin, a glycopeptide antibiotic widely used as a growth promoter in Western Europe and Australasia. Avoparcin is a fermentation product from a strain of *Streptomyces candidus* and is closely related to vancomycin (Aarestrup et al., 1996). Aarestrup et al (1996) showed that *E. faecium* isolates coresistant to vancomycin and avoparcin are commonly found in the feces of pigs and poultry in Denmark.

3.3 Others antimicrobials resistance

In Veterinary Medicine, clindamycin has been chosen as an antimicrobial alternative for the treatment of infections in dogs and cats caused by methicillin-resistant *Staphylococcus aureus* (MRSA) (Walther et al., 2008; Weese et al., 2006) and methicillin-resistant *Staphylococcus pseudintermedius* (MRSP) (Schwarz et al., 2008; Wettstein et al., 2008). However, an inducible form of clindamycin-resistance may be present in some staphylococci. These staphylococcal strains appear susceptible on routine antimicrobial susceptibility testing, but resistance can be induced during treatment, possibly resulting in treatment failure (Swenson et al., 2007; Yilmaz et al., 2007).

Azithromycin have a remarkable application due to its superior pharmacokinetics properties and broad spectrum activity, including Gram-positive and negative bacteria species, intracellular pathogens and protozoan parasites. The principal characteristic that supported its prescription and clinical significance is that it can be administrated by oral and parental routes, only by a single daily dose in short period of treatment facilitating veterinary therapy. Nevertheless, most of the knowledge that supports its use in veterinary therapy was based on studies that proved its therapeutic efficacy in human infections. Empirical antimicrobial chemotherapy without previous accomplishment of bacterial identification and antimicrobial susceptibility assays contributes to increase of antimicrobial resistance prevalence in pet animal reservoirs (Guardabassi et al., 2004; Morgan et al.; 2008).

Pereira et al. (2009) evaluated azithromycin resistance among 100 staphylococci isolates from pet animals infections. It was detected a percentual of resistant isolates of 54% to *Staphylococcus intermedius*, 67% of *S. aureus*, 38% of *S. hyicus*, 67% of coagulase-negative *Staphylococcus* spp through disc diffusion test. The variability of azithromycin susceptibility pattern is different to what is observed in humans infections whereas *Staphylococcus aureus* is the classical isolated pathogen. Broth dilution test detected azithromycin $MIC_{50/90}$ values of 16μg/mL, 64μg/mL in staphylococci isolates, respectively, and 256μg/mL in Gram-negative rods (GNR). Agar dilution azithromycin $MIC_{50/90}$ values corresponded to 32μg/mL and 256μg/mL in staphylococci and >512μg/mL in GNR. Crescent azithromycin resistance rate has been previously reported. A study from 90's decade, detected azithromycin $MIC_{50/90}$ >128 μg/mL of MRSA isolated from human clinical samples (Neu, 1991). When comparing human MIC values reported in literature to data obtained from pet animal samples in the present study, azithromycin activity pattern may vary from different bacteria species and hosts, leading to therapeutic failures when classical human pathogens are adopted as reference to calculate dose and drug concentration. This justify microbiologic and pharmacokinetic assays to determine the specific azithromycin susceptibility breakpoints and therapeutic drug concentration to different bacteria species detected from animal disease.

It is important to point that MIC_{50} values varied among different staphylococci species, such as, *Staphylococcus intermedius* (32μg/mL), *S. hyicus* (32μg/mL), CNS (32μg/mL), from that value detected in *S. aureus* (16μg/mL) isolated from pet animal specimens.

Pereira et al. (2009) also evaluated the genetic markers of *Staphylococcus* spp azithromycin resistance by PCR technique and detected a 39% prevalence of *erm* genes, being *ermC* gene the most detected, showing a prevalence of 24% among all *Staphylococcus* isolates, followed by 12% *ermA* and 3% of *ermB*. No isolates were positive to *mefA* gene, what may support the theory about methylase ribossomal modification as the principal resistance mechanism associated to macrolide resistance among staphylococci. The expression of *erm* genes can be inducible or constitutive. When expression is constitutive, the staphylococci are resistant to all macrolide, lincosamide and streptogramin B (MLS_B) antimicrobials (Schmitz et al., 2000). In this study, it was detected MLS_B resistance in 14% constitutive azithromycin-resistant *Staphylococcus* spp. Inducible resistance phenotype, expressed by a "D zone" next to clindamycin disc was available in 5% (5/100) of *Staphylococcus* spp.

Most of the knowledge applied to define microbiologic use and dose of azithromycin was based on *Staphylococcus aureus* assays, because this specie acts as classical pathogen of human infections, but the frame of etiology and antimicrobial susceptibility pattern change when animal pathogens are considered.

Gentamicin is one of the most used antibiotics in dairy farm cattle. It is especially used as a prophylactic measure of mastitis control through intramammary injection. Its principal resistance mechanism is mediated by the production of enzymes which transform aminoglycosides into inactive derivatives, such as acetyltranspherases, adenylyltranspherases and phosphotransferases. Modified aminoglycosides lose the ability to bind ribosomes and inhibit bacterial protein synthesis (Watanabe et al., 2009). Specific staphylococcal resistance to gentamicinis mediated by a bifuntional enzyme that acts as both acetyltranspherase and adenylyltranspherase. This enzyme is codified by the genes *aac* (6')-*Ie* + *aph* (2") which are transported in transposon Tn4001 located in plasmids of pSK1 family, conjugative plasmids pSK23 and in the chromosome (Udo & Dashti, 2000). Genetic elements Tn4001 are disseminated in *S. aureus* and CNSs. There is little information about its occurrence in staphylococci of animal origin (Lange et al., 2003).

3.4 Growth promoters

Antibiotic use in sub therapeutic levels as growth promoters is still common in Brazilian animal production. Defenders of this model believe that antimicrobial abolishment will result in higher morbidity, with a consequent raise of antimicrobial therapeutic use and consequently higher mortality. Also they think that it will directly implicate the efficiency of productivity as animals without growth promoters have a higher food consumer to achieve the same weight gain.

On the other hand, the European Economic Community established severe restrictions for products presenting antimicrobial residues defending the idea that this sub therapeutic use contributes to a positive selective pressure and to the spread of antimicrobial resistance genes between different pathogens. European Market defends that efficient animal handling is sufficient to control the infectious diseases and that avoid the probability of antimicrobial therapeutic failure. It is a highly controversial subject of extreme importance in a world concerned to the need of the improvement of food production. The experience of avoparcin use as growth promoter in some European countries and the consequent dissemination of a crossed-resistance to vancomycin in *Enterococcus faecium* and *E. faecalis* seems to be related to the adoption of these restrictive measures (Aarestrup et al., 1996)

Since 2003, Brazil instituted a work group in order to analyze and evaluate the use of substances such as carbadox, olaquindox, bacitracin zinc, spiramycin, virginiamycin and tylosin phosphate as animal feed additives products. In 2005, it also included the evaluation of avilamycin, flavomycin, enramycin, monensin and maduramycin.

The most efficient alternative to the antimicrobial indiscriminate use are probiotics. Probiotic acts in a significantly different mechanism from antimicrobials. They are thought to improve intestinal microbial balance through favoring the elimination of pathogenic bacteria and the proliferation of non pathogenic organisms. As a consequence it contributes to growth promotion without enhance antimicrobial resistance.

4. Advances in the field of nucleic acid-based techniques for the identification/typing and detection of antibiotic resistant *Staphylococcus* species

The importance of being able to identify staphylococci species routinely in clinical laboratories is increasing. However, the exact identification of CNS is not easy, because the biochemical traits of the species are very similar and many clinical isolates show intermediate traits. Additionally, the use of commercial identification kits to identify staphylococci does not include all *Staphylococcus* species, and their reliability for certain species is not sufficient. Molecular methods of identification seem to be the key to fulfill these spaces, as gene specific markers are being recognized. In the same way, molecular techniques have been developed in order to improve the detection of antibiotic resistant bacterial strains. So, nucleic acid-based detection systems offer rapid and sensitive methods to detect the presence of resistance genes and play a critical role in the elucidation of resistance mechanisms. This topic will discuss the variety of nucleic-based techniques used for diagnostic applications and demonstrate that no universal technique exists which is optimal for detection of specific genes. The choice of a particular technique is also dependent on the information required or the targets under consideration, but some techniques are more favored than others.

The advantages of genotypic detection of antibiotic resistance and bacterial characterization include: (i) The search for a defined resistance determinant; (ii) Independence upon phenotypic categories such as susceptibility, intermediate susceptibility and resistance for which breakpoints may vary between countries; (iii) Detection of low-level resistance which is difficult to detect using phenotypic methods; (iv) Reduction of the detection time through its performance directly with clinical specimens. This is particularly important for difficult-to-culture organisms; (v) Reduction in detection time of slow growth of the organism; (vi) More precise and fast therapeutic predictions; (vii) Minor biohazard risk once it is not necessary to propagate by culture of a microorganism (Sundsfjord et al., 2004).

On the other hand, the genotypic approach contains certain limitations and pitfalls: (i) It is based on screening for resistance determinants whereas antimicrobial therapy is preferably based on the detection of susceptibility; (ii) You can only screen for what you already know so it does not take into account new resistance mechanisms; (iii) There are silent genes and pseudogenes that may cause false-positive results. (iv) It may detect not clinically relevant resistance genotypes; (v) Mutations in primer binding sites can generate false-negative results; (vi) It presents low clinical sensitivity when performed directly on mixed microbial samples due to inhibition of nucleic acid amplification or a limited number of targets; (vii) Regulatory mutations that affect gene expression are not detected unless a quantitative measurement of the specific mRNA is targeted; (viii) Unlike for conventional culture-based susceptibility test methods, no standards exist for performing genetic testing methods (Sundsfjord et al., 2004).

Nucleic acid-based technology can be divided into hybridization systems and amplification systems, although most amplification technologies are also partly based on hybridization technology.

In hybridization, the DNA in a sample is rendered single stranded and allowed to combine with a single-stranded probe. Early hybridizations were performed with target DNA immobilized on a nitrocellulose membrane, but nowadays a variety of different solid supports are used. After binding of the target, the probe can hybridize. Probes can be labeled with a variety of reporters, including radioactive isotopes, antigenic substrates, enzymes or chemiluminescent compounds. Current modalities of hybridization DNA or RNA that have been used to detection of antimicrobial resistance in *Staphylococcus* spp. are Southern and Northern Blotting, FISH (Fluorescence *In Situ* Hybridization), microarray and Branched DNA (bDNA).

In Southern blotting, DNA becomes immobilized on a membrane and can be used as a substrate for hybridization analysis with labelled DNA or RNA probes that specifically target individual restriction fragments in the blotted DNA (Southern, 1975). The major difference between Southern and Northern blotting is that in the latter, RNA, rather than DNA, is immobilized in the membrane. The Southern blotting techniques was utilized to detect *mec*A gene in *Staphylococcus aureus* and to evaluate the efficiency of the techniques as PCR (Bignardi et al., 1996; Lan Mo & Qi-nan Wang, 1997).

Fluorescence *In Situ* Hybridization (FISH) is a technique originally developed for clinical diagnosis (Levsky & Singer, 2003). This approach applies the principle of hybridization involving the penetration of a fluorescent labeled sequence-specific nucleic acid probe into fixed cells, followed by specific binding to the complementary sequences of the target nucleic acid. It allows rapid simultaneous detection of structurally intact target genes while they are with the associated organism or particle (Bottari et al., 2006). It involves direct detection of the DNA without amplification of the target sequence and can be especially useful to detect specific bacterial community and antibiotic resistance gene (Rahube & Yost, 2010). A peptide nucleic acid fluorescence in situ hybridization (PNA FISH) (AdvanDx, Woburn, MA, USA) assay was development to rapidly detect *Staphylococcus aureus* (Forrest et al., 2006; Lawson et al., 2011). Peptide nucleic acid (PNA) molecules are pseudopeptides that obey Watson-Crick base-pairing rules for hybridization to complementary nucleic acid targets (RNA and DNA) (Nielsen et al., 1994). Due to their uncharged, neutral backbones, PNA probes exhibit favorable hybridization characteristics such as high specificities, strong affinities, and rapid kinetics, resulting in improved hybridization to highly structured targets such as rRNA. In addition, the relatively hydrophobic character of PNA compared to that of DNA oligonucleotides enables PNA probes to penetrate the hydrophobic cell wall of bacteria following mild fixation conditions that do not lead to disruption of cell morphology (Stefano & Hyldig-Nielsen, 1997).

DNA microarrays are based on the principle of hybridization which allow the mass screening of sequences. The method is based upon gene-specific probes (oligonucleotides or PCR amplicons) deposited on a solid surface like glass or a silicon chip. The test DNA is extracted, labelled and hybridized to the array. Target-probe duplexes are detected with a reporter system. Probe-target hybridization is usually detected and quantified by detection of fluorophore-, silver-, or chemiluminescence-labeled targets to determine relative abundance of nucleic acid sequences in the target (Schena et al., 1995). Microarray technology enables detection of a large number of resistance genes in a single experiment and has the potential for significant automation in a microchip format. However, a cost-effective and user-friendly format for application in antimicrobial susceptibility testing remains to be developed (Sundsfjord et al., 2004). There are many examples of the use of DNA microarray for detection of antibiotic resistance genes in staphylococcal (Cui et al., 2005; Frye et al., 2006; Garneau et al., 2010; Monecke et al., 2007; Zhu et al., 2007a). Recently, a team of scientists at the University of Dublin, the Irish National MRSA Reference Laboratory and the University of Dresden and Alere Technologies in Germany identified a new MRSA strain using high throughput DNA microarray screening. The new strain is not detected as MRSA by routine conventional and real time DNA-based polymerase chain reaction (PCR) assays commonly used to screen patients for MRSA (Shore et al., 2011).

Branched DNA (bDNA) was developed by Chiron Corp. and uses multiple hybridization sites for enzyme-coupled probes (Nolte, 1998). Target-specific probes bound to a solid surface are allowed to capture target ssDNA. A second probe is allowed to hybridize with the target. This probe has a 5′ extension that does not hybridize with the target. This extension can hybridize with a bDNA probe. This probe has a bristle-like structure. At least 15 bristles are attached to each probe, and as many as three alkaline phosphatase reporter molecules can bind to each bristle. A signal is generated by the addition of a chemiluminescent substrate. Branched DNA was used to detect *mecA* gene in *Staphylococcus* spp. culture and from blood (Kolbert et al., 1998; Zheng et al., 1999).

The amplification systems include, but are not limited to, simple and multiplex PCR, PCR-RFLP, PCR-single-strand conformation polymorphism (PCR-SSCP), DNA sequencing and real-time PCR. Amplification methods are more easily adapted in the laboratory compared to DNA probe assays and are the preferred methods for genetic detection of resistance determinants. An internal amplification control for both sample preparation and amplification is recommended to exclude false-negative results using consensus 16S rDNA primers or a more genus-or species-specific target; e.g. the *nuc* gene for *Staphylococcus aureus* (Brakstad et al., 1992; Hoorfar et al., 2004; Vannuffel et al., 1995). It is also critical that negative controls without template DNA and positive controls with defined targets be included to check for false-positive and false-negative results, respectively.

The Polymerase Chain Reaction (PCR) was first described by Mullis et al. (1987), and its first diagnostic application was published by Saiki et al. (1988). The technique became broadly used after the introduction of a thermostable DNA polymerase from *Thermus aquaticus* (Taq DNA polymerase) (Saiki et al., 1988) and the development of automated oligonucleotide synthesis and thermocyclers. PCR involves cycles of heating the sample for denaturing, annealing of the primers, and elongation of the primers. It has been the most commonly used nucleic acid amplification technique in the detection of antimicrobial genes, including *Staphylococcus aureus* (Simeoni et al., 2008).

Multiplex Polymerase Chain Reaction (Multiplex PCR) is a modification of PCR that have also been used to detection of antimicrobial genes in *Staphylococcus aureus* (Amghalia, et al., 2009; Braoios et al., 2009; Zhang et al., 2005) which consists of multiple primer sets within a single PCR mixture to produce amplicons of varying sizes that are specific to different DNA sequences. By targeting multiple genes at once, additional information may be gained from a single test run that otherwise would require several times the reagents and more time to perform.

The specificity of the amplicon can be confirmed by various methods such as restriction fragment length polymorphism (RFLP) analysis, single-strand conformational polymorphism (SSCP) analysis or DNA sequencing.

Restriction Fragment Length Polymorphism, or RFLP is a technique that exploits variations in homologous DNA sequences. It refers to a difference between samples of homologous DNA molecules that come from different locations of restriction enzyme sites. In PCR-RFLP analysis, the PCR product is digested by restriction enzymes and the resulting *restriction* fragments are separated according to their lengths by gel electrophoresis. It has been used to detect *groEL* gene in order to differentiate CNS species (Santos et al., 2007).

In PCR-single-strand conformation polymorphism (PCR-SSCP), the PCR amplication product is denatured into two single-stranded molecules and subjected to nondenaturing polyacrylamide gel electrophoresis. Under nondenaturing conditions, the single-stranded DNA (ssDNA) molecule has a secondary structure that is determined by the nucleotide sequence, buffer conditions, and temperature. PCR-SSCP is capable of detecting more than 90% of all single-nucleotide changes in a 200-nucleotide fragment (Hayashi, 1992).

DNA sequencing is almost universally performed by dideoxysequencing (Sanger et al., 1977) and is a well-known technique. Technological developments brought DNA sequencing within the capabilities of at least some diagnostic laboratories. The latest developments in nucleic acid sequence techniques, the pyrosequencing, have made the detection of mutational resistance easier by rapid DNA sequence analysis (Ronaghi et al., 1998). This technique has been used in the detection of linezolid resistance in enterococci, and to identify point mutations in 23S rRNA genes of linezolid-resistance *Staphylococcus aureus* and *Staphylococcus epidermis* (Sinclair et al., 2003; Zhu et al., 2007b) as well as rapid bacterial identification (Ronaghi et al., 2002).

The laborious post-PCR work and problems with carry-over contamination have been largely removed by the advent of real-time PCR, a powerful improvement on the basic PCR technique (Higuchi et al., 1993). The combination of fluorescent detection strategies with appropriate instrumentation enables a more accurate quantification of nucleic acids. This quantification is achieved by the measure ofthe increase in fluorescence during the exponential phase of PCR. The use of fluorescent agents and probes that only generate a fluorescence signal on binding to their target enables real-time amplification assays to be carried out in sealed tubes, eliminating the risk of carryover contamination. Different techniques are available to monitor real-time amplification. The amplification process can be monitored using nonspecific double-stranded deoxyribonucleic acid (DNA) binding dyes or specific fluorescent hybridization probes.

Four different chemistries, SYBR® Green (Molecular Probes), TaqMan® (Applied Biosystems, Foster City, CA, USA), Molecular Beacons and Scorpions® are available for real-time PCR.

Real-time PCR techniques have permitted the development of routine diagnostic applications for the microbiology laboratory (Espy et al., 2006; Mackay, 2004). Several reports have described the use of these techniques for detection of resistance determinants and surveillance of antimicrobial-resistant *Staphylococcus* spp. (Fang & Hedin, 2003; Huletsky et al., 2004; Palladino et al., 2003; Paule et al., 2005; Thomas et al., 2007; Volkmann et al., 2004). The ability to monitor the accumulating amplicon in real time is based on labelled primers, oligonucleotide probes and/or fluorescing amplicons producing a detectable quantitative signal related to the amount and specificity of the amplicon. Several improvements have been introduced. Reduced amplicon size, shorter cycling times and removal of separate post-PCR detection systems have allowed automation, reduced the detection time, and minimized the risk for carry-over contamination. Other significant technical developments include multiplex PCR assays using more than one primer set for simultaneous detection of several antimicrobial resistance genes (Depardieu et al., 2004; Martineau et al., 2000a; Sabet et al., 2006; Šeputienė et al., 2010; Suhaili et al., 2009).

4.1 Molecular Identification/Typing of *Staphylococcus* species

Earlier studies on the taxonomy of *Staphylococcus* species based on DNA-DNA reassociation indicated that in the genus there were nine distinct species groups, represented by *S. epidermidis*, *S. saprophyticus*, *S. simulans*, *S. intermedius*, *S. hyicus*, *S. sciuri*, *S. auricularis*, *S. aureus*, and *Staphylococcus caseolyticus* (Kloos & George, 1991). Several molecular targets have been exploited for the molecular identification of *Staphylococcus* species, including the 16S rRNA gene (De Buyser et al., 1992), the tRNA gene intergenic spacer (Maes et al., 1997), the heat shock protein 60 (HSP60) gene (Kwok et al., 1999), and the *femA* gene (Vannuffel et al., 1999). These targets, however, have been exploited through the technology of molecular probe hybridization, and therefore, they are useful only in laboratories that have the complete panel of probes and then only for identifying recognized *Staphylococcus* species. Further molecular targets that have been identified include the *nuc* gene, which occurs only in *S. aureus* (Brasktad et al., 1992), and a chromosomal DNA fragment specific for *Staphylococcus epidermidis* (Martineau et al., 1996).

The *rpoB*, gene encoding the highly conserved β subunit of the bacterial RNA polymerase, has previously been demonstrated to be a suitable target on which to base the identification of enteric bacteria (Mollet et al.,1997), spirochetes (Renesto et al.,2000), bartonellas (Renesto et al.,2001), and rickettsias (Drancourt & Raoult, 1999). The gene has been shown to be more discriminative than the 16S ribosomal DNA (rDNA) gene, which has also been used for identifying staphylococal bacteria (Mollet et al., 1997). In contrast to the probe hybridization technique and the RFLP approach, sequencing enables any isolate to be characterized, including new species by their phylogenetic relationships.

Other suitable targets for the molecular identification of *Staphylococcus* species that have been proposed include the *femA* gene, which was used in a multiplex PCR-reverse hybridization approach to identify 55 clinical isolates (Vannuffel et al.,1999). These, however, included only five *Staphylococcus* species, namely *S. aureus*, *S. epidermidis*, *S. hominis*, *S. saprophyticus*, and *S. simulans*. Finally, molecular identification methods for the identification of one or only a few *Staphylococcus* species have been reported for *S. saprophyticus* (Martineau et al., 2000b), *S. aureus* (Benito et al., 2000), and *S. epidermidis* (Wieser & Busse, 2000). Whole-genome DNA-DNA hybridization analysis (Svec et al., 2004) allows species identification, but the method is not suitable for routine use.

Accurate and rapid typing of *Staphylococcus aureus* is crucial to the control of infectious organisms (Naffa et al., 2005), and many different pheno- and genotyping methods have been used to distinguish their strains. Typing methods should have high and relevant discriminatory power and typeability, good reproducibility, applicability to all organisms of interest, ease of use, portability and low cost (Struelens et al., 1996). The common phenotyping techniques used for discriminating between bacteria from a single species are serotype, biotype, bacteriophage typing, or antibiogram. Techniques DNA-based such as pulsed field gel electrophoresis (PFGE), amplified fragment length polymorphism (AFLP), and multilocus sequence typing (MLST) have been many used (Melles et al., 2004; Murchan et al., 2003; Tenover et al., 1994). Other common techniques use the Polymerase Chain Reaction (PCR) targeted to specific sequences, for example ERIC-PCR; the resulting reactions yield fragments of different sizes, which can be used to discriminate between bacterial types. Sequencing an entire bacterial genome, and, using micro-array technologies, comparing strains to a reference strain (comparative genomic hybridization) is now technically feasible; however, the cost and time required limits the applicability for most epidemiologic studies (Foxman et al., 2005).

PFGE is the most commonly used method when studying local or short-term *S. aureus* epidemiology (Chung et al., 2000). PFGE involves embedding organisms in agarose, lysing the organisms in situ, and digesting the chromosomal DNA with restriction endonucleases that cleave infrequently (Finey, 1993; Goering & Winters, 1992). Slices of agarose containing the chromosomal DNA fragments are inserted into the wells of an agarose gel, and the restriction fragments are resolved into a pattern of discrete bands in the gel by an apparatus that switches the direction of current according to a predetermined pattern. The DNA restriction patterns of the isolates are then compared with one another to determine their relatedness. Multicentre studies using PFGE are now possible due to recent advances in the standardization of electrophoresis conditions (Chung et al., 2000; Oliveira et al., 2001) and the development of normalization and analysis software (Duck et al., 2003). Interpretative criteria for use in comparing complex PFGE patterns in outbreaks have been applied to non-outbreak situations to track the national and international dissemination of *S. aureus* clones (Tenover et al., 1995). The use of PFGE typing with adjusted interpretation criteria for grouping patterns with < 7 bands difference has been shown to correspond to clonal assignments made by other methods (Denis et al., 2004). The main criticisms of this technique for *S. aureus* are that PFGE may, on occasion, be too discriminatory for other than local or short-term epidemiological analyses, the arbitrary nature of the interpretive criteria used and the requirement for occasional subjective analysis of complex band patterns (Murchan et al., 2004).

Amplified fragment length polymorphism (AFLP) (Vos et al., 1995), a typing method, also documents the contribution of "accessory genetic elements" next to genome–core polymorphisms. AFLP scans for polymorphism in actual restriction sites and the nucleotides bordering these sites. As such it documents nucleotide sequence variation, insertions and deletions across entire genomes (Vos et al., 1995).

Multilocus sequence typing (MLST) (Maiden et al., 1998) has had a large impact on the field of bacterial typing and it has been used as an investigatory tool in many studies of *S. aureus* evolution and epidemiology (Aires de Sousa et al., 2003, Coombs et al., 2004, Enright et al., 2002; Mato et al., 2004). MLST characterizes bacterial isolates on the basis of sequence polymorphism within internal fragments of seven housekeeping genes, representing the stable "core" of the staphylococcal genome. Each gene fragment is translated into a distinct allele, and each isolate is classified as a sequence type (ST) by the combination of alleles of the seven housekeeping loci (Enright et al., 2002). MLST has a major advantage over PFGE as a reference method due to the unambiguous nature of DNA sequences which can be stored easily along with corresponding clinical information on each isolate in internet-linked databases. The *S. aureus* MLST website (www.mlst.net) currently contains information on > 1500 isolates from humans and animals from 40 different countries and represents a useful global resource for the study of the epidemiology of this species and the surveillance of hyper-virulent and / or antibiotic resistant clones.

The variety of molecular techniques used for diagnostic applications demonstrate that no universal technique exists which is optimal for detection of nucleic acids. The choice of a particular technique is also dependent on the information required or the targets under consideration, but some techniques are more favored than others. Hence, the genetic approach based on today's test principles cannot substitute for phenotypic methods in routine antimicrobial susceptibility testing. Novel resistance mechanisms will arise continuously or unknown pre-existing resistance genes will be mobilized from environmental reservoirs and spread under antimicrobial selection (Barlow et al., 2004). Thus, the role of traditional susceptibility testing will continue to be important. Rather the rationale for genetic assays is to complement conventional phenotypic analyses (Sundsfjord et al., 2004). Challenges that remain include the variety of point mutations or genes leading to resistance and the labor-intensive nature of current amplification methods. DNA chip technology combined with automated amplification techniques has the potential to meet these challenges. However, the development of DNA chips containing a broad range of resistance markers that are usable for many different species remains a formidable challenge and requires a broader knowledge of resistance markers than is currently available (Sundsfjord et al., 2004).

5. The relevance of surveillance for the prediction of antibiotic resistance

This topic discusses the relevance and limitations of surveillance initiatives in veterinary practice. Antibiotic resistance surveillance is based on the identification of new challenges, detection of new resistance mechanisms, monitoring the impact of new empiric antibiotic prescribing, identification of outbreaks of resistant organisms, detection of bacterial misidentification and promotion of the establishment of standards and **guidelines** for **education** and training for veterinaries, animal keepers, animal owners and the general public.

Cats and dogs represent potential sources of spread of antimicrobial resistance due to the extensive use of antimicrobial agents in these animals and their close contact with humans. Modern society has contributed to radical changes in the relationship between companion animals and humans through the years, with a significant raise in cats and dogs population and to a closer contact with humans (Guardabassi et al., 2004).

The introduction of a new drug, especially an antibiotic, has to be monitored in order to achieve its real benefit to the target audience. Recently, azithromycin was introduced to Brazilian pet market claiming to be an advantageous antimicrobial alternative to dogs and cats infections such as pyodermitis, external otitis, respiratory and urinary tract disturbs. Azithromycin have a remarkable application due to its superior pharmacokinetics properties and broad spectrum activity, including Gram-positive and negative bacteria species, intracellular pathogens and protozoan parasites Pereira et al. (2009) evaluated the resistance to azithromycin of 225 clinical samples from different infectious sites of pet animals in order to establish the benefits of introducing this drug in veterinary therapy in Brazil since it has already been used for human therapy. Azithromycin resistance can be caused by several mechanisms, such as target modification mediated by a 23S rRNA methylase, presence of efflux pumps and drug inactivation (Lim et al., 2002). These resistance mechanisms were identified in a wide range of Gram-positive and negative bacteria, such as, *Staphylococcus* spp, *Streptococcus* spp, *Enterococcus faecium*, *Corynebacterium* spp, *Pseudomonas aeruginosa*, *Escherichia coli* and *Bacteroides* spp, all of them implicated in the etiology of household pets infections. Among them, *Staphylococcus* spp, a resident member of the normal cutaneous and mucosal microbiota of humans and animals, stands out as an important pathogen involved in several animals infectious diseases due to its wide range of virulence factors and ability to overcome antimicrobial effects (Garber, 2001). Predominant staphylococci azithromycin resistance mechanisms are that mediated to *erm*(A) and *erm*(C) determinants of 23S rRNA methylase and *mef* genes that encode efflux pumps. The *erm*(A) genes are mostly spread in methicillin-resistant strains and are borne by transposons related to Tn*554*, whereas *erm*(C) genes are mostly responsible for macrolide resistance in methicillin-susceptible strains and are borne by plasmids (Lim et al., 2002). Most of the knowledge applied to define microbiologic use and dose of azithromycin was based on *Staphylococcus aureus* assays, because this specie acts as a classical pathogen of human infections, but the frame of etiology and antimicrobial susceptibility pattern change when animal pathogens are considered.

Otherwise, gentamicin, even being the most utilized antimicrobial in bases for intramammary use, keeps its effectiveness against staphylococci isolated from mastitic milk. Those data support the idea of the importance of monitoring the impact of new/old empiric antibiotic prescribing

6. Concluding remarks

- *Staphylococcus* species distribution considers that different animal species have a different staphylococcal microbiota divided into coagulase-positive and coagulase-negative groups. In veterinary medicine, besides *S. aureus*, others coagulase-positive species are reported as important pathogens, such as *Staphylococcus intermedius*, the new specie *S. pseudintermedius*, *S. delphini*, *S. schleiferi* subsp. *coagulans* and *S. aureus* subsp. *anaerobius*. Several Coagulase-negative Staphylococci have been isolated from animal clinical specimens such as *Staphylococcus epidermidis*, *Staphylococcus simulans*, *Staphylococcus xylosus*, *Staphylococcus chromogenes*, *Staphylococcus warneri*, *Staphylococcus haemolyticus*, *Staphylococcus sciuri*, *Staphylococcus saprophyticus*, *Staphylococcus hominis*, *Staphylococcus caprae*, *Staphylococcus cohnii* subsp. *cohnii*, *Staphylococcus cohnii* subsp. *urealyticus*, *Staphylococcus capitis* subsp. *capitis* and *Staphylococcus capitis* subsp. *urealyticus*.
- *Staphylococcus aureus* is considered the most pathogenic specie, especially due to its ability to produce a large range of virulence factors that enables it to colonize different tissues of a large range of animal species, such as coagulase, slime, protein A, hemolysins. Otherwise, like *S. aureus*, the *S. intermedius* strains isolated from animals have been reported to produce an array of virulence factors, including leukotoxin, enterotoxin, and hemolysins, together with elements essential for biofilm formation.
- The epidemiological and clinical importance of Staphylococcal species is not only because of its distribution and pathogenicity but especially due to its ability to overcome antimicrobial effects. So there is a need for continued vigilance and systematic study to enlarge the understanding of its dynamic. Considering the spread of MRSA strains it is necessary to determine risk factors for animal infections, especially for household pets that live in strict contact to men, the relationship between animal and human carriage, and the genetic relationship of animal and human strains.
- hVISA or VISA phenotype, mostly MRSA, have now been reported for many countries and it is considered to be related to the bacterial cell wall thickening, a passive resistance mechanism that reduces vancomycin access to its active site. Also MRSA strains that are also VRSA have been reported in the United States. VRSA phenotype is

due to acquisition from *Enterococcus* spp. of the *vanA* operon, carried by transposon Tn1546, resulting in high-level resistance. The emergence of enterococci vancomicin-resistant strains has been related to the use of avoparcin as growth promoter in swine culture and it seemed to arise in staphylococci due to the transfer of glycopeptide- and macrolide-resistance genes by transconjugation among enterococci and from *Enterococcus faecalis* to *S. aureus*.

- The large range of molecular techniques available for use demonstrates that no universal technique exists which is optimal for detection of nucleic acids. The choice of a particular technique is also dependent on the information required or the targets under consideration. Hence, the genetic approach based on today's test principles cannot substitute for phenotypic methods in routine identification and antimicrobial susceptibility testing.
- Antibiotic resistance surveillance is based on the identification of new challenges, detection of new resistance mechanisms, monitoring the impact of new empiric antibiotic prescribing, identification of outbreaks of resistant organisms, detection of bacterial misidentification and promotion of the establishment of standards and **guidelines** for **education** and training for veterinaries, animal keepers, animal owners and the general public.

7. Future challenges

Tenover (2008) in his article "Vancomicin-resistant *Staphylococcus aureus*: a Perfect but Geographically Limited Storm?" gives us a clue that antibitioc resistance issue is not so simple answer. Science is a creative activity that request exploration and gambling. We have to be open-minded to understand that some evolutionary steps are more successful than others and the pathways to resistance are not so predictable. As Tenover (2008) said: "Predicting which resistant strains will ultimately survive and disseminate is virtually impossible; predicting that at least some strains will disseminate broadly is a certainty." The biggest challenge is keep researching in order to enhance our knowledge of the mechanisms beyond resistance, the evolutionary pathways of resistance among microorganisms, and selective pressure factors that contribute to the expression of underlying genes.

8. Acknowledgments

We are grateful to FAPERJ for Grants No. E-26/103.076/2008 and E-26/111.147/20108 and CNPq for Grant No 473140/2008-0. We express our sincere thanks to Professor Cristina Bogni and Professor Mirta Demo, Department of Microbiology, University of Rio Cuarto, Cordoba, Argentina, for providing us with technical conditions for the development of part of this work. We have no words to express our deep gratitude to Professor Elina Reinoso, Department of Microbiology, University of Rio Cuarto, Cordoba, Argentina, and Dr. José Ivo Baldani, EMBRAPA – Agrobiologia, Brazil, for helping us performing the initial PCR experiments for Shana Coelho tesis.

9. References

Aarestrup, F. M. (1995). Occurrence of glycopeptide resistance among *Enterococcus faecium* isolates from conventional and ecological poultry farms. *Microbiological Drug Resistance*. Vol.1, pp. 255–257.

Aarestrup, F.M.; Ahrens, P.; Madsen,M.; Pallesen,L.V.; Poulsen, R.L. & Westh, H. (1996). Glycopeptide susceptibility among Danish *Enterococcus faecium* and Enterococcus faecalis isolates of animal and human origin and PCR identification of genes within the *VanA* cluster. *Antimicrobial Agents and Chemotherapy*. Vol. 40, No. 8, pp. 1938-1940.

Aires de Sousa, M.; Bartzavali, C.; Spiliopoulou, I.; Sanches, I.S.; Crisostomo, M.I. & H. de Lencastre. (2003). Two international methicillin-resistant *Staphylococcus aureus* clones endemic in a university hospital in Patras, Greece. *Journal of Clinical Microbiology*. Vol. 41, pp. 2027–2032.

Amghalia, E.; Nagi, A.A.; Shamsudin, M.N.; Radu, S.; Rosli, R.; Neela, V. & Rahim, R.A. (2009). Multiplex PCR Assays for the Detection of Clinically Relevant Antibiotic Resistance Genes in *Staphylococcccus aureus* Isolated from Malaysian Hospitals. *Research Journal of Biological Sciences*. Vol. 4, No. 4, pp. 444–448.

Arciola, C.R.; Baldassarri, L. & Montanaro, L. (2001). Presence of *icaA* and *icaD* genes and slime production in a collection of staphylococcal strains from catheter-associated infections. *Journal of Clinical Microbiology*. Vol.39, No.6, pp. 2151–2156.

Arthur, M.; Molinas, C.; Depardieu, F. & Courvalin, P. (1993). Characterization of Tn1546, a Tn3-related transposon conferring glycopeptide resistance by synthesis of depsipeptide peptidoglycan precursors in *Enterococcus faecium* BM4147. Journal of Bacteriology. Vol. 175, pp. 117-127.

Bannerman, T.M. *Staphylococcus, Micrococcus* and other catalase-positive cocci that grow aerobically. (2003). In: P. R. Murray (Ed.). *Manual of Clinical Microbiology*, Eighth Edition. Washington, DC: ASM Press, Vol. 1, pp. 384-404.

Baptiste, K.E.; Williams, K.; Willams, N.J.; Wattret, A.; Clegg, P.D.; Dawson, S.; Corkill, J.E. & O'Neill, T. (2005) Methicillin-resistant staphylococci in companion animals. *Emerging Infectious Disease Journal*. Vol. 11, pp. 1942-1944.

Barlow, R.S.; Pemberton, J.M.; Desmarchelier, P.M. & Gobius, K.S. (2004). Isolation and characterization of integron-containing bacteria without antibiotic selection. *Antimicrobial Agents and Chemotherapy*.Vol. 48, pp.838–842.

Benito, M.J.; Rodriguez, M.M.; Cordoba, M.G.; Aranda, E. & Cordoba, J.J. (2000). Rapid differentiation of *Staphylococcus aureus* from *Staphylococcus* spp. by arbitrarily primed-polymerase chain reaction. *Letters of Applied Microbiology*. Vol. 31, pp. 368-373.

Bes, V.; Guérin-Faublée, H.; Meugnier, J.; Etienne & Freney, J. (2000). Improvement of the identification of staphylococci isolated from bovine mammary infections using molecular methods, *Veterinary Microbiology*. Vol.71, pp. 287–294.

Bierbaum, G., Fuchs, K.; Lenz, W.; Szekat, C. & Sahl, H. G. (1999). Presence of *Staphylococcus aureus* with reduced susceptibility to vancomycin in Germany. *European Journal of Clinical Microbiology and Infectious Diseases*. Vol. 18, pp. 691–696.

Bignardi, G.E.; Woodford, N.; Chapman, A.; Johnson A.P. & Speller, D.C.E. (1996). Detection of the *mecA* gene and phenotypic detection of resistance *in Staphylococcus aureus* isolates with borderline or low-level methicillin Resistance. *Journal of Antimicrobial Chemotherapy*. Vol. 37, pp. 53-63.

Bottari, B.; Ercolini, D.; Gatti, M. & Neviani, E. (2006). Application of FISH technology for microbiological analysis: current state and prospects. *Applied Microbiology and Biotechnology*.Vol 73, pp. 485-494

Brakstad, O.G.; Aasbakk, K. & Maeland, J.A. (1992). Detection of *Staphylococcus aureus* by polymerase chain reaction amplification of the *nuc* gene. *Journal of Clinical Microbiology*. Vol. 30, pp. 1654-1660.

Braoios, A.; Fluminhan, J.A. & Pizzolitto, A.C. (2009) Multiplex PCR use for *Staphylococcus aureus* identification and oxacillin and mupirocin resistance evaluation. *Revista de Ciências Farmacêuticas Básica Aplicada*. Vol 30, No.3, pp. 303-307.

Brückler, J.; Schwarz, S. & Untermann, F. (1994) Staphylokokken-Infektionen und Enterotoxine Band II/I. *Handbuch der bakteriellen Infektionen bei Tieren, 2. Auflage,* Gustav Fischer Verlag Jena, Stuttgart.

CDC (1997). Reduced susceptibility of *Staphylococcus aureus* to vancomycin – Japan, 1996.*MMWR Morb Mortal Wkly Rep*. Vol. 46, pp. 624–626.

CDC (2004). Brief report: vancomycin-resistant *Staphylococcus aureus* – New York. *MMWR Morb Mortal Wkly Rep*. Vol. 53, pp. 322–323.

Chang, S.; Sievert, D.M.; Hageman, J.C.; Boulton, M.L.; Tenover, F.C.; Downes, F.P.; Shah, S.; Rudrik, J.T.; Pupp, G.R.; Brown, W.J.; Cardo, D. & Fridkin, S.K. (2003). Infection with vancomycin-resistant *Staphylococcus aureus* containing the *vanA* resistance gene. *The New England Journal of Medicine*. Vol. 348, pp. 1342-1347.

Chung, M., Lencastre, H.; Matthews, P.; Tomasz,A.; Adamsson,I.; Sousa, M.A.; Camou, T.; Cocuzza, C.; Corso,A.; Couto,I.; Dominguez, A.; Gniadkowski, M.; Goering,R.; Gomes,A.; Kikuchi, K.; Marchese,A.; Mato,R.; Melter,O.; Oliveira,D.; Palacio,R.; Sa-Leao, R.; Sanches, I.S.; Song, J.H.; Tassios, P.T. & Villari, P. (2000). Molecular typing of methicillin-resistant *Staphylococcus aureus* by pulsed-field gel electrophoresis: comparison of results obtained in a multilaboratory effort using identical protocols and MRSA strains. *Microbial Drug Resistance*. Vol. 6, pp.189-198.

Coelho, S.M.O.; Reinoso, E.; Pereira, I.A.; Soares, L.C.; Demo, M.; Bogni, C. & Souza, M.M.S. (2009). Virulence factors and antimicrobial resistance of *Staphylococcus aureus* isolated from bovine mastitis in Rio de Janeiro. *Pesquisa Veterinária Brasileira*. Vol. 29, No.5, pp. 369-374.

Coelho, S.M.O; Pereira, I.A.; Soares, L.C.; Pribul B.R. & Souza, M.M.S. (2011). Profile of virulence factors of *Staphylococcus aureus* isolated from subclinical bovine mastitis in the state of Rio de Janeiro, Brazil. *Journal of Dairy Science*. Vol. 94, No. 7, pp. 3305-3310.

Coombs, G. W.; Nimmo, G.R.; Bell, J.M.; Huygens, F.; O'Brien, G.; Malkowski, F. M. J.; Pearson, J. C. ; Stephens, A.J. & Giffard, P.M. (2004) Genetic diversity among community methicillin-resistant *Staphylococcus aureus* strains causing outpatient infections in Australia. *Journal of Clinical Microbiology*. Vol. 42, pp. 4735–4743.

Cui, L., Ma, X.; Sato, K.; Okuma, K.; Tenover, F.C.; Mamizuka, E.M.; Gemmell, C.G.; Kim, M.N.; Ploy, M. C.; El-Solh, N.; Ferraz, V. & Hiramatsu, K. (2003). Cell wall thickening is a common feature of vancomycin resistance in *Staphylococcus aureus*. *Journal of Clinical Microbiology*. Vol.41, pp. 5-14.

Cui, L.; Lian, J-Q.; Neoh, H.; Reyes, E. & Hiramatsu, K. (2005). DNA Microarray-Based Identification of Genes Associated with Glycopeptide Resistance in *Staphylococcus aureus*. *Antimicrobial Agents and Chemotherapy*. Vol. 49, No.8, pp. 3404–3413.

De Buyser, M. L.; Morvan, A.; Aubert, S.; Dilasser, F. & El Solh, N. (1992). Evaluation of ribosomal RNA gene probe for the identification of species and sub-species within the genus *Staphylococcus*. *Journal of Genetic Microbiology*. Vol. 138, pp. 889-899.

De Vliegher, S.; Laevens, H.; Devriese, L.A.; Opsomer, G.; Leroy, J.L.; Barkema, H.W. & De Kruif,A. (2003). Prepartum teat apex colonization with *Staphylococcus chromogenes* in dairy heifers is associated with low somatic cell count in early lactation. *Veterinary Microbiology*. Vol. 92, pp. 245–252.

Denis, O.; Nonhoff, C.; Byl, B.; Knoop, C.; Bobin-Dubreux, S. & Struelens, M. J. (2002). Emergence of vancomycin-intermediate *Staphylococcus aureus* in a Belgian hospital: microbiological and clinical features. *Journal of Antimicrobial Chemotherapy*. Vol.50, pp. 383–391.

Denis, O., Deplano, A.; Nonhoff, N.; De Ryck, R.; de Mendonca, R.; Rottiers, S.; Vanhoof, R. & Struelens, M.J. (2004). National surveillance of methicillin-resistant Staphylococcus aureus in Belgian hospitals indicates rapid diversification of epidemic clones. *Antimicrobial Agents of Chemotherapy*.Vol. 48, pp. 3625-3629.

Depardieu, F.; Perichon, B. & Courvalin, P. (2004). Detection of the *van* alphabet of enterococci and staphylococci at the species level by multiplex PCR. *Journal of Clinical Microbiology*. Vol. 42, pp. 5857–5860.

Devriese, L.A.; Vandamme, L.R. & Fameree, L. (1972). Methicillin-resistant *Staphylococcus aureus* strains isolated from bovine mastitis cases. *Zentralblatt fur Veterinarmedizin*. Vol.19, pp. 598-605.

Devriese, L.A.; Vancanneyt, M. & Baele, M. (2005). *Staphylococcus intermedius* sp. nov., a coagulase positive species from animals. *International Journal of Systematic and Evironmental Microbiology*, Vol. 55, pp. 1569-1573.

Drancourt, M. & Raoult, D. (1999). Characterization of mutations in the *rpoB* gene in naturally rifampin-resistant *Rickettsia* species. *Antimicrobial Agents of Chemotherapy*. Vol. 43, pp. 2400-2403.

Duck, W.M.; Steward, C.D.; Banerjee, S.N.; McGowan Jr., J.E. & Tenover, F. C. (2003). Optimization of computer software settings improves accuracy of pulsed-field gel electrophoresis macrorestriction fragment pattern analysis. *Journal of Clinical Microbiology*. Vol. 41, pp. 3035-3042.

Enright, M.C.; Robinson, D.A.; Randle, G.; Feil, E.; Grundmann, J.H. & Spratt B. G. (2002). The evolutionary history of methicillin-resistant *Staphylococcus aureus* (MRSA). *Proceedings of the National Academy of Sciences USA*. Vol. 99, pp. 7687–7692.

Espy, M.J.; Uhl, J. R.; Sloan, L. M.; Buckwalter, S.P.; Jones, M.F.; Vetter, E.A.; Yao, J.D.C.; Wengenack, N.L.; Rosenblatt, J.E.; Cockerill III, F.R. & Smith, T.F. (2006). Real-Time PCR in Clinical Microbiology: Applications for Routine Laboratory Testing. *Clinical Microbiology Reviews*. pp. 165–256.

Fang, H. & Hedin, G. (2003). Rapid screening and identification of methicillin-resistant *Staphylococcus aureus* from clinical samples by selective-broth and Real-Time PCR Assay. *Journal of Clinical Microbiology*. Vol.41, pp.2894–2899.

Ferraz, V.; Duse, A. G.; Kassel, M.; Black, A. D.; Ito, T. & Hiramatsu, K. (2000). Vancomycin-resistant *Staphylococcus aureus* occurs in South Africa. *South African Medical Journal*. Vol.90, pp.1113.

Forrest, G.N.; Mehta, S.; Weekes, E.; Lincalis, D.P.; Johnson, J.K. & Venezia, R.A. (2006). Impact of rapid in situ hybridization testing on coagulase-negative staphylococci positive blood cultures. *Journal of Antimicrobial Chemotherapy*. Vol. 58, pp.154–158.

Foxman, B.; Zhang, L.; Koopman.; James, S.K.; Manning, S.D. & Marrs, C.F. (2005). Choosing an appropriate bacterial typing technique for epidemiologic studies. *Epidemiologic Perspectives & Innovations*. Vol. 2, pp.10.

Frenay, H.M.E.; Theelen, J.P.G.; Schouls, L.M.; Vandenbroucke-Grauls, C.M.J.; Verhoef, J.; Van-Leeuwen, W.J. & Mooi, F.R. (1994). Discrimination of epidemic and nonepidemic methicillin-resistant *Staphylococcus aureus*, strains on the basis of protein A gene polymorphism. *Journal of Clinical Microbiology*. Vol.32, pp.846-847.

Frye, J.G.; Jesse, T.; Long, F.; Rondeau, G.; Porwollik, S.; McClelland, M.; Jackson, C.R.; Englen, M. & Fedorka-Cray, P.J. (2006). DNA microarray detection of antimicrobial resistance genes in diverse bacteria. *International Journal of Antimicrobial Agents*. Vol. 27, pp. 138–151.

Futagawa-Saito, K.; Ba-Thein, W.; Sakurai, N. &. Fukuyasu, T. (2006). Prevalence of virulence factors in *Staphylococcus intermedius* isolates from dogs and pigeons. *BMC Veterinary Research*. Vol. 2, p. 4.

Garber, R. (2001). In: Inteligência Competitiva de Mercado. Ed. Madras editora, pp. 248-249, São Paulo

García-Alvarez, L.; Holden, M.; Lindsay, H.; Webb, C.R.; Brown, D.F.J.; Curran, M.D.; Walpole, E.; Brooks, K.; Pickard, D.; Teale, M.; Parkhill, J.; Bentley, S.D.; Edwards, G.; Girvan, E.K.; Kearns, A.M.; Pichon, B.; Hill, R.L.R.; Larsen, A.R.; Skov, R.; Peacock S.J.; Maskell, D. & Holmes, M.A. (2011). Meticillin-resistant *Staphylococcus aureus* with a novel *mecA* homologue in human and bovine populations in the UK and Denmark: a descriptive study. *The Lancet Infectious Diseases*. Vol. 11, pp. 70126-70128.

Garneau, P.; Labrecque, O.; Maynard, C.; Messier, S.; Masson, L. & Harel, J. (2010). Use of a Bacterial Antimicrobial Resistance Gene Microarray for the Identification of Resistant *Staphylococcus aureus*. *Zoonoses and Public Health*. Vol. 57, pp. 94-99.

Gemmell, C. G. (2004). Glycopeptide resistance in *Staphylococcus aureus*: is it a real threat? Journal of Infectious Chemotherapy. Vol.10, pp. 69–75.

Goh, S.H.; Byrne, S.K.; Zhang, J.L. & Chow, A.W. (1992). Molecular typing of *Staphylococcus aureus* on the basis of coagulase gene polymorphisms. *Journal of Clinical Microbiology*. Vol. 30, pp. 1642-1645.

Goh, S.H.; Potter, S.; Wood, J.O.; Hemmingsen, S.M.; R Eynolds R.P. & Chow, A.W. (1996). HSP60 gene Sequences as Universal Targets for Microbial Species Identification: Studies with Coagulase-Negative Staphylococci. *Journal of Clinical Microbiology*. Vol. 34, No. 4, pp. 818-823.

Goni, P.; Vergara, Y.; Ruiz, J.; Albizu, I.; Vila,J. & Gomez-Lus, R. (2004). Antibiotic resistance and epidemiological typing of *Staphylococcus aureus* strains from ovine and rabbit mastitis. *International Journal of Antimicrobial Agents*. Vol. 23, pp. 268–272.

Griffeth, C. & Morris, D.O. (2008). Screening for skin carriage of methicillin-resistant coagulase-positive staphylococci and *Staphylococcus schleiferi* in dogs with healthy and inflamed skin. *Veterinary Dermatology*. Vol.19, pp. 142–149.

Guardabassi, L.; Loeber, M.E. & Jacobson, A. (2004) Transmission of multiple antimicrobial-resistant *Staphylococcus intermedius* between dogs affected by deep pyoderma and their owners. *Veterinary Microbiology*. Vol.98, pp. 23-27.

Hartmann, F.A.; Trostle, S.S. & Klohnen, A.A.O. (1997). Isolation of methicillin-resistant *Staphylococcus aureus* from a postoperative wound infection in a horse. *Journal of the American Veterinary Medical Association*. Vol. 211, No.5, pp. 590-592.

Hayashi, K. (1992). PCR-SSCP: a method for detection of mutations. *Genetic Analysis Techniques and Applications*. Vol. 9, pp. 73–79.

Higuchi, R.; Fockler, C.; Dollinger, G. & Watson, R. (1993). Kinetic PCR analysis: real-time monitoring of DNA amplification reactions. *Biotechnology*. Vol.11, pp.1026–1030.

Hiramatsu, K.; Aritaka, N.; Hanaki, H.; Kawasaki, S.; Hosoda, Y.; Kobayashi, I. (1997). Dissemination in Japanese hospitals of strains of *S.aureus* heterogeneously resistant to vancomycin. *The Lancet*. Vol. 350, pp. 1670-1673.

Hoorfar, J.; Malorny, B.; Abdulmawjood, A.; Cook, N.; Wagner, M. & Fach, P. (2004). Practical considerations in design of internal amplification controls for diagnostic PCR assays. *Journal of Clinical Microbiology*. Vol.42, pp.1863–1868.

Howden,B. P; Davies, J. K.; Johnson, P. D. R.; Stinear, T. P. & Lindsay Grayson, M. (2010). Reduced Vancomycin Susceptibility in *Staphylococcus aureus*, Including Vancomycin-Intermediate and Heterogeneous Vancomycin-Intermediate Strains: Resistance Mechanisms, Laboratory Detection, and Clinical Implications. *Clinical Microbiology Reviews*. Vol. 23, pp. 99–139

Huletsky, A.; Giroux, R.; Rossbach, V.; Gagnon, M.; Vaillancourt, M.; Bernier, M.; Gagnon, F.; Truchon, K.; Bastien, M.; Picard, F.J.; Van Belkum, A.; Ouellette, M.; Roy, P.H. & Bergeron, M.G.(2004). New Real-Time PCR assay for rapid detection of methicillin-resistant *Staphylococcus aureus* directly from specimens containing a mixture of staphylococci. *Journal of Clinical Microbiology*. Vol. 42, pp.1875–84.

Huxley, J.N.; Greent, M.J.; Green, L.E. & Bradley, A.J. (2002). Evaluation of the efficacy of an internal teat sealer during the dry period. *Journal of Dairy Science*. Vol. 85, pp. 551–561.

Ito, T.; Ma, X.X.; Takeuchi, F.; Okuma, K.; Yuzawa, H.; Hiramatsu, K. (2004). Novel type V staphylococcal cassette chromosome *mec* driven by a novel cassette chromosome recombinase, *ccrC*. *Antimicrobial Agents of Chemotherapy*. Vol. 48, pp.2637-2651.

Juhász-Kaszanyitzky, E.; Janosi, S.; Somogyi, P.; Dan, A.; Van Der, L.; Bloois, G.; Van Duijkeren, E. & Wagenaar, J.A. (2007). MRSA Transmission between Cows and Humans. *Emmerging Infection Disease*. Vol.13, pp. 630–632.

Katayama, Y.; Ito, T.; Hiramatsu, K. (2000). A new class of genetic element, staphylococcus cassette chromosome *mec*, encodes methicillin resistance in *Staphylococcus aureus*. *Antimicrobial Agents of Chemotherapy*. Vol. 44, No.6, pp. 1549-55.

Kim M.N.; Pai C.H. & Woo JH (2000). Vancomycin intermediate *Staphylococcus aureus* in Korea. *Journal of Clinical Microbiology*. Vol.38, pp. 3879-3881.

Kloos, W.E. & George, C.G. (1991). Identification of *Staphylococcus* species and subspecies with the Microscan Pos ID and rapid Pos ID panel systems. *Jounal of Clinical Microbiology*. Vol. 29, pp. 738-744.

Kolbert, C.P.; Arruda, J.; Varga-Delmore, P.; Zheng, X.; Lewis, M.; Kolberg, J. & Persing, D.H. (1998) Branched-DNA assay for detection of the *mecA* gene in oxacillin-resistant and oxacillin-sensitive staphylococci. *Journal of Clinical Microbiology*. Vol.36, pp.2640–2644.

Koreen L.; Ramaswamy, S.V.; Graviss, E.A.; Naidich, S.; Musser, J.M. & Kreiswirth, B.N. (2004). *Spa* typing method for discriminating among *Staphylococcus aureus* isolates: implications for use of a single marker to detect genetic micro- and macrovariation. *Journal of Clinical Microbiology*. Vol. 42, pp.792-799.

Kwok, A.Y., Su, S.C. ; Reynolds, R .P. ; Bay, S.J.; Av-Gay, Y. ; Dovichi, N. J. & Chow, A.W. (1999). Species identification and phylogenetic relationships based on partial HSP60 gene sequences within the genus *Staphylococcus*. *International. Journal of Systematic Bacteriology*. Vol. 49, pp. 1181-1192.

Lan Mo, M.D. & Qi-nan Wang, M.D. (1997). Rapid Detection of Methicillin-Resistant Staphylococci Using Polymerase Chain Reaction. *International Journal of Infectious Disease*. Vol. 2, pp.15-20.

Lange, C. C.; Werckenthin, C. & Schwarz, F. (2003). Molecular analysis of the plasmid-borne *aacA/aphD* resistance gene region of coagulase-negative staphylococci from chickens. *Journal of Antimicrobial Chemotherapy* . Vol. 51, pp.1397–1401.

Lawson, T.; Connally, R.E.; Iredell, Jonathan, R. Vemulpad, S. & Piper, J.A. (2011). Detection of *Staphylococcus aureus* With a Fluorescence In Situ Hybridization That Does Not Require Lysostaphin. *Journal of Clinical Laboratory Analysis*. Vol. 25, pp. 142–147.

Lee, J. H. (2003). Methicillin (oxacillin)-resistant *Staphylococcus aureus* strains isolated from major food animals and their potential transmission to humans. *Applied Environmental Microbiology*. Vol. 69, pp. 6489–6494.

Levsky, J.M. & Singer, R.H. (2003). Fluorescence in situ hybridization: past, present and future. *Journal of Cell Science*. Vol.116, pp. 2833-2838.

Lilenbaum, W.; Veras, M.; Blum, E. & Souza, G.N. (2000) Antimicrobial susceptibility of staphylococci isolated from otitis externa in dogs. *Letters of Applied Microbiology*. Vol 31, pp. 42-45.

Lim, J.A.; Kwon, A.R.; Kim, S.K.; Chomg, Y.; Lee, K. & Choi, E.C. (2002). Prevalence of resitance to macrolide, lincosamide and streptrogramine antibiotics in Gram-positive cocci isolated in Koream hospital. *Journal of Antimicrobial Chemotheraty*. Vol.49, pp. 489-495.

Linehan, D.; Etienne, J. & Sheehan D. (2003). Relationship between haemolytic and sphingomyelinase activities in a partially purified β-like toxin from *Staphylococcus schleiferi*. *FEMS Immunology and Medical Microbiology*. Vol. 36, No.1, pp. 95-102.

Ludwig, W.; Schleifer, K-H. & Whitman, W. B. 2009. Revised Road Map to the Phylum *Firmicutes*. http://www.bergeys.org/outlines/Bergeys_Vol_3_Outline.pdf, pp. 1-32

Lyon, G. J.; Mayville, P.; Muir, T.W.R. & Novick, P. (2000). Rational design of a global inhibitor of virulence response in *Staphylococcus aureus*, based in part on localization of the site of inhibition to the receptor-histidine kinase, AgrC. *The Proceedings of the National Academy of Sciences of the United States of America*.Vol. 97, pp. 13330-13335.

Mackay, I.M. (2004). Real-time PCR in the microbiology laboratory. *Clinical Microbiology and Infection*. Vol.10, pp.190–212.

Maes, N.; De Gheldre, Y.; DeRyck, R.; Vaneechoutte, M.; Meugnier, H.; Etienne, J. & Struelens, M. J. (1997). Rapid and accurate identification of *Staphylococcus* species by tRNA intergenic spacer length polymorphism analysis. *Jounal of Clinical Microbiology*. Vol 35, pp. 2477-2481.

Maiden, M.C.; Bygraves, J.A.; Feil, E.; Morelli, G.; Russell, J.E.; Urwin, R.; Zhang, Q.; Zhou, J.; Zurth, K.; Caugant, D.A; Feavers, I.M.; Achtman, M. & Spratt, B.G. (1998). Multilocus sequence typing: a portable approach to the identification of clones within populations of pathogenic microorganisms. *Proceedings of the National Academy of Sciences* USA. Vol. 95, pp. 3140–3145.

Martineau, F.; Picard, F.J. & Lansac, N. (2000). Correlation between resistance genotype determined by multiplex PCR assays and the antibiotic susceptibility patterns of *Staphylococcus aureus* and *Staphylococcus epidermidis*. *Antimicrobial Agents of Chemotherapy*. Vol. 44, pp.231–238.

Martineau, F.; Picard, F. J.; Menard, C.; Roy, P. H.; Ouellette, M. & Bergeron, M. G. (2000). Development of a rapid PCR assay specific for *Staphylococcus saprophyticus* and application to direct detection from urine samples. *Journal of Clinical Microbiology*. Vol. 38, pp. 3280-3284.

Martineau, F.; Picard, F.J.; Roy, P. H.; Ouellette, M. & Bergeron, M.G. (1996). Species-specific and ubiquitous DNA-based assays for rapid identification of *Staphylococcus epidermidis*. *Journal of Clinical Microbiology*. Vol. 34, pp. 2888-2893.

Mato, R.; Campanile, F.; Stefani, S.; Crisostomo, M.I.; Santagati, M.; Sanches, S.I. & Lencastre, H. (2004). Clonal types and multidrug resistance patterns of methicillin-resistant *Staphylococcus aureus* (MRSA) recovered in Italy during the 1990s. *Microbial Drug Resistance*. Vol. 10, pp. 106–113.

Melles, D.C.; Gorkink, R.F.; Boelens, H.A.; Snijders, S.V.; Peeters, J.K.; Moorhouse, M.J.; Van Der Spek, P.J.; Van Leeuwen, W.B.; Simons, G.; Verbrugh, H.A. & Van Belkum, A. (2004). Natural population dynamics and expansion of pathogenic clones of *Staphylococcus aureus*. *The Journal of Clinical Investigation*. Vol. 114, pp. 1732–1740.

Młynarczyk, A.; Młynarczyk, G. & Łuczak, M. (2002). Conjugative transfer of glycopeptide and macrolide resistant genes among enterococci and from *Enterococcus faecalis* to *Staphylococcus aureus*. *Med Dosw Mikrobiol*. Vol. 54, pp. 21–28.

Mollet, C.; Drancourt, M. & Raoult, D. (1997). *rpoB* gene sequence analysis as a novel basis for bacterial identification. *Molecular Microbiology*. Vol. 26, pp. 1005-1011.

Monecke, S.; Kuhnert, P.; Hotzel, H.; Slickers, P. & Ehricht, R. (2007). Microarray based study on virulence-associated genes and resistance determinants of *Staphylococcus aureus* isolates from cattle. *Veterinary Microbiology*. Vol.125, pp. 128–140.

Montesinos I.; Salido, E.; Delgado, T.; Cuervo, M. & Sierra, A. (2002). Epidemiological genotyping of methicillin resistant *Staphylococcus aureus* by pulsed field gel electrophoresis at a university hospital and comparison with antibiotyping and protein A and coagulase gene polymorphisms. *Journal of Clinical Microbiology*. Vol. 40, pp. 2119–2125.

Moon, J.S.; Lee, A.R.; Kang, H.M.; Lee, E.S.; Kim, M.N.; Paik, Y.H.; Park, Y.H.; Joo, Y.S. & Koo, H.C. (2007). Phenotypic and genetic antibiogram of methicillin-resistant staphylococci isolated from bovine mastitis in Korea. *Journal of Dairy Science*. Vol. 90, pp. 1176-1185.

Morgan, M. (2008). Methicillin-resistant *Staphylococcus aureus* and animals: zoonotic or humanosis. *Journal of Antimicrobial Chemotherapy* 62, 1181-1187.

Mullis, K.B. & Faloona, F. A. (1987). Specific synthesis of DNA *in vitro* via a polymerase-catalyzed chain reaction. *Methods in Enzymology*. Vol.155, pp. 335–350.

Murchan, S.; Kaufmann, M.E.; Deplano, A.; De Ryck, R.; Struelens, M.; Zinn, C.E.; Fussing, V.; Salmenlinna, S.; Vuopio-Varkila, J.; El Solh N.; Cuny, C.; Witte, W.; Tassios, P.T.; Legakis N.; Van Leeuwen, W.; Van Belkum, A.; Vindel A.; Laconcha, I.; Garaizar, J.; Haeggman, S.; Olsson-Liljequist, B.; Ransjo, U.; Coombes G. & Cookson, B. (2003). Harmonization of pulsed-field gel electrophoresis protocols for epidemiological typing of strains of methicillin-resistant *Staphylococcus aureus*: a single approach developed by consensus in 10 European laboratories and its application for tracing the spread of related strains. *Journal of Clinical Microbiology*. Vol 41, pp. 1574–1585.

Murchan, S.; Aucken, H.M.; O'Neill, G.L.; Ganner, M. & Cookson, B.D. (2004). Emergence, spread, and characterization of phage variants of epidemic methicillin-resistant *Staphylococcus aureus* 16 in England and Wales. *Journal of Clinical Microbiology*. Vol. 42, pp. 5154-5160.

Naffa, R.G.; Bdour, S.M.; Migdadi, & Shehabi, A.A. (2006). Enterotoxicity and genetic variation among clinical *Staphylococcus aureus* isolates in Jordan. *Journal of Medical Microbiology*. Vol. 55, No. 2, pp.183-187.

Neu, H.C. (1991). Clinical Microbiology of Azithromycin. *The American Journal of Medicine*. 91(3A), 3A-12S.

Nielsen, P. E.; Egholm, M. & Buchard, O. (1994). Peptide nucleic acids (PNA). A DNA mimic with a peptide backbone. *Bioconjugate Chemestry.* Vol. 5, pp. 3–7.

Nolte, F. S. (1998). Branched DNA signal amplification for direct quantitation of nucleic acid sequences in clinical specimens. *Advances in Clinical Chemistry.* Vol. 33, pp. 201–235.

Novick, R.P. (2000). Pathogenicity factors and their regulation. In Gram-Positive Pathogens. Fischetti, V.A., Novick, R.P.; Ferreti, J.J.; Portnoy, D.A. & Rood, J.I. (eds). *Washington, DC: American Society for Microbiology Press.* pp. 392–407.

O'Mahony, R.; Abbott, Y.; Leonard, F.C.; Markey, B.K.; Quinn, P.J.; Pollock, P.J.; Fanning, S. & Rossney, A.S. (2005) Methicillin-resistant *Staphylococcus aureus* (MRSA) isolated from animals and veterinary personnel in Ireland. *Veterinary Microbiology.* Vol. 109, pp. 285-296.

Oliveira, D.C.; Tomasz, A. & Lencastre, H. (2001). The evolution of pandemic clones of methicillin-resistant *Staphylococcus aureus*: identification of two ancestral genetic backgrounds and the associated *mec* elements. Microbial Drug Resistance. Vol. 7, pp.349-361.

Palladino, S.; Kay, I.D.; Flexman, J.P.; Boehm, I.; Costa, A.M.G; Lambert, E.J. & Christiansen, K.J. (2003). Rapid detection of *vanA* and *vanB* genes directly from clinical specimens and enrichment broths by Real-Time multiplex PCR assay. *Journal of Clinical Microbiology.* Vol. 41, pp. 2383–2386.

Palma M,; Haggar A. & Flock J. (1999). Adherence of *Staphylococcus aureus* is enhanced by an endogenous secreted protein with broad binding activity. *Journal of Bacteriology.* Vol.181, pp. 2840–2845.

Patel, R.; Uhl, J.R.; Kohner, P.; Hopkins, M.K. & Cockerill, F.R. (1997). Multiplex PCR detection of *vanA*, *vanB*, *vanC-1*, and *vanC2/3* genes in enterococci. *Journal of Clinical Microbiology.* Vol. 35, pp. 703–707.

Paule, S.M.; Pasquariello, A.C.; Thomson, R.B.; Kaul, K.L. & Peterson, L.R. (2005). Real-Time PCR Can Rapidly Detect Methicillin-Susceptible and Methicillin-Resistant *Staphylococcus aureus* Directly From Positive Blood Culture Bottles. *American Journal of Clinical of Pathology.* Vol. 124, pp. 404-407.

Pereira, I.A.; Soares, L.C.; Coelho, S.M.O.; Pribul, B.R. & Souza, M.M.S. (2009). Suscetibilidade à azitromicina de isolados bacterianos de processos infecciosos em cães e gatos. *Pesquisa Veterinária Brasileira.* Vol. 29, No. 2, pp.153-159.

Perichon, B. & Courvalin, P. (2006). Synergism between beta-lactams and glycopeptides against vanA-type methicillin-resistant *Staphylococcus aureus* and heterologous expression of the *vanA* operon. *Antimicrobial Agents of Chemotherapy.* Vol.50, pp. 3622–3630.

Pyorala,S. & Taponen, S. (2009). Coagulase-negative staphylococci: Emerging mastitis pathogens. *Veterinary Microbiology,* Vol. 134, pp. 3-8.

Rahube, T.O. & Yost, C.K. (2010). Antibiotic resistance plasmids in wastewater treatment plants and their possible dissemination into the environment. *African Journal of Biotechnology.* Vol. 9, No.54, pp 9183-9190.

Reinoso, E.B.; El-Sayed, A.; Lämmler, C.; Bogni, C. & Zschöck M. (2006). Genotyping of *Staphylococcus* aureus isolated from humans, bovine subclinical mastitis and food samples in Argentina. *Microbiological Research.* Vol. 163, pp. 314-22.

Renesto, P.; Lorvellec-Guillon, K.; Drancourt, M. & Raoult, D. (2000). *rpoB* gene analysis as a novel strategy for identification of spirochetes from the genera *Borrelia*, *Treponema*, and *Leptospira*. *Journal of Clinical Microbiology.* Vol. 38, pp. 2200-2203

Renesto, P.; Gouvernet, J.; Drancourt, M.; Roux, V. & Raoult, D. (2001). Use of *rpoB* gene analysis for detection and identification of *Bartonella* species. *Journal of Clinical Microbiology*. Vol. 39, pp. 430-437.

Rich, M. & Roberts, L. (2004). Methicillin-resistant *Staphylococcus aureus* isolates from companion animals. *Veterinary Research*. Vol.154, pp.310.

Ronaghi, M.; Uhlen, M. & Nyren, P. (1998). A sequencing method based on real-time pyrophosphate. *Science*, Vol. 281, pp. 363–365.

Ronaghi, M. & Elahi, E. (2002). Pyrosequencing for microbial typing. *Journal of Chromatography*. Vol. 782, pp. 67–72.

Sabet, N.S.; Subramaniam, G.; Navaratnam, P. & Sekaran, S.D. (2006). Simultaneous species identification and detection of methicillin resistance in staphylococci using triplex real-time PCR assay. *Diagnostic Microbiology and Infectious Disease*. Vol.56, pp. 13–18.

Saiki, R.K.; Gelfand, D.H.; Stoffel, S.; Scharf, S.J.; Higuchi,R.; Horn, G.T.; Mullis, K.B. & Ehrlich, H.A. (1988). Primer-directed enzymatic amplification with a thermostable DNA polymerase. *Science* Vol. 239, pp. 487–491.

Sanger, F.; Nicklen, S. & Coulson, A.R. (1977). DNA sequencing with chain-terminating inhibitors. *Proceedings of the National Academy of Sciences*. Vol. 74, pp. 5463–5467.

Santos, O.C.S.; Barros,E.M.; Bastos, M.C.F.; Santos,K.R.N.; Giambiagi-Demarval, M. (2008). Identification of coagulase-negative staphylococci from bovine mastitis using RFLP-PCR of the *groEL* gene. *Veterinary Microbiology*. Vol.130, N°1-2, pp. 134-140.

Sasaki, S.; Kikuchi,K.; Tanaka,Y.; Takahashi, N.; Kamata, S. & Hiramatsu, K. (2007). Methicillin-resistant *Staphylococcus pseudintermedius* in a veterinary teaching hospital. *Journal of Clinical Microbiology*. Vol.45, pp. 1118–1125.

Schena, M.; Shalon, D.; Davis, R.W. & Brown, P.O. (1995). Quantitative monitoring of gene expression patterns with a complementary DNA microarray. *Science*. Vol. 270, pp. 467–470.

Schmitz, F.J.; Sadurski, R.; Kray, A.; Boos, M.; Geisel, R.; Köhrer, K.; Verhoef, J.; Fluit, A.C. (2000). Prevalence of macrolide-resistance genes in *Staphylococcus aureus* and *Enterococcus faecium* isolates from 24 european University hospitals. *Journal of Antimicrobial Chemotherapy*. Vol. 45, pp. 891-894.

Schwarz, S.; Kadlec, K. & Strommenger, B. (2008). Methicillin-resistant *Staphylococcus aureus* and *Staphylococcus pseudintermedius* detected in the BfT-GermVet monitoring programme 2004–2006 in Germany. *Journal of Antimicrobial Chemotherapy*. Vol. 61, pp. 282–285.

Segal & Ron, E.Z. (1996). Regulation and organization of the *groE* and *dnaK* operons in eubacteria, *FEMS. Microbiology Letters*. Vol.138, pp. 1–10.

Šeputienė, V.; Vilkoicaitė, A.; Armalytė, J.; Pavilonis, A. & Sužiedėlienė, E. (2010). Detection of Methicillin-Resistant *Staphylococcus aureus* using Double Duplex Real-Time PCR and Dye Syto 9. *Folia Microbiologica*. Vol. 55 , No.5, pp. 502–507.

Shore,A.C.; Deasy, E.C.; Slickers, P.; Brennan,G.; O'Connell, B.; Monecke,S.; Ehricht,R. & Coleman, D.C. (2011). Detection of Staphylococcal Cassette Chromosome *mec* Type XI Carrying Highly Divergent *mecA*, *mecI*, *mecR1*, *blaZ*, and *ccr* Genes in Human Clinical Isolates of Clonal Complex 130 Methicillin-Resistant *Staphylococcus aureus*. *Antimicrobial Agents and Chemotherapy*. Vol. 55, No. 8, pp. 3765-3773.

Simeoni, D.; Rizzottia, L.; Cocconcelli, P.; Gazzola, S.; Dellaglio, F. & Torriani, S. (2008). Antibiotic resistance genes and identification of staphylococci collected from the production chain of swine meat commodities. *Food Microbiology*. Vol. 25, pp. 196–201.

Sinclair, A.; Arnold, C. & Woodford, N. (2003). Rapid detection and estimation by pyrosequencing of 23S rRNA genes with a single nucleotide polymorphism conferring linezolid resisistance in enterococci. *Antimicrobial Agents of Chemotherapy.* Vol. 47, pp. 3620-3622.

Sng, L. H.; Koh, T. H.; Wang, G. C.; Hsu, L. Y.; Kapi, M. & Hiramatsu, K. (2005). Heterogeneous vancomycin-resistant *Staphylococcus aureus* (hetero-VISA) in Singapore. *International Jounal of Antimicrobial Agents.* Vol. 25, pp. 177-179.

Soares, L. C.; Pereira, I. A.; Coelho, S.M.O.; Cunha, C.M.M.; Oliveira, D.F.B.; Miranda, A.F. & Souza, M.M.S. (2008). Caracterização fenotípica da resistência a antimicrobianos e detecção do gene *mecA* em *Staphylococcus* spp. coagulase-negativos isolados de amostras animais e humanas. *Ciência Rural.* Vol. 38, No. 5, pp. 1346-1350.

Song, J. H., Hiramatsu, K.; Suh, J. Y.; Ko, K. S. ; Ito, T.; Kapi, M.; Kiem, S.; Kim, Y. S.; Oh, W. S.; Peck, K. R. & Lee, N. Y. (2004). Emergence in Asian countries of *Staphylococcus aureus* with reduced susceptibility to vancomycin. *Antimicrobial Agents Chemotherapy.* Vol. 48, pp. 4926-4928.

Southern, E.M. (1975) Detection of specific sequences among DNA fragments separated by gel electrophoresis. *Journal of Molecular Biology.* Vol. 98, pp. 503-517.

Stefano, K. & J. J. Hyldig-Nielsen. (1997). Diagnostic applications of PNA oligomers. *In* S. A. Minden & L. M. Savage (ed.), Diagnostic gene detection & quantification technologies. IBC Library Series, Southborough, Mass.

Struelens, M. J. (1996). Consensus guidelines for appropriate use and evaluation of microbial epidemiologic typing systems. *Clinical Microbiology Infectious.* Vol.2, pp.2-11.

Suhaili, Z.; Johari, S.A.; Mohtar, M.; Abdullah, A.R.T.; Ahmad, A. & Ali, A.M. (2009). Detection of Malaysian methicillin-resistant *Staphylococcus aureus* (MRSA) clinical isolates using simplex and duplex real-time PCR. *World Journal of Microbiology & Biotechnology.* Vol. 25, pp. 253-258.

Sundsfjord, A.; Simonsen, G.S.; Haldorsen, B.C.; Haaheim, H.; Hjelmevoll, S.O.; Littauer, P. & Dahl, K.H. (2004) Genetic methods for detection of antimicrobial resistance. *Acta Pathologica, Microbiologica. et Immunologica Scandinavica.* Vol. 112, No. 11-12, pp. 815-837.

Svec, P.; Vancanneyt,M.; Sedlacek, I.; Engelbeen, K.; Stetina, V.; Swings, J. & Petras, P. (2004). Reclassification of *Staphylococcus pulvereri* Zakrzewska-Czerwinska et al. 1995 as a later synonym of *Staphylococcus vitulinus* Webster et al. 1994. *Internartional Journal of Systematic and Evolutionary Microbiology.* Vol.54, pp. 2213-2215.

Swenson, J.M.; Lonsway, D.; McAllister, S.; Thompson, A.; Jevitt, L. & Patel, J.B. (2007). Detection of *mecA*-mediated resistance using cefoxitin disk diffusion (DD) in a collection of *Staphylococcus aureus* expressing *borderline* oxacillin MICs. *Diagnostic Microbiology and Infectious Disease.* Vol. 58, pp. 33-39.

Takahashi, T.; Satoh, I. & Kikuchi, N. (1999). Phylogenetic relationships of 38 taxa of the genus *Staphylococcus* based on 16S rRNA gene sequence analysis. *International Journal of Systematic Bacteriology* Vol. 49, pp. 725-728.

Taponen, S.; Simojoki, H.; Haveri, M.; Larsen, H.D. & Pyorala, S. (2006). Clinical characteristics and persistence of bovine mastitis caused by different species of coagulase-negative staphylococci identified with API or AFLP. *Veterinary Microbiology.* Vol. 115, pp. 199-207.

Tenover, F.C.; Arbeit, R.; Archer G.; Biddle, J.; Byrne, S.; Goering, R.; Hancock, G.; Hebert, G.A.; Hill, B. & Hollis, R. (1994). Comparison of traditional and molecular methods of typing isolates of Staphylococcus aureus. Journal of Clinical Microbiology. Vol. 32, pp. 407-415.

Tenover, F.C.; Arbeit, R.D.; Goering, R.V.; Mickelsen, P.A.; Murray, B.E.; Persing, D.H. & Swaminathan, B. (1995). Interpreting chromosomal DNA restriction patterns produced by pulsed-field gel electrophoresis: criteria for bacterial strain typing. Journal of Clinical Microbiology. Vol. 33, pp. 2233-2239.

Tenover, F.C.; Weigel, L.M.; Appelbaum, P.C.; McDougal, L.K.; Chaitram, J.; McAllister, S.; Clark, N. Killgore, G.; O'Hara, C.M.; Jevitt,L.; Patel, J.B. & Bozdogan, B. (2004). Vancomycin-resistant Staphylococcus aureus isolate from a patient in Pennsylvania. Antimicrobial Agents and Chemotherapy. Vol. 48, pp. 275-280.

Tenover, F. C. (2008). Vancomycin-resistant Staphylococcus aureus: a perfect but geographically limited storm? Clinical Infection Disease; Vol. 46, pp. 675-677.

Thomas, L.C.; Gidding, H.F.; Ginn, A.N.; Olma, T. & Iredell, J. (2007). Development of a real-time Staphylococcus aureus and MRSA (SAM-) PCR for routine blood culture. Journal of Microbiological Methods. Vol.68, pp. 296-302.

Tiwari, H.K. & Sen, M.R. (2006). Emergence of vancomycin resistant Staphylococcus aureus (VRSA) from a tertiary care hospital from northern part of India. Infection Disease, Vol.6, pp. 156.

Udo, E.E., & Dashti, A.A. (2000). Detection of genes encoding aminoglycoside-modifying enzymes in staphylococci by polymerase chain reaction and dot blot hybridization. International Journal of Antimicrobial Agents. Vol. 13, pp. 273-279.

Vannuffel, P., Heusterspreute, M.; Bouyer, M.; Vandercam, B.; Philippe, M. & Gala, J.L. (1999). Molecular characterization of femA from Staphylococcus hominis and Staphylococcus saprophyticus, and femA-based discrimination of staphylococcal species. Research Microbiology. Vol. 150, pp. 129-141.

Vannuffel, P.; Gigi, J.; Ezzedine, H.; Vandercam, B.; Delmee, M. & Wauters, G.; Gala, J.L. (1995). Specific detection of methicillin-resistant Staphylococcus species by multiplex PCR. Journal of Clinical Microbiology. Vol. 33, pp.2864-2867.

Velasco, D.; Tomas, M.M.; Cartelle, M.; Beceiro, A.; Perez, A.; Molina, F.; Moure, R.; Villanueva, R. & Bou, G. (2005). Evaluation of different methods for detecting methicillin (oxacillin) resistance in Staphylococcus aureus. J. Antimicrobial Chemotherapy. Vol.55, No.3, pp. 379-382.

Volkmann, H.; Schwartz, T.; Bischoff, P.; Kirchen, S. & Obst, U. (2004). Detection of clinically relevant antibiotic-resistance genes in municipal wastewater using real-time PCR (TaqMan). Journal of Microbiological Methods. Vol.56, pp.277- 286.

Vos, P.R.; Hogers, M.; Bleeker, M.; Van De Lee Reijans, T.; Hornes, M.; Fritjers, A.; Pot, J.; Peleman, J.; Kuiper, M.; Zabeau, M. (1995). AFLP: A new concept for DNA fingerprinting. Nucleic Acids Research. Vol. 23, pp. 4407-4414.

Walther, B.; Wieler, L.; Friedrich, A.; Hanssen, A.; Kohn, B.; Brunnberg, L. & Lübke-Becker, A. (2008). Methicillin-resistant Staphylococcus aureus (MRSA) isolated from small and exotic animals at a university hospital during routine microbiological examinations. Veterinary Microbiology. Vol. 127, pp. 171-178.

Watanabe, S.; Kobayashi, N.; Quiñones, D.; Nagashima, S.; Uehara, N. & Watanabe, N. (2009). Genetic diversity of enterococci harboring the high-level gentamicin resistance gene aac(6')-Ie-aph(2'')-Ia or aph(2'')-Ie in a Japanese hospital. Microbial Drug Resistance. Vol.15, pp.185-94.

Weese, J.S. (2005) Methicillin-resistant *Staphylococcus aureus*: An emerging pathogen in small animals. *Journal of the American Animal Hospital Association*. Vol.41, pp. 150-157.

Weese J.; Caldwell, F.; Willey, B.; Kreiswirth, B.; McGeer, A.; Rousseau J. & Low, D. (2006). An outbreak of methicillin-resistant *Staphylococcus aureus* skin infections resulting from horse to human transmission in a veterinary hospital. *Veterinary Microbiology*. Vol. 114, pp. 160–164.

Weese, J.S. & Van, Duijkeren, E. (2010). Methicillin-resistant *Staphylococcus aureus* and *Staphylococcus pseudintermedius* in veterinary medicine. *Veterinary Microbiology*. Vol. 140, pp. 418-29.

Weigel, L.M.; Donlam, R.M.; Shin, D.H.; Jensen,B.; Clark, N.C.; McDougal, L.K.; Zhu, W.; Musser, K.A.; Thompson, J.; Kohlerschmidt, D.; Dumas, N.; Limberger, R.J. & Patel, J.B. (2007). High-level vancomycin resistant *Staphylococcus aureus* isolates associated with a polymicrobial biofilm. *Antimicrobial Agents of Chemotherapy*.Vol. 51, pp. 231–238

Werckenthin, C.; Cardoso, M.; Martel, J.L. & Schwarz, S. (2001). Antimicrobial resistance in staphylococci from animals with particular reference to bovine *Staphylococcus aureus*, porcine *Staphylococcus hyicus*, and canine *Staphylococcus intermedius*. *Veterinary Research*. Vol. 32, pp. 341–362.

Wettstein, K.; Descloux, S.; Rossano, A. & Perreten, V. (2008). Emergence of methicillin-resistant *Staphylococcus pseudintermedius* in Switzerland: three cases of urinary tract infection in cats. *Schweiz Arch Tierheilk*. Vo.150, pp. 339–343.

Wieser, M. & Busse, H.J. (2000). Rapid identification of *Staphylococcus epidermidis*. *International Journal of Systematic and Evolutionary Microbiology*. Vol. 50, pp. 1087-1093.

Witte, W.; Pasemann, B.; Cuny, C. (2007). Detection of low-level oxacillin resistance in *mec*A-positive *Staphylococcus aureus*. *Clinical Microbiological and Infection*. Vol. 13, No. 4, pp. 408-412.

Yilmaz, G.; Aydin, K.; Iskender, S.; Caylan, R. & Koksal, I. (2007). Detection and prevalence of inducible clindamycin resistance in staphylococci. *Journal of Medical Microbiology*. Vol. 56, pp. 342–345.

Zhang, K.; McClure, J.; Elsayed, S.; Louie, T. & Conly, J.M. (2005). Novel Multiplex PCR Assay for Characterization and Concomitant Subtyping of Staphylococcal Cassette Chromosome mec Types I to V in Methicillin-Resistant *Staphylococcus aureus*. *Journal of Clinical Microbiology*. pp. 5026–5033.

Zheng, X.; Kolbert, C.P.; Varga-Delmore, P.; Arruda, J.; Lewis, M.; Kolberg, J.; Cockerill, F.R. & Persing, D. H. (1999). Direct *mecA* Detection from Blood Culture Bottles by Branched-DNA Signal Amplification. *Journal of Clinical Microbiology*. Vol.37, pp. 4192-4193.

Zhu, L.X.; Zhang, Z.-W.; Wang, C.; Yang, H.-W.; Jiang, D.; Zhang, Q.; Mitchelson, K. & Cheng, J. (2007). Use of a DNA microarray for simultaneous detection of antibiotic resistance genes among staphylococcal clinical isolates. *Journal of Clinical Microbiology*. Vol.45, pp. 3514–3521.

Zhu, W.; Tenover, F.C.; Limor, J.; Lonsway, D.; Prince, D.; Dunne, W.M. Jr & Patel, J.B. (2007). Use of pyrosequencing to identify point mutations in domain V of 23S rRNA genes of linezolid-resistant *Staphylococcus aureus* and *Staphylococcus epidermidis*. *European Journal of Clinical Microbiology Infection Disease*. Vol. 26, No.3, pp.161-165.

Permissions

The contributors of this book come from diverse backgrounds, making this book a truly international effort. This book will bring forth new frontiers with its revolutionizing research information and detailed analysis of the nascent developments around the world.

We would like to thank Dr. Marina Pana, for lending her expertise to make the book truly unique. She has played a crucial role in the development of this book. Without her invaluable contribution this book wouldn't have been possible. She has made vital efforts to compile up to date information on the varied aspects of this subject to make this book a valuable addition to the collection of many professionals and students.

This book was conceptualized with the vision of imparting up-to-date information and advanced data in this field. To ensure the same, a matchless editorial board was set up. Every individual on the board went through rigorous rounds of assessment to prove their worth. After which they invested a large part of their time researching and compiling the most relevant data for our readers. Conferences and sessions were held from time to time between the editorial board and the contributing authors to present the data in the most comprehensible form. The editorial team has worked tirelessly to provide valuable and valid information to help people across the globe.

Every chapter published in this book has been scrutinized by our experts. Their significance has been extensively debated. The topics covered herein carry significant findings which will fuel the growth of the discipline. They may even be implemented as practical applications or may be referred to as a beginning point for another development. Chapters in this book were first published by InTech; hereby published with permission under the Creative Commons Attribution License or equivalent.

The editorial board has been involved in producing this book since its inception. They have spent rigorous hours researching and exploring the diverse topics which have resulted in the successful publishing of this book. They have passed on their knowledge of decades through this book. To expedite this challenging task, the publisher supported the team at every step. A small team of assistant editors was also appointed to further simplify the editing procedure and attain best results for the readers.

Our editorial team has been hand-picked from every corner of the world. Their multi-ethnicity adds dynamic inputs to the discussions which result in innovative outcomes. These outcomes are then further discussed with the researchers and contributors who give their valuable feedback and opinion regarding the same. The feedback is then collaborated with the researches and they are edited in a comprehensive manner to aid the understanding of the subject.

Apart from the editorial board, the designing team has also invested a significant amount of their time in understanding the subject and creating the most relevant covers. They scrutinized every image to scout for the most suitable representation of the subject and create an appropriate cover for the book.

The publishing team has been involved in this book since its early stages. They were actively engaged in every process, be it collecting the data, connecting with the contributors or procuring relevant information. The team has been an ardent support to the editorial, designing and production team. Their endless efforts to recruit the best for this project, has resulted in the accomplishment of this book. They are a veteran in the field of academics and their pool of knowledge is as vast as their experience in printing. Their expertise and guidance has proved useful at every step. Their uncompromising quality standards have made this book an exceptional effort. Their encouragement from time to time has been an inspiration for everyone.

The publisher and the editorial board hope that this book will prove to be a valuable piece of knowledge for researchers, students, practitioners and scholars across the globe.

List of Contributors

Maimoona Ahmed
King Abdul Aziz University Hospital, Jeddah, Saudi Arabia

Wilfried Rozhon, Mamoona Khan and Brigitte Poppenberger
Max F. Perutz Laboratories, University of Vienna, Austria

Giorgio Ricci, Lucia Maria Barrionuevo, Paola Cosso and Patrizia Pagliari
Residenza Sanitaria Assistenziale Villa San Clemente,
Segesta Group Korian, Villasanta (MB), Italy

Aladar Bruno Ianes
Medical Direction, Segesta Group Korian, Milan, Italy

Sloane Ritchey, Siva Gandhapudi and Mark Coyne
University of Kentucky, USA

Patricia Munsch-Alatossava, Vilma Ikonen and Tapani Alatossava
Department of Food and Environmental Sciences, Division of Food Technology, University
of Helsinki, Finland

Jean-Pierre Gauchi
Unité de Mathématiques et Informatique Appliquées (UR 341), Institut National de la
Recherche Agronomique, Centre de Jouy en Josas, France

K.C.A. Jalal, B. Akbar John and B.Y. Kamaruzzaman
Department of Biotechnology, Kulliyyah of Science, International Islamic University
Malaysia, India

K. Kathiresan
Centre of Advanced Studies in Marine Biology, Annamalai University, Malaysia

Castrillón Rivera Laura Estela and Palma Ramos Alejandro
Universidad Autónoma Metropolitana, Departamento de Sistemas Biológicos, México

K. Prashanth, T. Vasanth, R. Saranathan, Abhijith R. Makki and Sudhakar Pagal
Laboratory No. 6, Department of Biotechnology, Pondicherry University, India

Ranginee Choudhury, Sasmita Panda and Durg V. Singh
Infectious Disease Biology, Institute of Life Sciences, Bhubaneswar, India

Savitri Sharma
Ocular Microbiology Service, LV Prasad Eye Institute, Bhubaneswar, India

M.M. Ehlers, J.M. Hughes and M.M. Kock
University of Pretoria/NHLS, South Africa

Miliane Moreira Soares de Souza, Shana de Mattos de Oliveira Coelho, Bruno Rocha Pribul and Irene da Silva Coelho
Institute of Veterinary, Microbiology and Immunology Department, Federal Rural University of Rio de Janeiro, Brazil

Ingrid Annes Pereira
Institute Osvaldo Cruz Foundation, Rio de Janeiro, Brazil

Lidiane de Castro Soares
University Severino Sombra, Rio de Janeiro, Brazil